Fundamentals of Phonetics

A Practical Guide for Students

Fundamentals
of Phonetics

A Practical Guide for Students

Third Edition

Larry H. Small

Bowling Green State University

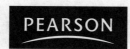

Boston   Columbus   Indianapolis   New York   San Francisco   Upper Saddle River
Amsterdam   Cape Town   Dubai   London   Madrid   Milan   Munich   Paris   Montreal   Toronto
Delhi   Mexico City   São Paulo   Sydney   Hong Kong   Seoul   Singapore   Taipei   Tokyo

Vice President and Editorial Director: Jeffery W. Johnston
Executive Editor and Publisher: Stephen D. Dragin
Editorial Assistant: Jamie Bushell
Vice President, Director of Marketing: Margaret Waples
Marketing Manager: Weslie Sellinger
Senior Managing Editor: Pamela D. Bennett
Senior Project Manager: Linda Hillis Bayma
Senior Operations Supervisor: Matthew Ottenweller

Senior Art Director: Diane C. Lorenzo
Cover Designer: Diane C. Lorenzo
Cover Image: iStock
Full-Service Project Management: Walsh & Associates, Inc.
Composition: S4Carlisle Publishing Services
Printer/Binder: Edwards Brothers Malloy
Cover Printer: Edwards Brothers Malloy
Text Font: Charis SIL

Credits and acknowledgments for materials borrowed from other sources and reproduced, with permission, in this textbook appear on appropriate page within text.

Every effort has been made to provide accurate and current Internet information in this book. However, the Internet and information posted on it are constantly changing, so it is inevitable that some of the Internet addresses listed in this textbook will change.

Library of Congress Cataloging-in-Publication Data
Small, Larry H.
   Fundamentals of phonetics: a practical guide for students / Larry H. Small.—3rd ed.
      p. cm.
   Includes bibliographical references and index.
   ISBN-13: 978-0-13-258210-0
   ISBN-10: 0-13-258210-4
   1. English language—Phonetics—Problems, exercises, etc.   I. Title.
   PE1135.S49 2012
   421'.58—dc22

                                        2011004916

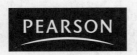

www.pearsonhighered.com

10 9 8
ISBN-13: 978-0-13-258210-0
ISBN-10:   0-13-258210-4

*for
dB
and
my parents*

Contents

Preface

As in the first two editions, I hope that *Fundamentals of Phonetics: A Practical Guide for Students* will continue to help students become skilled experts in phonetic transcription of American English. The third edition has been thoroughly revised. Although the basic format of the text has not veered from the previous editions, all chapters have been modified. While some chapters have been reorganized with the addition of new material, others have been thoroughly reworked.

Supplemental recordings of many of the exercises in the text are available on supplemental audio CDs from Pearson. These recordings are essential in helping students learn the subtleties of pronunciation, in relation to both the segmental and suprasegmental characteristics of speech. A list of the recordings appears in the Appendix of this text.

New to This Edition

- Chapter 1, *Phonetics: A "Sound" Science*, has been expanded in scope. Information relating to the use of computer fonts in phonetic transcription has also been added.

- New exercises have been added to Chapter 3, *Anatomy and Physiology of the Speech Mechanism*.

- In response to many reader comments, information on speech acoustics has been added to both Chapter 4, *Vowels*, and Chapter 5, *Consonants*. Both chapters contain dedicated sections that focus on spectrographic analysis of vowels and consonants, helping students better understand the relationship between acoustics and production of speech.

- Chapter 7, *Clinical Phonetics: Transcription of Speech Sound Disorders*, has a stronger emphasis on transcription of speech sound disorders. More information related to the use of diacritics and non-English IPA symbols in transcription of disordered speech is provided.

- Chapter 8, *Dialectal Variation*, has been largely reshaped and revised. Updates reflect current trends and philosophies related to our current understanding of regional and ethnic dialects. In addition, the section on language transfer and the learning of English as a second language has been completely rewritten.

■ *Online Resources* have been provided at the end of each chapter in order to help students supplement their learning of phonetics.

■ *Learning Objectives* have been added at the beginning of each chapter.

■ The references have all been updated to reflect current philosophies and best practices in the field of communication disorders.

New! CourseSmart eTextbook Available

CourseSmart is an exciting new choice for students looking to save money. As an alternative to purchasing the printed textbook, students can purchase an electronic version of the same content. With a CourseSmart eTextbook, students can search the text, make notes online, print out reading assignments that incorporate lecture notes, and bookmark important passages for later review. For more information, or to purchase access to the CourseSmart eTextbook, visit www.coursesmart.com.

Instructor's Resource Manual and Test Bank

Each chapter in the *Instructor's Resource Manual and Test Bank* contains Key Terms and Learning Objectives. Each chapter also includes Multiple Choice, True/False, and Matching questions. The supplement is available online or you can contact your Pearson representative. To download and print the *Instructor's Resource Manual and Test Bank*, go to www.pearsonhighered.com and then click on "Educators."

Acknowledgments

I would like to express my sincere appreciation to Rob Fox and Ewa Jacewicz at The Ohio State University for their assistance in the creation of the recordings and spectrograms used in Chapters 4 and 5. Some of the spectrograms were produced at Ohio State with the TF32 time-frequency analysis software program (Paul Milenkovic, Department of Electrical and Computer Engineering, University of Wisconsin-Madison). The rest of the spectrograms were produced using Praat software (P. Boersma, and D. Weenink, University of Amsterdam), retrieved from www.fon.hum.uva.nl/praat/download_win.html.

A special thank you goes to the reviewers of this third edition. They were quite instrumental in the revisions you see before you. Thank you to Eva Fernandez, Queens College, City University of New York; Iona Johnson, Towson University; Solveig Sperati Korte, The University of South Dakota; Bonnie Lorenzen, Indiana University; and H. S. Venkatagiri, Iowa State University.

Finally, I would like to thank my project manager for the third edition of *Fundamentals of Phonetics*, Kathy Whittier (of Walsh & Associates). She has been a huge help, seeing me through all three editions. Also, hats off to Jamie Bushell and the rest of the editorial staff at Pearson. Last, but certainly not least, I wish to thank my editor Steve Dragin for his continued friendship, wisdom, humor, patience, and overwhelming support since the creation of the first edition more than 10 years ago.

Phonetics:
A "Sound" Science

Learning Objectives

After reading this chapter you will be able to:

1. Explain the importance of the study of phonetics.
2. Name and define the various branches of phonetics.
3. Explain the importance of the *International Phonetic Alphabet* (IPA) in phonetic transcription.
4. State reasons for variation in phonetic transcription practice.
5. State the benefits of using a Unicode font for phonetic transcription.

As adults, you are all familiar with the speaking process. Speaking is something you do every day. In fact, most people find speech to be quite automatic. It is safe to say that most of us are experts at speaking. We probably have been experts since the time we were 3 or 4 years old. Yet we never really think about the process of speech. We do not, as a rule, sit around thinking about how ideas are formed and how their encoded forms are sent from the brain to the speech organs, such as the teeth, lips, and tongue. Nor do we think about how the speech organs can move in synchrony to form words. Think about the last party you attended. You probably did not debate the intricacies of the speech process while conversing with friends. Speaking is something we learned during infancy, and we take the entire process for granted. We are not aware of the speech process; it is involuntary—so involuntary that we often are not conscious of what we have said until after we have said it. Those of you who have "stuck your foot in your mouth" know exactly how automatic the speech process is. Often we have said things and we have no idea why we said them.

Phonetics is the study of the production and perception of speech sounds. During your study of phonetics, you will begin to think about the process of speech production. You will learn how speech is formulated by the speech organs. You also will learn how individual speech sounds are created and how they are combined during the speech process to form syllables and words. You will need to learn to *listen* to the speech patterns of words and sentences to become familiar with the sounds of speech that comprise spoken language. A large part of any course in phonetics also involves how speech sounds are transcribed, or written. Therefore, you also will be learning a new alphabet that will enable you to transcribe speech sounds.

The idea of studying speech sounds may be an odd idea to understand at first. We generally think about words in terms of how they appear in print or how they are spelled. We usually do not take the time to stop and think about how words are spoken and how spoken words sound to a listener. Look at the word "phone" for a moment. What comes to mind? You might consider the fact that it contains the five letters: p-h-o-n-e. Or you might think of its definition. You probably did not say to yourself that there are only three speech sounds in the word ("f"-"o"-"n"). The reason you do not consider the sound patterns of words when reading is simple—it is not something you do daily. Nor is it something you were taught to do. In fact, talking about the sound patterns of words and being able to transcribe them is an arduous task; it requires considerable practice.

As you soon will find out, the way you believe a word sounds may not be the way it sounds at all. First, it is difficult to forget our notions of how a word is spelled. Second, our conception of how a word sounds is usually wrong. Consider the greeting, "How are you doing?" We rarely ask this question with such formality. Most likely, we would say, "How ya doin'?" What happens to the word "are" in this informal version? It disappears! Now examine the pronunciation of the words "do" and "you" in "Whatcha want?" (the informal version of "What do you want?"). Neither of these words is spoken in any recognizable form. Actually, these words become the non-English word "cha" in "whatcha." With these examples, you can begin to understand the importance of thinking about the sounds of speech in order to be able to discuss and transcribe speech patterns.

EXERCISE 1.1

The expressions below are written two separate ways: (1) formally and (2) casually. Examine the differences between the two versions. What happens to the production of the *individual* words in the casual version?

Formal	Casual
1. Are you going to eat now?	Ya gonna eat now?
2. Can't you see her?	Cantcha see 'er?
3. Did you go?	Ja go?

Phonetics is a skill-based course much like taking a foreign language or sign language course. In many ways, it *is* like learning a new language because you will be learning new symbols and new rules to represent spoken language. However, the new symbols you will be learning will be representative of the sounds of English, not their spelling. As with the learning of any new language, phonetics requires considerable practice in order for you to become proficient in its use when transcribing speech patterns. This textbook is designed to promote practice of phonetic transcription principles.

At the beginning of each chapter, several *Learning Objectives* will be listed. By reading through the Learning Objectives, you will have a clear idea of the material contained in each chapter and what you should expect to learn as you read through the text and complete the exercises.

By now, you have noticed that exercises are embedded in the text. It is important that you complete the exercises as you go along instead of waiting until after you have completed the chapter. These exercises emphasize particular points, highlighting the material you just completed, assisting in the learning process. If you are unsure of an answer, simply look in the back of the book for assistance in completing the embedded exercises.

At the end of each chapter, you will find a series of *Review Exercises* so that you may gain expertise with the material presented. The Review Exercises help drive home much of the material discussed in each chapter. All of the answers to the Review Exercises are located at the back of the book. Similar to the embedded exercises, providing the correct answers for the Review Exercises will provide you with immediate feedback, helping you learn from your mistakes. There is no better way to learn! To aid in the learning process, all new terms will be in bold letters the first time they are used. In addition, all new terms can be found in the *Glossary* at the back of the book.

Study Questions at the end of each chapter will help you explore the major concepts presented. *Online Resources* also are provided in order to supplement the material presented in the text. *Assignments* at the end of the chapters were designed to be collected by your instructor to test your comprehension of the material. Therefore, the answers for Assignments are not given in the text.

There are several conventions that will be adopted throughout the text. When there is a reference to a particular Roman alphabet letter, it will be enclosed with a set of quotation marks: for example, the letter "m." Likewise, references to a particular word will also be enclosed with quotation marks: for example, "mail." Individual speech sounds will be referenced with the traditional slash marks: for example, the /m/ sound. When a word and its transcription are given together, they will appear in the following format: "mail" /meɪl/.

A set of three optional audio CDs provide listening exercises to accompany the text. Clinical practice generally requires phonetic transcription of recorded speech samples. Reading words on paper and transcribing them is not the same as transcribing spoken words. The audio CDs are designed to increase your listening skills and your ability to transcribe spoken English. Exercises requiring the audio CDs will be indicated with a CD icon in the margin of the text. There also will be a notation indicating the CD track number where the recorded exercise may be found. A complete listing of the audio tracks is given in the Appendix.

Phonetics as a Field of Study

Phonetics is a multifaceted field of study, containing several interrelated branches. **Historical phonetics** involves the study of sound changes in words. There is a constant mutation over time in the pronunciation of words in all languages. The way we pronounce words in English today is vastly different from the pronunciation of English from C.E. 300 to 1700. For instance, between the fourteenth and seventeenth centuries, there was a marked evolution in the pronunciation of English long vowels. This change in vowel pronunciation is known as the *Great Vowel Shift*. Due to this shift in vowel pronunciation, the words we know today as "bite," "beet," "bait," and "boot" were pronounced (prior to 1700) as "beet," "bait," "bet," and "boat," respectively (Stevick, 1968). Believe it or not, vowel production is still in a state of flux in the United States. In Chapter 8, we will see how northern and southern speech patterns especially are being affected by ongoing changes in vowel pronunciation.

When saying a word, such as "phonetics," there is an intricate interaction between the lips, the tongue, and the other speech organs. **Physiological phonetics** involves the study of the function of the individual speech organs during the process of speaking. The knowledge of the muscles and innervation of the speech organs is especially important in fully understanding their operation during the production of speech. **Acoustic phonetics,** on the other hand, focuses on the differences in the frequency, intensity, and duration of the various consonants and vowels. Differences in the acoustic attributes of speech sounds allow listeners to be able to perceive how sounds, syllables, and words differ from one another. For instance, it is the specific acoustic attributes of the initial consonants in the words "mug," "hug," "rug," and "thug" that allow listeners to tell them apart. **Perceptual phonetics** is the study of a listener's psychoacoustic response (perception) of speech sounds in terms of loudness, pitch, perceived length, and quality. **Experimental phonetics** entails the laboratory study of physiological, acoustic, and perceptual phonetics. Laboratory equipment is used to measure the various attributes of the speech organs during speech production as well as to measure the acoustic characteristics of speech. The scope of **clinical phonetics** involves the study and transcription of speech sound disorders. Disordered speech can be found in children or adults who may have experienced a hearing impairment, fluency disorder, head trauma, stroke, or phonological disorder.

EXERCISE 1.2

Match each branch of phonetics with the description given.

_____ 1. the study of a listener's psychoacoustic response to speech sounds

_____ 2. the study and transcription of speech sound disorders

_____ 3. the laboratory study of phonetics

_____ 4. the study of the function of the speech organs during the process of speaking

_____ 5. the study of sound changes in words

_____ 6. the study of the frequency, intensity and duration of the various consonants and vowels

a. historical phonetics

b. physiological phonetics

c. acoustic phonetics

d. perceptual phonetics

e. experimental phonetics

f. clinical phonetics

Another "sound" science related to phonetics is **phonology.** Phonology is the systematic organization of speech sounds in the production of language. The major distinction between the fields of phonetics and phonology is that *phonetics* focuses on the study of speech sounds, their acoustic and perceptual characteristics, and how they are produced by the speech organs. *Phonology* focuses on the linguistic (phonological) rules that are used to specify the manner in which speech sounds are organized and combined into meaningful units, which are then combined to form syllables, words, and sentences. Phonological rules, along with syntactic/morphological rules (for grammar), semantic rules (for utterance meaning), and pragmatic rules (for language use), are the major rule systems used in production of language.

Once you have mastered the concepts in this text, you will be able to transcribe the speech patterns of your clients using the **International Phonetic Alphabet (IPA).** This alphabet is different from most alphabets because it is designed to represent the *sounds* of words, not their spellings. Without such a systematic phonetic alphabet, it would be virtually impossible to capture on paper an accurate representation of the speech sound disorders of individuals seeking professional remediation. Using the IPA also permits consistency among professionals in their transcription of typical or atypical speech.

Variation in Phonetic Practice

Although the IPA was developed for consistency, not everyone transcribes speech in the same manner. The IPA does allow for some flexibility in actual practice. If you were to pick up another phonetics textbook, you would find some definite differences in transcription symbols. Therefore, alternate transcription schemes will be introduced throughout this text.

One reason transcription practice differs from individual to individual is due to personal habit or the method learned. For instance, the word "or" (or "oar") could be transcribed reliably in all of the following ways:

/ɔr/, /or/, /ɔɚ/, /oɚ/, /ɔɚ/

All of these forms have appeared in other phonetics textbooks and have been adopted by professionals through the years.

Several years ago, I was assigned to a jury trial that lasted two weeks. Due to the length of the trial, the judge allowed us to take notes. So that no one could read my notes, I decided to use the IPA! Because I had to write quickly, my transcription habits changed. At the beginning of the trial, I transcribed the word "or" as /ɔɚ/ due to personal preference. By the middle of the trial, I had switched to /ɔr/, simply because it was easier to write and was more time efficient.

Another difference in use of transcription symbols related to ease of use involves the symbol /r/, traditionally used to transcribe the initial sound in the word "red." According to the IPA, this sound actually should be transcribed with the symbol /ɹ/. The IPA symbol /r/ represents a *trill*, a sound found in Spanish and other languages, but not part of the English speech sound system. Because /r/ and /ɹ/ both do not exist in English, /r/ routinely has been substituted simply because it is easier to write. Since most speech and hearing professionals have continued to use the symbol /r/ instead of /ɹ/ in written transcription, the tradition will be continued in this textbook.

As future speech and hearing professionals, you will be using the IPA to transcribe clients with speech sound disorders. Because the IPA was not originally designed for this purpose, clinicians have varied in their choice of symbols in transcription of speech sound disorders. In 1990, an extended set of phonetic symbols (known as the extIPA) was created as a supplement to the IPA in order to provide a more standard method for transcription of speech sound disorders (see Chapter 7). Similar to the original IPA, the extIPA has not been used consistently among phoneticians, linguists, and speech and hearing professionals.

Is one method of transcription "better" or more correct than another? Some linguists and phoneticians might argue that one form is superior to another based on linguistic, phonological, or acoustic theory. The form of transcription you adopt is not important as long as you understand the underlying rationale for your choice of symbols. In addition, you need to make sure that you are consistent and accurate in the use of the symbols you adopt. Throughout this book, variant transcriptions will be introduced to increase your familiarity with the different symbols you may encounter in actual clinical practice in the future.

IPA Fonts

Historically, the typical typewriter or computer keyboard did not lend itself well to the IPA. Some keyboard symbols were routinely substituted for IPA symbols simply because typewriters and computer keyboards did not have keys for many of the IPA symbols. For example, the word "dot" was typically transcribed (i.e., typed) as /dat/ instead of the correct form /dɑt/ because it simply was not possible to type the vowel symbol /ɑ/.

You may not know it, but you already may have the ability to type IPA symbols with one of the fonts located on your computer. For instance, the Arial Unicode MS and Lucida Sans Unicode fonts (Windows) provide the ability to type IPA symbols, as does the Lucida Grande font (Macintosh).

In 1991, the Unicode Consortium was established in order to develop a universal character set that would represent all of the world's languages. The Consortium continues to publish the Unicode Standard, which in its most recent version, version 5.2, covers 90 different writing systems, including the IPA. The current version of the Standard allows for over 100,000 characters, each mapped to a unique alphanumeric sequence called a *code point*. A code point is a hexadecimal sequence of four numbers (0 through 9) and/or letters ("a" through "f") that uniquely identify each of the characters in the set. Since each character in the universal set is linked to an alphanumeric sequence, the word processor and font you select will determine the "look" of each individual character, that is, what appears on your monitor and what is reproduced by your printer. Keep in mind that any one particular Unicode font does not contain all of the code points from the universal set.

The nice thing about Unicode fonts is that they can be used on multiple platforms (e.g., Macintosh, Windows, or Linux) and can be used with most word processing software packages. In the past, cross-platform fonts did not exist. Also, there was a limit to the number of characters contained in any one font package; most fonts were limited to 256 characters. Also, fonts of different languages existed separately, making it difficult to switch between writing systems in the same document.

Another advantage of using a Unicode font with IPA symbols is that once the symbols have been typed into a particular document, you can switch to a different Unicode font and all of the symbols will remain intact. The only difference in appearance between fonts would be related to a particular font's size and shape, and whether it is a serif or sans serif font. Prior to the utilization of Unicode, it was not possible to switch fonts without obliterating all of the IPA symbols in a document. Trust me, I know!

A large number of Unicode phonetic fonts are available online. Many are available for free and are really quite easy to download and use. The phonetic symbols in this book were created with *Charis SIL*, a Unicode font available from SIL International (see "Online Resources" at the end of this chapter). This font contains over 2000 characters. *Doulos SIL* and *Gentium* are two other Unicode phonetic fonts available for free from the SIL International website.

There are three ways to enter IPA symbols from a Unicode font into a document: (1) make use of software that creates an alternate keyboard layout;

(2) enter the code point for each IPA symbol; or (3) insert each symbol individually by using character maps available as part of the Windows and Macintosh operating systems.

The easiest method is to use an alternate keyboard layout. I used a specialized keyboard for entering the IPA symbols in this text. For instance, to enter the symbol /ʃ/, I simply had to type SHIFT + "s." Without such a keyboard, it would be necessary to type the unique code point for each character (which is a tedious and time-consuming task). For instance, in Microsoft Word (Windows), you would have to type the four-character code point, followed by the sequence of ALT + "x," for entry of a particular symbol. For instance, typing the sequence "0283" followed by ALT + "x," will yield the IPA symbol /ʃ/ (without the slash marks). With a Macintosh, you would hold down the OPTION key and then type the code point. Alternatively, you also could use the "insert symbol" function (Windows) or use "keyboard viewer" (Macintosh) to enter the symbols individually from a character map that shows all of the symbols associated with a particular font. This process is also very tedious and time-consuming.

EXERCISE 1.3

Configure your computer so that you can enter code points into a text document (see "Online Resources" at the end of the chapter for help). Then, enter the following code points and write the corresponding IPA symbol in the blanks provided.

Code Point	IPA Symbol
1. 0259	_____
2. 03B8	_____
3. 028A	_____
4. 0271	_____
5. 0279	_____

A Note on Pronunciation and Dialect

As you read this book, and as you attempt to answer the various exercises, please keep in mind that English pronunciation varies depending upon individual speaking style as well as on **dialect.** A dialect is a variation of language based on geographical area as well as social and ethnic group membership. Dialect not only involves pronunciation of words, but also grammar (syntax) and vocabulary usage. As you will see in Chapter, 8, there is no one fixed standard of English in the United States as is the case in other countries. Instead, Americans speak several different varieties of English.

Knowledge of dialects is extremely important when establishing a treatment plan for individuals whose speech patterns reflect regional or ethnic dialectal variation. Because a dialect should not be considered a substandard form of English, a speech-language pathologist will be concerned with remediation of clients' speech sound errors, not their dialects.

The pronunciations used in this book often reflect the author's Midwest (northern Ohio) pronunciation patterns. This does not mean that alternate pronunciations are wrong! The numerous text and recorded examples, as well as the answer key, may not be indicative of the way *you* pronounce a particular word or sentence. Always check with your instructor for alternate pronunciations of the materials found in this book and on the supplemental CDs.

Study Questions

1. What is a *phonetic alphabet*?
2. Why is it important to use a phonetic alphabet in transcription of individuals with speech sound disorders?
3. Why is there variation in phonetic transcription from person to person?
4. List and define the branches of phonetics.
5. What is the difference between *phonetics* and *phonology*?
6. What is a Unicode font? What are the advantages of using such a font?
7. What are three ways you can enter phonetic symbols into a document using a Unicode font?

Online Resources

Penn State Teaching and Learning with Technology (2009). *Computing with Accents, Symbols and Foreign Scripts—Typing with Non-English Keyboards*. Retrieved from:
http://tlt.its.psu.edu/suggestions/international/keyboards/index.html
(information regarding phonetic font keyboards)

SIL International (2010). *IPA Unicode Keyboards*. Retrieved from
http://scripts.sil.org/UniIPAKeyboard
(keyboarding information)

SIL International (2010). *Welcome to Computers and Writing Systems*. Retrieved from
http://scripts.sil.org/Home
(phonetic fonts)

University College London (UCL) Speech, Hearing and Phonetic Sciences (2010). *Phonetic Symbols, Keyboards and Transcription*. Retrieved from
www.phon.ucl.ac.uk/resource/phonetics.php
(phonetic font keyboard)

Wells, John (2008). University College London (UCL) Speech, Hearing and Phonetic Sciences, *The International Phonetic Alphabet in Unicode*. Retrieved from
www.phon.ucl.ac.uk/home/wells/ipa-unicode.htm
(Unicode code points for the IPA symbols)

Wood, Alan (2010). *Alan Wood's Unicode Resources: Unicode and Multilingual Support in HTML, Fonts, Web Browsers and Other Applications*. Retrieved from
www.alanwood.net/unicode/
(information about Unicode fonts)

Phonetic Transcription of English

Learning Objectives

After reading this chapter you will be able to:

1. Contrast the differences between spelling and sound in English.
2. Describe the various sections of the IPA chart.
3. Define and contrast the terms *phoneme, allophone,* and *morpheme.*
4. Define and describe the components of a syllable.
5. Identify primary stress in words.
6. Contrast between systematic and impressionistic transcription schemes.

As you begin your study of phonetics, it is extremely important to think about words in terms of how they sound and *not* in terms of how they are spelled. As you begin your study of phonetics, it is extremely important to think about words in terms of how they sound and *not* in terms of how they are spelled. *The repetition of this first sentence is not a typographical error.* The importance of this concept cannot be stressed enough. You *must* ignore the spelling of words and concentrate only on speech sounds. If you have been troubled in the past with your inability to spell, do not fear—phonetics is the one course where spelling is highly discouraged.

For many, ignoring spelling and focusing only on the sounds of words will be a difficult task. Most of us started to spell in kindergarten or in first grade as we learned to read. It was drilled into our heads that "cat" was spelled C-A-T and "dog" was spelled D-O-G. Consequently, we learned to connect the spoken (or printed) words with their respective spellings. Imagine the following fictitious scenario between a parent and a child reading along together before bedtime:

> "O.K., Mary. Now, let's think about the word 'cat.' It's spelled C-A-T, but the first speech sound is a /k/ as in 'king,' the second sound is an /æ/ as in 'apple' and the third sound is a /t/ as in 'table.' Notice that the first sound is really a /k/ not a letter 'c.' Words that begin with the letter 'c' may sound like /k/ or may sound like /s/, as in the word 'city.' Actually, Mary, there is no phonetic symbol in English that uses the printed letter 'c' . . ."

Obviously, this type of interchange would cause children to lose any desire to read!

The Difference Between Spelling and Sound

Examine the word "through." Although there are seven printed letters, or **graphemes,** in the word, there are only three speech sounds: "th," "r," and "oo." Now examine the word "phlegm." How many sounds (not letters) do you think are in this word? If you answered four, you are correct—"f," "l," "e," and "m." Obviously, letters do not always adequately represent the number of sounds in a word. Letters only tell us about spelling; they give no clues as to the actual pronunciation of a word. It is imprecise to talk about a sound that may be associated with a particular alphabet letter (or letters) because the letters may not be an accurate reflection of the sound they represent. For instance, the grapheme "s" represents a different sound in the word "size" than it does in the word "vision." What do you think is the sound associated with the letter "g" in the word "phlegm"?

EXERCISE 2.1

Say each of the following words out loud to determine the number of sounds that comprise each one. Write your answer in the blank. Hint: You may want to refer to Table 2.1 for help.

Examples:

3	reed	4	frog	4	wince
___	lazy	___	smooth	___	cough
___	spilled	___	driven	___	oh
___	comb	___	why	___	raisin
___	thrill	___	judge	___	away

An alphabet that contains a separate letter for each individual sound in a language is called a **phonetic alphabet.** A phonetic alphabet maintains a one-to-one relationship between a sound and a particular letter. Our (Roman) alphabet is not phonetic because it contains only 26 alphabet letters to represent approximately 42 English speech sounds. In elementary school we all learned that the English vowels were "a, e, i, o, u, and sometimes y." In actuality, there are approximately fourteen vowel sounds in our language, but we don't have fourteen different letters to represent them.

Because the Roman alphabet contains fewer letters than the number of speech sounds in English, one alphabet letter often represents more than one speech sound. For instance, the grapheme "c," in the words "cent" and "car," represents two different sounds. Likewise, the grapheme "o" represents *six* different sounds in the words "cod," "bone," "women," "bough," "through," and "above." Sometimes, the same sequence of letters represents different sounds in English. For instance, the letter sequence "ough" represents four different vowel sounds in the words "through," "bough," "cough," and "rough." (Note that the spelling "ough" also represents the inclusion of the consonant /f/ in the last two words.) These examples provide further evidence why it is inappropriate to discuss sounds in association with letters. After reading the information above, how would you answer the question, What is the sound of the letter "o" or the letters "ough"?

Another way sound and spelling differ is the fact that the same sound can be represented by more than one letter or sequence of letters. **Allographs** are different letter sequences or patterns that represent the same sound. The following groups of words contain allographs of a particular sound, represented by the underlined letters. You will see that the sound associated with some allographs is predictable, while the sound associated with others is not. Keep in mind that for each example, although the spelling is different, *the sounds they represent are the same.*

> l<u>oo</u>p, thr<u>ough</u>, thr<u>ew</u>, fr<u>ui</u>t, can<u>oe</u>
> m<u>ai</u>l, conv<u>ey</u>, h<u>a</u>te, st<u>ea</u>k
> tr<u>i</u>te, tr<u>y</u>, tr<u>ie</u>d, <u>ai</u>sle, h<u>ei</u>ght
> <u>f</u>or, lau<u>gh</u>, <u>ph</u>oto, mu<u>ff</u>in
> <u>sh</u>oe, <u>S</u>ean, cau<u>ti</u>on, pre<u>ci</u>ous, ti<u>ss</u>ue
> <u>e</u>ked, v<u>i</u>sa, h<u>ee</u>d, m<u>ea</u>t

Note in some of the examples that *pairs* of letters often represent one sound because there are simply not enough single alphabet letters to represent all of the sounds of English. These pairs of letters are called **digraphs.** Digraphs may be the same two letters (as in "h<u>oo</u>t," "h<u>ee</u>d," or "ti<u>ss</u>ue") or two completely different letters (as in "<u>sh</u>oe," "st<u>ea</u>k," or "tr<u>ie</u>d").

EXERCISE 2.2

Examine the underlined sounds (letter combinations) in the words in each row. Place an "X" in front of the one word that does not share an allograph with the others.

Example:

_____	r<u>ai</u>d	_____	c<u>a</u>ke	_____	h<u>ey</u>	X	b<u>a</u>ck
1. _____	<u>sh</u>oe	_____	mea<u>s</u>ure	_____	o<u>c</u>ean	_____	suffi<u>ci</u>ent
2. _____	<u>ch</u>ord	_____	li<u>qu</u>or	_____	bis<u>c</u>uit	_____	ra<u>g</u>
3. _____	m<u>oo</u>n	_____	thr<u>ough</u>	_____	th<u>ou</u>gh	_____	s<u>ui</u>t
4. _____	w<u>oo</u>d	_____	d<u>o</u>ne	_____	fl<u>oo</u>d	_____	r<u>u</u>b
5. _____	<u>i</u>ce	_____	wa<u>s</u>	_____	pre<u>ss</u>	_____	<u>s</u>cissors

---

Another oddity of the spelling of words involves *silent letters.* Although the word "plumb" has five graphemes, the final letter has no connection to the pronunciation of the word. Consequently, "plumb" has only four speech sounds. These "silent" letters also can be found in the words "gnome," "psychosis," "rhombus," and "pneumonia."

Many oddly spelled English words, and those that contain silent letters, are often related to the origin of a word, and usually reflect a spelling common to the language from which it was borrowed. For example, words such as "pneumonia," "rhombus," and "cyst" are derived from the Greek language, helping to explain their particular spellings. In addition, we borrow entire words from other languages, keeping their spelling intact. This only adds to our spelling irregularities. Examples of some words borrowed from other languages include:

savoir faire (French)	karaoke (Japanese)
kielbasa (Polish)	chutzpah (Yiddish)
kindergarten (German)	taekwondo (Korean)
tequila (Spanish)	lasagna (Italian)

Morphemes

If our system of spelling is so irregular, how are we ever able to learn the complexities of the English language? How do we learn to read and write? Actually, our English spelling system is not as odd as it appears. In fact, only about 25 percent of the words in English have irregular spellings (Crystal, 1987). Unfortunately, many of the irregularly spelled words tend to be the ones used often in our language.

One key to the regularity of oddly spelled words can be found if we study the spelling patterns among words that share similar meaningful linguistic units, or morphemes. A **morpheme** is the smallest unit of language capable of carrying meaning. For instance, the word "book" is a morpheme. The word "book" carries meaning because it connotes an item that is composed of pages with print, binding, two covers, and so on. The word "chair" is also a morpheme; it conveys meaning.

Now consider the word "books." It contains two morphemes, the morpheme "book" and the plural morpheme, represented by -s. The -s ending indicates the plural form of the word, that is, more than one book. Since -s carries meaning, it is a morpheme. Other examples of morphemes include regular verb endings (such as -ed and -ing as in the words "walk<u>ed</u>" and "call<u>ing</u>"), prefixes (such as pre- and re- as in "prepaid" and "reread"), and suffixes (such as -tion in "constitution" and -ive as in "talkative"). Notice that syllables and morphemes are not the same thing. It is possible for a one-syllable word, such as "books" or "walked" to have more than one morpheme. Also, it is possible for a two- or three-syllable word to be comprised of only one morpheme (e.g., "carrot" and "celery").

Take a moment to examine the three pairs of words below. Notice that each word pair shares the same morpheme. Say each pair aloud. What do you notice?

*music music*ian   *phlegm phlegm*atic   *press press*ure

Hopefully, you noted that although each pair shares the same morpheme, the pronunciation of the morphemes in each pair is different. English morphemes tend to be spelled the same even though the words that share them are pronounced in a different manner. English spelling may not appear to be so odd if one considers the spelling of the morphemes that form the roots of many irregularly spelled English words (MacKay, 1987).

Morphemes that can stand alone and still carry meaning, such as "book," "phlegm," "music," or "press," are called **free morphemes.** Morphemes (bold) such as **pre**(date), **re**(tread), (book)**s**, (music)**ian**, and (press)**ure** are called **bound morphemes** because they are bound to other words and carry no meaning when they stand alone.

EXERCISE 2.3

For each item below, think of another word that shares the same morpheme.

Example:

create   <u>   creation   </u>

1. deduce	_____	6. great	_____
2. protect	_____	7. honest	_____
3. potent	_____	8. decent	_____
4. scrutiny	_____	9. late	_____
5. labor	_____	10. magnet	_____

EXERCISE 2.4

Indicate the number of morphemes in each of the following words.

Examples:

1	cucumber	2	reading	3	reworked		
_____	caution	_____	running	_____	lived	_____	relistened
_____	warmly	_____	finger	_____	talker	_____	kangaroo
_____	prorated	_____	clarinetist	_____	sharply	_____	swarming

Phonemes

Because it is difficult to use the Roman alphabet to represent speech sounds, the IPA has been adopted by linguists, phoneticians, and speech and hearing professionals for the purpose of speech transcription. The IPA was created for adoption by languages worldwide by the International Phonetic Association, formed in 1886. The IPA symbols are consistent from language to language. For example, the English word "sit" and the German word "mit" (meaning "with") both have the same vowel. Therefore, we would use the same vowel symbol to transcribe these words (/sɪt/ and /mɪt/, respectively). If you were familiar with all of the IPA symbols, you would be capable of transcribing languages other than English. Keep in mind that you would need to know the IPA symbols for speech sounds that are not part of the English language. A list of all of the common IPA symbols used in English is located in Table 2.1. The complete IPA chart (revised to 2005) is located in Figure 2.1. Take some time to examine the IPA chart. There are several sections of the chart that need to be highlighted. The large area at the top, labeled "consonants (pulmonic)," shows all the consonants of the world's languages that are produced with an airstream from the lungs. All English consonants are pulmonic consonants. Many of these symbols may appear foreign to you. Compare the IPA pulmonic consonants with the English consonant symbols given in Table 2.1. You will see that many of the symbols in the IPA chart represent sounds not present in spoken English. However, some of the non-English symbols are used in transcription of disordered speech. This will be discussed in some detail in Chapter 7. Also, call your attention to the section of "non-pulmonic" consonants that are produced without the need for airflow from the lungs. Non-pulmonic consonants include the "clicks" often heard in some African languages.

A very important section of the IPA chart is labeled "vowels." You will note that the vowels are placed in various locations around a four-sided figure. This *quadrilateral* is a schematic drawing of a speaker's mouth, or oral cavity. The placement of the vowel symbols within the quadrilateral is roughly based on where the tongue is located during production of the various vowels. As with the consonants, many of the IPA vowel symbols are representative of speech sounds not found in English.

The area marked "diacritics" presents another array of symbols that are used in conjunction with the IPA consonant and vowel symbols. The use of

TABLE 2.1 The IPA Symbols for American English Phonemes

	Symbol	Key Word
Vowels	/i/	key
	/ɪ/	win
	/e/	reb<u>a</u>te
	/ɛ/	red
	/æ/	had
	/u/	moon
	/ʊ/	wood
	/o/	<u>o</u>kay
	/ɔ/	law
	/ɑ/	cod
	/ə/	<u>a</u>bout
	/ʌ/	bud
	/ɚ/	butt<u>er</u>
	/ɜ/	bird
Diphthongs	/aʊ/	how
	/aɪ/	tie
	/ɔɪ/	boy
	/eɪ/	bake
	/oʊ/	rose
Consonants	/p/	pork
	/b/	bug
	/t/	to
	/d/	dog
	/k/	king
	/g/	go
	/m/	mad
	/n/	name
	/v/	vote
	/ŋ/	ri<u>ng</u>
	/f/	for
	/θ/	<u>th</u>ink
	/ð/	<u>th</u>em
	/s/	say
	/z/	zoo
	/ʃ/	<u>sh</u>ip
	/ʒ/	beige
	/h/	hen
	/tʃ/	<u>ch</u>ew
	/dʒ/	join
	/w/	wise
	/j/	<u>y</u>et
	/r/	row
	/l/	let

THE INTERNATIONAL PHONETIC ALPHABET (revised to 2005)

CONSONANTS (PULMONIC)

© 2005 IPA

	Bilabial	Labiodental	Dental	Alveolar	Post alveolar	Retroflex	Palatal	Velar	Uvular	Pharyngeal	Glottal
Plosive	p b			t d		ʈ ɖ	c ɟ	k g	q ɢ		ʔ
Nasal	m	ɱ		n		ɳ	ɲ	ŋ	N		
Trill	ʙ			r					R		
Tap or Flap		ⱱ		ɾ		ɽ					
Fricative	ɸ β	f v	θ ð	s z	ʃ ʒ	ʂ ʐ	ç ʝ	x ɣ	χ ʁ	ħ ʕ	h ɦ
Lateral fricative				ɬ ɮ							
Approximant		ʋ		ɹ		ɻ	j	ɰ			
Lateral approximant				l		ɭ	ʎ	L			

Where symbols appear in pairs, the one to the right represents a voiced consonant. Shaded areas denote articulations judged impossible.

CONSONANTS (NON-PULMONIC)

Clicks		Voiced implosives		Ejectives	
ʘ	Bilabial	ɓ	Bilabial	ʼ	Examples:
ǀ	Dental	ɗ	Dental/alveolar	pʼ	Bilabial
ǃ	(Post)alveolar	ʄ	Palatal	tʼ	Dental/alveolar
ǂ	Palatoalveolar	ɠ	Velar	kʼ	Velar
ǁ	Alveolar lateral	ʛ	Uvular	sʼ	Alveolar fricative

OTHER SYMBOLS

ʍ	Voiceless labial-velar fricative	ɕ ʑ	Alveolo-palatal fricatives
w	Voiced labial-velar approximant	ɺ	Voiced alveolar lateral flap
ɥ	Voiced labial-palatal approximant	ɧ	Simultaneous ʃ and x
ʜ	Voiceless epiglottal fricative		
ʢ	Voiced epiglottal fricative		Affricates and double articulations can be represented by two symbols joined by a tie bar if necessary. k͡p t͡s
ʡ	Epiglottal plosive		

VOWELS

Where symbols appear in pairs, the one to the right represents a rounded vowel.

SUPRASEGMENTALS

ˈ	Primary stress
ˌ	Secondary stress ˌfoʊnəˈtɪʃən
ː	Long eː
ˑ	Half-long eˑ
˘	Extra-short ĕ
ǀ	Minor (foot) group
‖	Major (intonation) group
.	Syllable break ɹi.ækt
‿	Linking (absence of a break)

DIACRITICS

Diacritics may be placed above a symbol with a descender, e.g. ŋ̊

̥	Voiceless	n̥ d̥	̤	Breathy voiced	b̤ a̤	̪	Dental	t̪ d̪
̬	Voiced	s̬ t̬	̰	Creaky voiced	b̰ a̰	̺	Apical	t̺ d̺
ʰ	Aspirated	tʰ dʰ	̼	Linguolabial	t̼ d̼	̻	Laminal	t̻ d̻
̹	More rounded	ɔ̹	ʷ	Labialized	tʷ dʷ	̃	Nasalized	ẽ
̜	Less rounded	ɔ̜	ʲ	Palatalized	tʲ dʲ	ⁿ	Nasal release	dⁿ
̟	Advanced	u̟	ˠ	Velarized	tˠ dˠ	ˡ	Lateral release	dˡ
̠	Retracted	e̠	ˤ	Pharyngealized	tˤ dˤ	̚	No audible release	d̚
̈	Centralized	ë	̴	Velarized or pharyngealized	ɫ			
̽	Mid-centralized	e̽	̝	Raised	e̝ (ɹ̝ = voiced alveolar fricative)			
̩	Syllabic	n̩	̞	Lowered	e̞ (β̞ = voiced bilabial approximant)			
̯	Non-syllabic	e̯	̘	Advanced Tongue Root	e̘			
˞	Rhoticity	ɚ a˞	̙	Retracted Tongue Root	e̙			

TONES AND WORD ACCENTS

LEVEL			CONTOUR		
e̋ or ˥	Extra high		ě or ꜛ	Rising	
é ˦	High		ê	Falling	
ē ˧	Mid		e᷄	High rising	
è ˨	Low		e᷅	Low rising	
ȅ ˩	Extra low		e᷈	Rising-falling	
↓	Downstep		↗	Global rise	
↑	Upstep		↘	Global fall	

FIGURE 2.1 The International Phonetic Alphabet (revised to 2005). Reprinted with permission from The International Phonetic Association. Copyright 2005 by International Phonetic Association. www.langsci.ucl.ac.uk/ipa/

diacritics indicates an alternate way of producing a certain sound. The use of diacritical markings is explained in more detail in Chapter 7.

The last section of the IPA chart most important for our purposes is labeled "suprasegmentals." The suprasegmental symbols are used to indicate the stress, intonation pattern, and tempo of any particular utterance in a language.

As you look over the entire chart, you will notice that many of the unfamiliar symbols appear similar to the letters of the Roman alphabet. This was one of the guiding principles of the International Phonetic Association when creating the symbols for the IPA. That is, all symbols of the IPA were designed to blend in with the letters of the Roman alphabet (*Handbook of the International Phonetic Association,* 1999).

Initially, the IPA chart will be confusing to you. As you progress through this text, the IPA chart will become less confusing and more meaningful in your study of phonetics. Some good websites that will help you become acquainted with all of the sounds and symbols of the IPA can be found in the "Online Resources" at the end of the chapter.

EXERCISE 2.5

Examine the vowel symbols in Table 2.1. Which vowel symbol would be used to transcribe each vowel in the following words?

Example:

    beast   _i_

1. lend	_____		4. should	_____
2. man	_____		5. rude	_____
3. flick	_____		6. week	_____

EXERCISE 2.6

Examine the consonant symbols in Table 2.1. Which consonant symbol would be used to transcribe the *last* consonant in each of the following words? Hint: Listen to the last sound in each word as you say it aloud. Remember: Forget about spelling!

Examples:

    dog   _g_
    rich   _tʃ_

1. ram	_____		4. sung	_____
2. laugh	_____		5. bath	_____
3. wish	_____		6. leave	_____

EXERCISE 2.7

Which vowel or consonant IPA symbol would you use when transcribing the sounds represented by the digraphs (underlined) in the following words? Write your answer in the blank. (Consult Figure 2.1 and Table 2.1 to assist in completing this exercise.)

1. <u>sh</u>oe _____
2. <u>th</u>em _____
3. <u>ch</u>ew _____
4. g<u>ui</u>lt _____
5. w<u>oo</u>d _____
6. rou<u>gh</u> _____

7. mock<u>ed</u> _____
8. wi<u>ng</u> _____
9. e<u>xa</u>ggerate _____
10. bis<u>cu</u>it _____
11. vi<u>si</u>on _____
12. lab<u>or</u> _____

Since the IPA is a phonetic alphabet, each symbol represents one specific speech sound, or **phoneme.** A phoneme is a speech sound that is capable of differentiating morphemes, and therefore is capable of distinguishing meaning. Note that a morpheme (such as "look") is composed of a string of individual phonemes. A change in a single phoneme always will change the identity and meaning of the morpheme. For example, by changing the initial phoneme from /l/ to /b/, the morpheme "look" becomes "book." Using our definition of phoneme, we can say that the phoneme /l/ (or the phoneme /b/) differentiates the two morphemes "look" and "book." By changing the final phoneme from /t/ to /b/ the morpheme "cat" is distinguished from the morpheme "cab." In these two examples, a change of only one phoneme results in the creation of two morphemes (words, in this case) with completely different meaning. Words that vary by only one phoneme (in the same word position) are called **minimal pairs** or **minimal contrasts.** "Look"/"book" and "cat"/"cab" are examples of minimal pairs because they vary by only one phoneme. In "look"/"book," the phoneme variation occurs at the beginning of the word, and in "cat"/"cab" the phonemes vary at the end of the word. Other examples of minimal pairs include "hear"/"beer," "through"/"brew," "clip"/"click," and "brine"/"bright." Notice that these words differ by only *one speech sound* even though spelling shows more than one letter change.

EXERCISE 2.8

For each word below, create a minimal pair by writing a word in the blank. The first five minimal pairs should reflect a change in the initial phoneme; the second five should involve a change in the final phoneme.

Examples: initial phoneme change   seal   <u>meal</u>
final phoneme change   card   <u>cart</u>

initial phoneme change

1. tame _____
2. late _____
3. call _____
4. could _____
5. boil _____

final phoneme change

6. heart _____
7. tone _____
8. web _____
9. cheap _____
10. rub _____

Complete Assignment 2-1.

Allophones: Members of a Phoneme Family

Up to this point, the term *phoneme* has been discussed as a speech sound that can distinguish one morpheme from another. However, there is another way to define *phoneme*. We could also say that a phoneme is a family of sounds. Speech sounds are not always produced the same way in every word. For example the /l/ in the word "lip" is different from the /l/ in the word "bottle." You might say to yourself: "How are they different? They are both /l/s." You need to consider how these /l/ sounds are produced in the mouth when saying these two words. In "lip," the /l/ is produced with the tongue toward the front of the mouth, and in the word "bottle" the /l/ is produced in the back of the mouth. Say them to yourself and you will discover that this is indeed true. These are but two examples of the /l/-family of sounds.

Members of a phoneme family are actually variant pronunciations of a particular phoneme. These variant pronunciations are called **allophones.** The front (or light)/l/ and the back (or dark) /l/ are allophones or variant productions of the phoneme /l/. These two variants both can be found in the word "little" (the first /l/ is light, the second is dark). Try saying "little" by using the dark /l/ at the beginning of the word. Although the word may sound funny to you, it is still recognizable as the word "little." For this reason, the variants of /l/ are not individual phonemes. Saying the word "little" with either the front or back /l/ at the beginning of the word *does not change the identity or meaning of the original word.* That is, it does not result in the creation of a minimal pair.

EXERCISE 2.9

Try saying the /p/ sound in the word "keep" two different ways:

1. exploding (or releasing) the /p/

2. not exploding the /p/

(These are two allophones of the /p/ phoneme.)

Certain allophones must be produced a particular way due to the constraints of the other sounds in a word, that is, the phonetic context. For instance, the /k/ sound in the word "kid" is produced close to the front of the mouth because the vowel that follows it is a "front vowel," that is, a vowel produced toward the front of the mouth. On the other hand, the /k/ sound in "could" is produced farther back in the mouth, because the vowel following /k/ is a "back vowel," that is, produced toward the back of the mouth. Say the two words, paying attention to the position of your lips and tongue as you pronounce them. Hopefully, you will see that there is a difference in the position of your speech organs. These two allophones of /k/ are *not* interchangeable due to the phonetic constraints of the vowel in each word. These allophones are said to be in **complementary distribution.** That is, these two allophones of /k/ are found in distinctly different phonetic environments and are not free to vary in terms of where in the mouth they may be produced.

Another example of complementary distribution involves production of /p/ in the words "pit" and "spit." In English, when /p/ is produced at the beginning of a word, a small puff of air occurs after its release. The puff of air is called *aspiration*. Say the word "pit," holding your hand in front of your mouth. You should be able to feel the puff of air escaping from your lips following the production of /p/. Whenever the phoneme /p/ follows the phoneme /s/, as in the word "spit," it will always be *unaspirated*. Say the word "spit," holding your hand in front of your mouth. You should feel less air than when you said the word "pit." Hold your hand in front of your mouth, alternating the productions of these two words. You should be able to feel the variance in the airstream on your hand. These two allophones of /p/, aspirated and unaspirated, are in complementary distribution. In English, unaspirated phonemes never occur at the beginning of a word. However, unaspirated phonemes do occur at the beginning of words in many other languages including Russian, Spanish, Mandarin Chinese, and Tagalog.

In contrast to the examples just given, some allophones are not linked to phonetic context and therefore can be exchanged for one another; they are free to vary. In Exercise 2.9 you were asked to say the word "keep" two different ways, either releasing the /p/ or not. In this case, it is up to the speaker to decide. The phonetic environment has no bearing on whether the /p/ will be exploded. In this case, the allophones of /p/ are said to be in **free variation.** Likewise, the final /t/ in the word "hit" may be released or unreleased, depending on the speaker's individual production of the word. These two variant productions (released or unreleased) are allophones of /t/ that are in free variation.

Syllables

In conversational speech, it is often difficult to determine where one phoneme ends and the next one begins. This is due to the fact that in connected speech, phonemes are not produced in a serial order, one after the other. Instead, phonemes are produced in an overlaid fashion due to overlapping movements of the articulators (speech organs) during speech production. Because there is considerable overlap in phonemes during the production of speech, many phoneticians and linguists suggest that the smallest unit of speech production is not the allophone or phoneme, but the **syllable.**

As you know, words are composed of one or more syllables. We all have a general idea of what a syllable is. If you were asked how many syllables were in the word "meatball," you would have little difficulty determining the correct answer—two. Even though you have a general idea of what a syllable is, in actuality it is quite difficult to answer the seemingly simple question, *What is a syllable?* The reason for this difficulty is that a syllable may be defined in more than one way. Also, phoneticians and linguists often do not agree on the actual definition of a syllable.

We will begin our definition by stating that a syllable is a basic building block of language that may be composed of either one vowel alone, or a vowel in combination with one or more consonants. This is the definition typically found in a dictionary or in a junior high school language arts textbook. However, for our purposes, this definition is not adequate. This definition is based on vowel and consonant letters, not vowel and consonant phonemes.

In most cases, it is easy to identify the number of syllables in a word. For instance, we would agree that the words "control," "intend," and "downtown" all have two syllables. Likewise, it is easy to determine that the words "contagious," "alphabet," and "tremendous" each have three syllables. However, it is not always so easy to determine the number of syllables in a word. Using our simple dictionary definition, the words "feel" and "pool" would be one-syllable words. That is, they each contain a vowel in combination with one or more consonant letters. Many individuals, however, pronounce these words as two syllables. On the other hand, some people pronounce these words as one syllable depending on their individual speaking style and dialect. The word "pool" is pronounced by many as "pull," as in "swimming pull." Likewise, some southern speakers pronounce the word "feel" as "fill," as in "I fill fine."

Another example involves the words "prism" and "chasm." According to the basic definition, these words would be considered one syllable, because they contain only one vowel. However, most speakers would probably consider these words to consist of two syllables. One last example involves the pronunciation of words like "camera" or "chocolate." These words have three vowels, but can be pronounced as either two or three syllables, depending on whether the speaker pronounces the middle vowel (i.e., "camra" or "choclate"). Both pronunciations would be considered to be appropriate for either word.

Obviously, a better definition of "syllable" is necessary to help overcome these difficulties. One way to refine our definition might be to more fully describe a syllable's internal structure, using terms other than consonant and vowel. It is possible to divide English syllables into two components: **onset** and **rhyme.** The onset of a syllable consists of all the consonants that precede a vowel, as in the words "**spl**it," "**tr**ied," and "**f**ast" (onset in bold letters). Note that the onset may consist of either a single consonant or a **consonant cluster** (two or three contiguous consonants in the same syllable).

In syllables with no initial consonant, there would be no onset. Examples of words with no onset would be "eat," "I," and the first syllable in the word "afraid." Note that the second syllable of "afraid" has an onset consisting of the consonants /f/ and /r/.

EXERCISE 2.10

Circle the syllables in the following one-syllable and two-syllable words containing an onset. (For the two-syllable words, circle *any* syllable with an onset.)

ouch	crab	hoe	oats	elm	your
react	cargo	beware	atone	courage	eating

The rhyme of a syllable is divided into two components, the **nucleus** and the **coda.** The nucleus is typically a vowel. The nuclei of the words "spl**i**t," "tr**ie**d," and "f**a**st" are indicated in bold letters. However, several *consonants* in English may be considered to be the nucleus of a syllable in certain instances. In the words "chasm" and "feel," the /m/ and /l/ phonemes would be considered to be the nucleus of the second syllable of each word (if "feel" is pronounced as a two-syllable word). In these words, the consonants /m/ and /l/ assume the role of the vowel in the second syllable. When consonants take on the role of vowels, they are called **syllabic consonants.**

The coda includes either single consonants or consonant clusters that follow the nucleus of a syllable, as in the words "split," "tried," and "fast." In some instances, the coda may in fact have no elements at all, as in the words "me," "shoe," "oh," and "pry."

EXERCISE 2.11

Circle the letters that make up the nucleus in the following words. Some of the words have more than one nucleus.

shrine	scold	plea	produce	schism	away
elope	selfish	auto	biceps	flight	truce

EXERCISE 2.12

Circle the word(s) (or syllables) that have a coda.

through	spa	rough	bough	row	spray
lawful	funny	create	inverse	candy	reply

To further illustrate the nomenclature associated with syllables, the structure of the one-syllable words "scrub," "each," and "three" are detailed in "tree diagrams" (Figure 2.2). The onset, rhyme, nucleus, and coda of each word are labeled appropriately. The Greek letter sigma (σ) is used to indicate a syllable division. Note the null symbol (φ), which indicates the absence of the onset and coda in two of the examples. Diagrams of the two-syllable words "behave" and "prism" follow the diagrams of the one-syllable words (see Figure 2.3). Notice in Figure 2.3 that the consonant /m/ in "prism" forms the nucleus of the second syllable.

Syllables that end with a vowel phoneme (no coda) are called **open syllables.** Examples include "the" and both syllables of the word "maybe." Words that consist solely of a vowel nucleus, as in the words "I," "oh," and "a," also are considered to be open syllables. Syllables with a coda—that is, those that end with a consonant phoneme—are called **closed syllables.** Examples of closed syllables are "had," "keg," and both syllables in the word "contain." When determining whether a syllable is open or closed, you need to pay attention to the phonemic specification of the syllable, not its spelling. More examples of open and closed syllables are given below.

Words with Open Syllables		*Words with Closed Syllables*	
One-Syllable	*Two-Syllable*	*One-Syllable*	*Two-Syllable*
he	allow	corn	captive
bow	daily	suave	chalice
may	belie	wish	dentist
rye	zebra	charge	English
through	hobo	slammed	invest

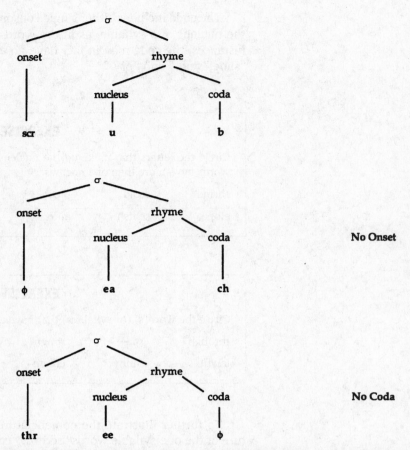

FIGURE 2.2 Syllable structure of the one-syllable words "scrub," "each," and "three."

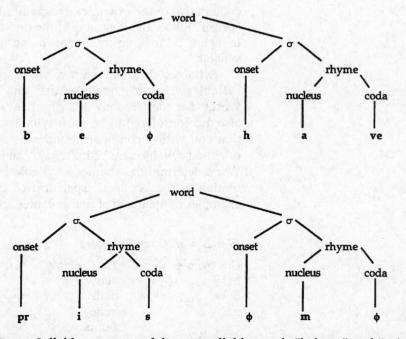

FIGURE 2.3 Syllable structure of the two-syllable words "behave" and "prism."

EXERCISE 2.13

Examine the following two-syllable words. Indicate whether the *first* syllable is open (O) or closed (C) by filling in the blank with the appropriate letter.

Example: __O__   around   __C__   blistered

____ pliant   ____ comply   ____ coerced   ____ minutes

____ decree   ____ encase   ____ flatly   ____ preface

EXERCISE 2.14

Examine the same two-syllable words as those in the previous exercise. Indicate whether the *second* syllable is open (O) or closed (C) by filling in the blank with the appropriate letter.

Example: __C__   around   __C__   blistered

____ pliant   ____ comply   ____ coerced   ____ minutes

____ decree   ____ encase   ____ flatly   ____ preface

Word Stress

In words with more than one syllable, there will be one syllable that will be produced with the greatest force or greatest muscular energy. The increased muscular energy will cause the syllable to stand apart from the others due to greater emphasis of the syllable. This increased emphasis in the production of one syllable is commonly referred to as **word stress** or **lexical stress.** The increase in muscular force or emphasis results in a syllable that is perceived by listeners as longer in duration, higher in pitch, and, to a lesser extent, louder (i.e., greater in intensity). The rise in pitch is particularly important in alerting listeners to the stressed syllable in a word (Lehiste, 1970). Phoneticians also refer to word stress, or lexical stress, as *word accent* (Calvert, 1986; Cruttenden, 2001).

Stress is not a trivial matter in learning and understanding spoken language. When we hear a word such as "confuse," we recognize it not only because of the particular phonemes that comprise it, but also because of the inherent stress pattern of the word. Try saying this word by changing the stress to the first syllable, that is, CONfuse. The word now sounds somewhat odd to you because the string of phonemes does not coincide with the new stress pattern. The unique combination of these individual phonemes and this particular stress pattern does not match any item stored in your mental dictionary. As language is developed, children (not just those learning English) must master not only the phonemes that make up individual words, but also their associated stress patterns. However, the stress patterns of different languages vary remarkably. One major reason why foreign speakers of English (or any second language) have difficulty with pronunciation is due to lack of knowledge of the stress patterns of the new language being learned. Second-language learners will often sound "foreign," that is, have an "accent," when using the stress pattern of their native language while speaking a second language.

In English, words that have more than one syllable will always have one particular syllable that will receive *primary stress* (i.e., the greatest emphasis). For example, the bisyllabic (two-syllable) word "SISter" has primary stress on the first syllable. The multisyllabic (more than two-syllable) word "courAgeous" has primary stress on the second syllable. Syllables in bisyllabic and multisyllabic words that do not receive primary stress may receive *secondary stress* or no stress, depending on the level of emphasis given to the individual syllable.

Word (lexical) stress is extremely important in learning the phonetic transcription of English because some of the IPA symbols indicate which syllable in a word receives primary stress. Although it is possible to learn how to mark levels of stress in multisyllabic words (i.e., primary versus secondary stress), for now, we will focus primarily on indicating whether a syllable receives primary stress.

Some students will experience little difficulty in identifying the syllable with primary stress in bisyllabic and multisyllabic words. Unfortunately, for many this ability is extremely trying. Part of the reason for this difficulty is that although we know how to use stress correctly in *production of speech,* we are not accustomed to thinking about stress patterns in the *perception of speech.* As communicators, we simply are not used to listening to speech and identifying stressed syllables in words. Researchers have been successful in enumerating the rules that govern the location of primary stress in words (Chomsky & Halle, 1968; Cruttenden, 2001; Jones, 1967). However, the rules do have exceptions, and they are also difficult to remember. During transcription of speech, there is simply not enough time to think about the rules governing stress in words. For purposes of phonetic transcription, what is important is the ability to hear the location of primary stress in words, not the rules that govern how stress is assigned to syllables. Fortunately, the ability to identify (hear) the location of primary stress in words can be developed in time with much listening practice.

Examine the following bisyllabic words. Say them aloud. What do you notice about the stress patterns of these words? (**Hint:** They all have the *same* stress pattern.)

contain	aware	berserk	charade
inspect	reveal	suppose	detain

Hopefully, you determined that the *second* syllable of each of these words receives primary stress. Say the words again, paying careful attention to the increased pitch associated with the second syllable:

conTAIN	aWARE	berSERK	chaRADE
inSPECT	reVEAL	supPOSE	deTAIN

The IPA symbol used for indicating the primary stress of a word is a raised mark (') placed at the initiation of the stressed syllable. The words above would be marked in the following manner to indicate second-syllable stress:

con'tain	a'ware	ber'serk	cha'rade
in'spect	re'veal	sup'pose	de'tain

Now, examine the following bisyllabic words. Each of these words contain *first* syllable primary stress:

'teacher	'certain	'careful	'practice
'plural	'larynx	'primate	'contact

EXERCISE 2.15

One word in each row does not have the same stress pattern as the others. Circle the word that does not have the same stress pattern.

1. dandruff shampoo bottle fragrance
2. cologne   soufflé   surreal careful
3. always   never   okay   maybe
4. Marie   Sarah   April   Lizzie
5. intrude   instruct   invade   injure

Word stress, in addition to its role in pronunciation, also helps differentiate words that are spelled the same but vary in part of speech, or **word class** (i.e., whether a word is a noun, verb, adjective, adverb, etc.). For instance, the words "'contract" (noun) and "con'tract" (verb), although spelled the same, have different stress patterns. The noun form 'contract has stress placed on the first syllable, whereas the verb form con'tract has word stress on the second syllable. Note that the change in the stress pattern not only changes the meaning of the word, but also changes its pronunciation. Say these two words aloud. How do the two words differ in pronunciation? You probably noted that as stress changes, vowel pronunciation changes in one or both syllables. Other examples of two-syllable noun/verb pairs differing in word stress include:

Noun	*Verb*	*Noun*	*Verb*
'conflict	con'flict	'permit	per'mit
'record	re'cord	'subject	sub'ject
'digest	di'gest	'rebel	re'bel
'convert	con'vert	'conduct	con'duct

Note that in these word pairs, the noun form always receives first-syllable stress, and the verb form always receives second-syllable stress.

EXERCISE 2.16

Circle the words that can be spoken as both a noun *and* a verb by shifting the stress pattern between the first and second syllables.

propose contest protest congress research

project   consume compress reasoned confines

CD #1
Track 1

Because identifying the primary stress in bisyllabic and multisyllabic words is a difficult chore, the following 12 word lists will provide you with some practice in listening for primary stress in words. These word lists (and accompanying exercises) are designed to make you focus on one particular stress pattern at a time. The lists begin with bisyllabic words and progress to multisyllabic words. As you examine each list, say the words aloud, focusing on the particular stress pattern being demonstrated. Listen to each list several times until you are comfortable with the stress pattern being demonstrated. If you experience any difficulty with Exercises 2.17, 2.18, and 2.19, review the word lists until you understand your errors.

**CD #1
Track 2**

List 1: Bisyllabic words; first-syllable stress (words beginning with "e")

edict	easy	eager	Easter
Egypt	ether	either	even
Ethan	eagle	eater	ego

Note: Keep in mind that words beginning with the letter "e" do not always have first-syllable stress. Examine the words in List 2.

**CD #1
Track 3**

List 2: Bisyllabic words; second-syllable stress (words beginning with "e")

eclipse	elapse	efface	effect
elate	elect	ellipse	elude
Elaine	emote	enough	erupt

**CD #1
Track 4**

List 3: Bisyllabic words; first-syllable stress (words beginning with "o")

over	ocean	omen	owner
Oprah	onus	oboe	ogre
okra	open	ozone	odor

Note: Keep in mind that words beginning with the letter "o" do not always have first-syllable stress. Examine the words in List 4.

**CD #1
Track 5**

List 4: Bisyllabic words; second-syllable stress (words beginning with "o")

overt	obey	oppress	olé
okay	oblique	obese	oblige

**CD #1
Track 6**

List 5: Bisyllabic words; first-syllable stress (words beginning with "in")

invoice	instant	inbred	insect
inner	inches	ingrate	infant
income	index	infield	inlay

Note: Keep in mind that words beginning with the letters "in" do not always have first-syllable stress. Examine the words in List 6.

**CD #1
Track 7**

List 6: Bisyllabic words; second-syllable stress (words beginning with "in")

inspire	instead	induce	inject
infect	inflict	indeed	inept
infer	inscribe	intrude	involve

**CD #1
Track 8**

List 7: Bisyllabic words; second-syllable stress (words beginning with "a")

around	abuse	abort	amass	avoid	abode
away	aware	arise	alike	afloat	avenge
abrupt	adorn	accost	atone	aloof	aghast
alas	akin	avow	adapt	afraid	anoint

Note: There are many words in English (such as those in List 7) that begin with the letter "a." The vowel phoneme associated with the sound at the beginning of these words is called *schwa*, represented with the IPA symbol /ə/. This unstressed vowel constitutes its own syllable in all of the words in List 7.

CD #1
Track 9

List 8: Bisyllabic words; first-syllable stress

engine	master	caring	lucky	staples	Harold
plastic	rowing	neither	happen	Dayton	careful
forest	whisper	quandary	listless	tantrum	nacho
siphon	solo	hidden	trophy	panda	Pittsburgh

Note: Most, but not all, two-syllable words in English have first-syllable primary stress. Examine List 9 for two-syllable words with second-syllable primary stress.

CD #1
Track 10

List 9: Bisyllabic words; second-syllable stress

remove	control	serene	carafe	pertain	repulse
arranged	remain	caffeine	repute	suppose	untrue
perspire	beside	react	Brazil	invoke	humane
manure	discrete	compress	admire	assist	beguile

CD #1
Track 11

List 10: Three-syllable words; first-syllable stress

realize	horrible	circulate	fidgety	element	hypnotize
hydrogen	insulin	character	mediate	critical	Michigan
premium	rivalry	sacrifice	tolerant	verbalize	readable
yesterday	xylophone	mystify	glorious	caraway	terrible

CD #1
Track 12

List 11: Three-syllable words; second-syllable stress

Missouri	insipid	metallic	Ohio	betrayal	inscription
confusion	diploma	abortion	courageous	erosion	contagious
awareness	preparing	computer	neurotic	palatial	morphemic
repulsive	reminded	semantics	charisma	aroma	transistor

CD #1
Track 13

List 12: Three-syllable words; third-syllable stress

interrupt	indiscreet	Illinois	prearrange	disrespect	contradict
minuet	intervene	buccaneer	decompose	interfere	masquerade
reprehend	obsolete	readjust	disinfect	reapply	connoisseur
reimburse	introduce	predispose	disenchant	represent	nondescript

Note: It is possible to pronounce some of words in List 12 with stress on the *first* syllable, depending on your own speaking habit and dialect. In addition, the location of stress in a multisyllabic word may change, depending on the message the speaker wishes to convey.

CD #1
Track 14

EXERCISE 2.17

Circle the words that have *second*-syllable stress.

decoy	mirage	pastel	puzzle	regret	platoon
stipend	thesis	undo	reason	falter	Maureen
timid	planted	derail	virtue	restricts	peon
transcend	parade	circus	suspend	movie	shoulder
lucid	cajole	devoid	cassette	provide	merchant

CD #1
Track 15

EXERCISE 2.18

Circle the three-syllable words that have *first*-syllable stress.

pondering	edited	consequent	misery	calendar	ebony
plentiful	asterisk	pharyngeal	persona	distinctive	example
surrounded	December	caribou	underling	Barbados	lasagna
terrified	hydrangea	telephoned	contended	perfected	India
musical	skeletal	courageous	umbrella	Philistine	perusal

CD #1
Track 16

EXERCISE 2.19

Circle the three-syllable words that have *second*-syllable stress.

stupendous	pliable	creative	carefully	elevate	magical
corporal	answering	spectacle	presumption	placenta	bananas
plantation	clarinet	murderer	predisposed	decorum	horribly
heroic	violin	integer	discover	clavicle	majestic
daffodil	subscription	expertise	immoral	muscular	Hawaii

Complete Assignment 2-2.

Broad Versus Narrow Transcription

Throughout the book, we will be referring to different forms of phonetic transcription. Therefore, it is important to say a brief word regarding these different forms of transcription now. Transcription of speech, making no attempt at transcribing allophonic variation is called **systematic phonemic transcription.** Systematic phonemic transcription also is referred to as *broad transcription,* or simply *phonemic transcription.* Virgules (or slash marks) always are used with phonemic transcription. All forms of "systematic" transcription require knowledge of the phonological patterns, or sound system, of a language prior to analysis of a speech sample (*Handbook of the International Phonetic Association,* 1999). An example of broad transcription would be transcribing the word "pull" as /pʊl/. The final /l/ is a *dark* /l/. However, broad transcription does not make that distinction since the intent of phonemic (broad) transcription is to capture on paper the transcription of phonemes, with no reference to allophonic variation.

Systematic narrow transcription (*allophonic transcription*), on the other hand, relies on specialized symbols, called **diacritics,** to show modifications in the production of a vowel or consonant phoneme during transcription. As with systematic phonemic transcription, knowledge of the phonological system of a language is required when using systematic narrow (allophonic) transcription. Allophonic transcription of the word "ball" with a velarized or *dark* /l/ would be [bɑɫ]. Notice that brackets, not virgules, are used with narrow transcription. Narrow transcription also would allow for differentiation between the released (exploded) /p/ and the unreleased /p/ in production of the words "keep" [kip] and [kip̚], respectively.

There are times when transcription of an *unknown* sound system may be necessary. Suppose you were asked to analyze the phonological system of someone who spoke a language with which you were not familiar. You would need to listen very carefully and would need to put down on paper every phonemic and allophonic detail associated with that person's speech production. Every detail would be important, because you would be interested in trying to understand the rules that explain how the speech sound system is structured. This type of transcription, where nothing is known about a particular speech sound system prior to analysis, is termed an **impressionistic transcription,** another form of narrow transcription. Impressionistic transcription also may be employed when working with a child who has a severe speech sound disorder affecting the rules associated with typical speech development. Brackets always are used when performing an impressionistic transcription.

EXERCISE 2.20

Match the terms that can be associated with *phonemic, allophonic,* or *impressionistic* transcription. There will be more than one correct answer for each term.

_____ phonemic	1. broad transcription
_____ allophonic	2. narrow transcription
_____ impressionistic	3. use of virgules
	4. use of brackets
	5. systematic transcription

Review Exercises

A. How many phonemes are there in each of the following words? Circle the words that have the same number of phonemes as letters.

1. bread _____	5. plot _____	9. fat _____
2. coughs _____	6. stroke _____	10. tomb _____
3. throw _____	7. fluid _____	11. walked _____
4. news _____	8. spew _____	12. last _____

B. How many morphemes are there in the following words?

1. clueless _____	6. rewrite _____
2. tomato _____	7. winterized _____
3. pumpkin _____	8. edits _____
4. likable _____	9. thoughtlessness _____
5. cheddar _____	10. coexisting _____

C. Listed below are three columns of words. Decide if the words in columns 2 or 3 *end* in the same phoneme as the words in the first column. *Circle* the correct matches.

1. box	flack	puss
2. buzz	dogs	fits
3. flag	lounge	league
4. cooked	pant	nagged

5. throw	cow	beau
6. through	chow	flew
7. tomb	limb	bob
8. fleas	wheeze	mice
9. laugh	giraffe	bough
10. path	bathe	cloth

D. When the sounds in the words below are reversed, they make another word. What is the new word in each case, after reversing the sounds?

1. net	_____	6. main	_____
2. sell	_____	7. pin	_____
3. pots	_____	8. ban	_____
4. gnat	_____	9. tack	_____
5. need	_____	10. tune	_____

E. For the following set of items, circle the one that *begins* with a sound *different* from the other two.

1. church	chef	chop
2. see	cent	cut
3. think	this	these
4. knee	came	nut
5. phone	please	frost
6. song	sure	sheep
7. gnat	grim	groan
8. cup	choir	chore
9. gerbil	goat	George
10. their	thanks	thing

F. Give a minimal pair for each of the following words by changing the underlined phoneme.

1. spit	_____	6. fan	_____
2. hand	_____	7. think	_____
3. pink	_____	8. had	_____
4. sin	_____	9. took	_____
5. pail	_____	10. rob	_____

G. Circle the following pairs of words that are *minimal pairs*.

1. maybe, baby	6. bribe, tribe
2. plaid, prod	7. smart, dart
3. looks, lacks	8. dinner, runner
4. mail, snail	9. window, minnow
5. prance, prince	10. lumpy, bumpy

H. Indicate, for the underlined syllables, whether they are open (O) or closed (C).

| 1. marble | _____ | 3. patron | _____ |
| 2. previous | _____ | 4. trifle | _____ |

5. <u>so</u>dium   _____   8. <u>luck</u>y   _____

6. <u>awe</u>some   _____   9. <u>pro</u><u>fit</u>   _____

7. mi<u>stake</u>   _____   10. <u>sys</u>tem   _____

I. Examine the following words. Indicate whether the *first* syllable has an *onset* and/or a *coda* by placing an "X" in the appropriate column.

Examples:

	Onset		Coda	
	Yes	*No*	*Yes*	*No*
social	X	____	____	X
picture	X	____	X	____
1. mentions	____	____	____	____
2. icon	____	____	____	____
3. camper	____	____	____	____
4. instinct	____	____	____	____
5. able	____	____	____	____
6. lotion	____	____	____	____
7. charming	____	____	____	____
8. asterisk	____	____	____	____
9. Japan	____	____	____	____
10. aloof	____	____	____	____

J. Indicate the primary stress for each of the following two-syllable words. Write "1" if the first syllable has primary stress or "2" if the second syllable has primary stress.

CD #1
Track 17

____ 1. loser	____ 6. provoke	____ 11. plastic
____ 2. unsure	____ 7. stagnant	____ 12. divorce
____ 3. anxious	____ 8. beside	____ 13. western
____ 4. disturb	____ 9. germane	____ 14. language
____ 5. Grecian	____ 10. gourmet	____ 15. defer

K. Indicate the primary stress for each of the following three-syllable items. Write "1", "2," or "3" to indicate the syllable with primary stress.

CD #1
Track 18

____ 1. provincial	____ 6. hypocrite	____ 11. picturesque
____ 2. sorceress	____ 7. indisposed	____ 12. relegate
____ 3. indigent	____ 8. uncertain	____ 13. foundation
____ 4. commander	____ 9. magenta	____ 14. contagious
____ 5. arabesque	____ 10. platypus	____ 15. constable

L. Indicate the primary stress for each of the following four-syllable words. Write "1," "2," "3," or "4" to indicate the syllable with primary stress.

CD #1
Track 19

_____ 1. problematic   _____ 6. correlation   _____ 11. protozoan

_____ 2. mercenary   _____ 7. catamaran   _____ 12. contradiction

_____ 3. statistical   _____ 8. continuant   _____ 13. protoplasm

_____ 4. ecosystem   _____ 9. allegory   _____ 14. Argentina

_____ 5. gregarious   _____ 10. carnivorous   _____ 15. obstructionist

Study Questions

1. What is a phonetic alphabet?

2. What is the difference between a *digraph* and an *allograph?*

3. Discuss three ways in which English spelling principles deviate from the ways words are pronounced.

4. Define the following terms:
    a. *morpheme*
    b. *phoneme*
    c. *grapheme*

5. Why are *allophones* not considered to be *phonemes?*

6. Contrast the terms *complementary distribution* and *free variation.*

7. What is the purpose of the IPA?

8. Why is the term *syllable* difficult to define?

9. Define the following terms: *onset, rhyme, coda, nucleus.*

10. What is the difference between an *open* and a *closed* syllable?

11. Why are the words "spread" and "bread" not *minimal pairs?*

12. What is the difference between *phonemic* (broad), *allophonic* (narrow), and *impressionistic* transcription?

Online Resources

International Phonetics Association Home Page (nd). Retrieved from:
   www.langsci.ucl.ac.uk/ipa/
   (numerous resources including charts, sounds, and fonts)

SIL International (2010). *IPA Help.* Retrieved from:
   www.sil.org/computing/ipahelp/index.htm
   (downloadable computer program for learning sounds of the IPA)

UCLA Phonetics Lab Archive (2009). Retrieved from:
   http://archive.phonetics.ucla.edu/
   (provides information and audio recordings regarding the sounds of the world's languages)

UCLA Phonetics Lab Data Web Page (Peter Ladefoged) (nd). Retrieved from:
   www.phonetics.ucla.edu/
   (provides recorded samples of the sounds of the world's languages)

The University of Victoria Department of Linguistics: Linguistics IPA Lab (nd). *Public IPA Chart.* Retrieved from:
   http://web.uvic.ca/ling/resources/ipa/charts/IPAlab/IPAlab.htm
   (interactive IPA chart with pronunciations of all IPA symbols)

Assignment 2-1   Name _____

1. Indicate the number of phonemes in the following words.

   a. ____ queen   e. ____ treats   i. ____ window
   b. ____ Christine   f. ____ rough   j. ____ Toledo
   c. ____ thought   g. ____ diskette   k. ____ received
   d. ____ ripped   h. ____ extra   l. ____ sprints

2. Indicate the number of morphemes in the following words.

   a. ____ lasting   e. ____ paper   i. ____ currently
   b. ____ wonders   f. ____ speedy   j. ____ unchanging
   c. ____ ideas   g. ____ monkeys   k. ____ cantaloupe
   d. ____ misplaced   h. ____ devalue   l. ____ reapplied

3. For the following set of items, circle the words that *begin* with a sound different from the other two.

   a. train   think   Thomas
   b. Janet   genie   gaunt
   c. them   Theo   that
   d. capture   chaos   chowder
   e. fathom   phone   push
   f. chasm   king   chastity
   g. knot   gnu   guru
   h. genre   judge   gym
   i. chance   chortle   chord
   j. sail   candy   centipede

4. For the following set of items, circle the words that *end* with a sound different from the other two.

   a. wreath   breathe   breath
   b. coop   coup   flew
   c. keys   gnats   wheeze
   d. catch   splash   mesh
   e. blue   flow   chew
   f. rapt   rad   caulked
   g. was   floss   causes
   h. tract   trapped   trailed
   i. wax   laws   wicks
   j. below   brow   crow

Assignment 2-2   Name _____

1. Give a minimal pair for each of the following words by changing the underlined phonemes.

   a. b<u>i</u>nd _____   f. w<u>i</u>n _____

   b. lea<u>n</u> _____   g. pa<u>th</u> _____

   c. r<u>e</u>d _____   h. <u>j</u>ob _____

   d. wi<u>sh</u> _____   i. <u>t</u>rash _____

   e. <u>l</u>ook _____   j. f<u>oa</u>m _____

2. Circle the following pairs of words that are *not* minimal pairs.

   a. one, sun   f. respire, perspire

   b. clasp, grasp   g. large, charge

   c. learn, turn   h. feud, rude

   d. slice, nice   i. thrash, crash

   e. spite, spot   j. gerbil, journal

3. Indicate, for the underlined syllables, whether they are open (O) or closed (C).

   a. grue<u>some</u> _____   f. con<u>spire</u> _____

   b. la<u>zy</u> _____   g. set<u>tee</u> _____

   c. <u>pre</u>dict _____   h. <u>sev</u>eral _____

   d. con<u>fuse</u> _____   i. <u>sui</u>table _____

   e. <u>suc</u>cess _____   j. <u>thy</u>roid _____

4. Indicate (with an "X") the words that have an onset in the *second* syllable.

   a. concern _____   f. preempt _____

   b. inaugurate _____   g. request _____

   c. gigantic _____   h. earring _____

   d. bulkhead _____   i. barley _____

   e. cocoa _____   j. coaxial _____

5. Examine the following words. Indicate whether the *first* syllable has an onset and/or a coda by placing an "X" in the appropriate column.

Examples:	*Onset*		*Coda*	
	Yes	*No*	*Yes*	*No*
social	X	___	___	X
picture	X	___	X	___
a. sandbag	___	___	___	___
b. deactivate	___	___	___	___

Assignment 2-2 (cont.)

	Onset		Coda	
	Yes	*No*	*Yes*	*No*
c. auspicious	_____	_____	_____	_____
d. enunciate	_____	_____	_____	_____
e. sycamore	_____	_____	_____	_____
f. toxic	_____	_____	_____	_____
g. reflective	_____	_____	_____	_____
h. overtly	_____	_____	_____	_____
i. encapsule	_____	_____	_____	_____
j. fusion	_____	_____	_____	_____

6. Indicate the primary stress for each of the following multisyllable words. Write "1", "2", "3," or "4" to indicate the syllable with primary stress.

_____ a. intestinal	_____ f. devaluated	_____ k. unaccompanied
_____ b. demarcation	_____ g. maniacal	_____ l. orthodontist
_____ c. statuary	_____ h. sociology	_____ m. trigonometric
_____ d. monetary	_____ i. coriander	_____ n. confederation
_____ e. superfluous	_____ j. elasticity	_____ o. begrudgingly

7. For each of the following, indicate whether the underlined letters represent the onset (O), the nucleus (N), or the coda (C). Write O, N, or C in the blank.

a. <u>o</u>vert	_____	f. <u>h</u>andsome	_____
b. <u>r</u>evered	_____	g. sean<u>ce</u>	_____
c. spiri<u>ts</u>	_____	h. <u>gr</u>asped	_____
d. wh<u>y</u>	_____	i. con<u>f</u>ined	_____
e. le<u>dg</u>er	_____	j. st<u>oic</u>	_____

8. On a separate piece of paper, draw tree diagrams of the syllable structure for the following words.

a. own

b. crust

c. lonely

d. undo

CHAPTER

3

Anatomy and Physiology of the Speech Mechanism

Learning Objectives

After reading this chapter you will be able to:

1. Describe the role of the three major biological systems in production of speech: *respiratory, laryngeal,* and *supralaryngeal.*
2. Describe the role of the individual speech organs in the production of the English phonemes.

To fully understand the production of English phonemes, it is essential to have a basic understanding of the role of the speech organs. When you hear the term "speech organs," what comes to mind? Most likely, you think of the tongue, and perhaps the teeth and lips. If you already have taken an introductory course in speech-language pathology and audiology, you also may be familiar with the role of the alveolar ridge and the hard and soft palates. Speech production is, however, quite a complex process involving many other anatomical structures. For instance, the lungs are important in generating the breath stream for speech, and the larynx is important for generating voice. In this chapter we will explore the function of the various components of the speech mechanism and also discuss their role in respiration, phonation, and articulation. To understand these processes we will explore three major biological systems, namely the *respiratory, laryngeal,* and *supralaryngeal* systems, respectively.

The Respiratory System and Respiration

Generally, when we think of respiration, we think of breathing for vegetative, or for life, purposes. As a matter of fact, that *is* the primary role of the respiratory system. However, respiration is vital in the production of speech, because speech could not occur without a steady supply of air from the lungs. We tend to think primarily of the lungs when we think of respiration. The respiratory system involves not only the lungs, but also the trachea, the rib cage, the thorax, the abdomen, the diaphragm, and other major muscle groups. Examine Figure 3.1, which displays the airway involved in respiration.

The process of speech production begins with the lungs. When a person begins to speak, a preparatory breath is taken (usually unconsciously) in order to have enough air to create an utterance (i.e., a word, phrase, or sentence). This preparatory breath uses more air volume than is needed when sleeping, or when sitting quietly reading a book, or watching a DVD. More air volume is necessary

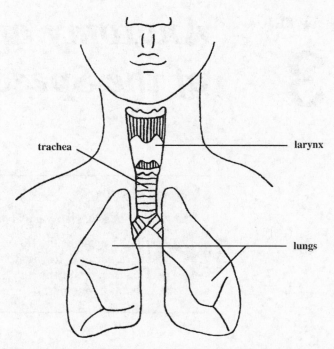

FIGURE 3.1   The anatomical relationship among the human larynx, trachea, and lungs.

in order to speak. Try speaking without taking a preparatory breath—you will run out of air very quickly. You probably have tried to speak when you are "out of breath"—your speech is choppy and characterized by gasps for air. Therefore, good breath support is essential during speech production. Singers also need good breath support to sustain their notes while performing.

When sitting quietly, the period of time devoted to inhalation and exhalation is fairly equal. That is, inhalation and exhalation each comprise about 50 percent of one inhalation/exhalation cycle. When we breathe for speech, this 50-50 relationship drastically changes. For speech purposes, inhalation only takes up approximately 10 percent of the inhalation/exhalation cycle. The other 90 percent is devoted to exhalation (Borden, Harris, & Raphael, 1994). This is necessary to have enough breath support to sustain the airstream for speech.

During inhalation, the **thoracic cavity** (chest cavity) must expand in order to make room for the expansion of the lungs. This is accomplished, in part, by lowering the **diaphragm.** The diaphragm is a major muscle that separates the abdominal cavity from the thoracic cavity. The diaphragm contracts, thereby lowering, during inhalation. As the diaphragm lowers, the rib cage expands, enlarging the thoracic cavity and creating extra space for the inflating lungs. These actions are accomplished by several sets of muscles, most notably (but not limited to) the **external intercostal muscles,** located between the ribs. As the muscles of inhalation contract, the **sternum,** or breast bone, and the rib cage are also raised.

What causes the lungs to fill with air during inhalation? As the lungs expand, the air pressure in the lungs becomes less than the air pressure in the environment. This results in what is called a *negative pressure,* relative to atmospheric pressure, inside the lungs. That is, there is a drop in air pressure. To equalize the air pressure between the lungs and the environment, air rushes into the lungs.

During exhalation, the lungs deflate because they are composed of elastic tissue (not unlike letting the air out of a balloon). Simultaneously, the diaphragm begins to relax and rise, returning to its original position. Also, the rib cage becomes smaller as it lowers due to both the relaxation of the inhalation muscles and the contraction primarily of the **internal intercostal muscles** and the abdominal muscles. The internal intercostal muscles are located between the ribs, but are located *deep* to (beneath) the external intercostals. The end result is the expulsion of the airstream through the **trachea,** or windpipe. The trachea, which connects the lungs with the larynx, is a tube comprised of cartilaginous rings embedded in muscle tissue (see Figure 3.1).

The Laryngeal System and Phonation

The laryngeal system consists primarily of the **larynx,** or "voice box." The larynx is composed mainly of muscle and cartilages. It attaches *inferiorly* to (below) the trachea, and *superiorly* (above), by a broad curtain-like ligament, to a "floating" bone known as the **hyoid bone** (see Figures 3.2 and 3.3). This is the only bone in the human body that does not attach to another bone. The hyoid also has muscular attachments to the tongue and to the **mandible** (lower jaw).

Figure 3.2 displays the major structures of the larynx from the *anterior* (front) and *posterior* (rear) viewpoints. Located in the larynx are the vocal cords, or **vocal folds.** The vocal folds are elastic folds of tissue, primarily composed of muscle. They attach anteriorly to the **thyroid cartilage.** The thyroid cartilage is more sharply angled in males than in females, explaining why males have more prominent thyroid cartilages. The vocal folds attach posteriorly to the **arytenoid cartilages.** Each vocal fold connects to a separate arytenoid cartilage. The arytenoid cartilages attach to the superior portion of the **cricoid cartilage,** which encircles the larynx. The cricoid looks somewhat like a class ring, with

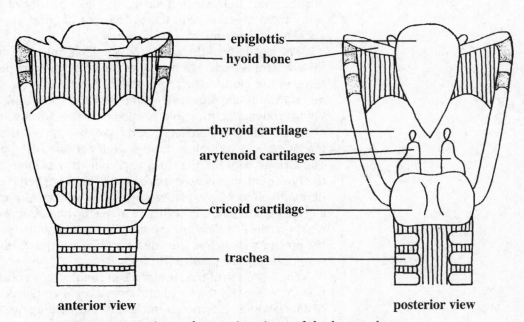

epiglottis
hyoid bone
thyroid cartilage
arytenoid cartilages
cricoid cartilage
trachea

anterior view   **posterior view**

FIGURE 3.2 Anterior and posterior views of the human larynx.

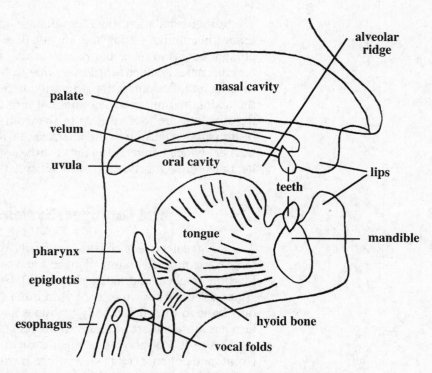

FIGURE 3.3   The vocal tract and related supralaryngeal structures.

the band facing anteriorly and the ring's features facing posteriorly. The thyroid cartilage attaches *laterally* to (at the sides of) the cricoid.

When the airstream enters the larynx, it exerts a pressure on the vocal folds from below. Actually, the pressure is applied to the **glottis,** the space between the vocal folds. For this reason, the air pressure is referred to as **subglottal pressure.** When the subglottal pressure is great enough, the vocal folds are pushed apart, releasing an air burst. The elasticity of the vocal folds helps to bring them together, and the action repeats, thus creating the process called vocal fold vibration.

The elasticity of the vocal folds explains only part of the picture in bringing the vocal folds back together. Once the vocal folds are pushed apart, air is forced through the glottis. The rapid flow of air through the glottis causes a simultaneous drop in air pressure, resulting in the vocal folds being sucked together. This aerodynamic principle is known as the **Bernoulli effect.** You may have observed this phenomenon if you have ever driven too close to a truck on the interstate, and you felt as though your car was being pulled toward the truck. The airflow between the truck and your car has increased, and the increase in the flow of air has caused a drop in air pressure between the two vehicles. The Bernoulli effect also explains how planes become airborne. Due to wing design, a pressure difference exists between the top and bottom of the wing as the plane picks up speed. As airflow increases across the wing (as the plane gains speed), the air pressure below the wing becomes greater than the pressure above the wing, causing the plane to lift off.

The vibration of the vocal folds in creation of a vocal sound is called **phonation.** You can feel the vocal folds vibrating if you place your fingertips on your "Adam's apple" (the notch in the thyroid cartilage in the front of your neck) while sustaining, or prolonging, the phoneme /z/ ("zzzzzzzz"). You should be able to feel the vocal fold vibration. The phoneme /z/ is called a **voiced** sound due to vocal fold vibration during its production. Some other examples of voiced phonemes include all of the vowels and several of the consonants, for example, /b/, /r/, /m/, /v/, and /g/.

Now place your fingers on your larynx while sustaining the phoneme/s/ ("sssssssss"). The production of the phoneme /s/ does *not* involve phonation. Because the vocal folds do not vibrate, the phoneme /s/ is called a **voiceless** phoneme. It is important to keep in mind that not all speech sounds require participation of the vocal folds. Many sounds such as /s/ and /f/ are formed by forcing the airstream through a narrow constriction formed by the speech organs in the oral cavity, without participation of the vocal folds.

EXERCISE 3.1

Think of at least two other phonemes that are voiced and two others that are voiceless.

voiced _____   *voiceless* _____

During quiet breathing (when not speaking), the vocal folds remain apart, that is, in a state of **abduction,** to allow air to flow from the lungs through the glottis to the oral and nasal cavities. The vocal folds also remain apart during the production of voiceless sounds. However, when producing voiced phonemes, the vocal folds are in a state of **adduction,** that is, they are brought together. The vocal folds then alternate during phonation between periods of abduction and adduction.

During phonation, the vocal folds open and close at the rate of approximately 125 times per second in the male larynx and approximately 215 times per second in the female larynx (Boone & McFarlane, 1994). This basic rate of vibration of the vocal folds is called the **fundamental frequency** of the voice. The fundamental frequency is responsible for the inherent voice pitch, or **habitual pitch,** of an individual. The pitch of the male voice is usually perceived to be lower than the pitch of the female voice due to the lower fundamental frequency. The pitch of the voice is largely dependent on the size of the individual larynx. Because the vocal fold tissue in the male larynx has greater mass than that of the female larynx, the male vocal folds vibrate more slowly. Hence, the male voice is perceived as being lower in pitch. Because children have smaller larynges than adults, their vocal pitch is the highest of all.

The fundamental frequency of the voice is not constant; voice pitch changes continually over time during speech production. When a word is given stress for emphasis (i.e., the *blue* car), the fundamental frequency rises. When someone asks a question, his or her voice pitch also rises, *doesn't it?* Singers change the fundamental frequency of their voices to sing a scale. Individuals who speak in a *monotone* ("one tone") rarely change the pitch of their voice. If you have ever had a professor who spoke in a monotone, you know how *monotonous* it was for the class. The pitch of the voice also conveys information regarding our moods, that is, whether we are happy, sad, excited, bored, or angry.

In addition to phonation, the larynx serves other important purposes. During a meal, the **epiglottis,** another cartilage of the larynx, diverts food away from the trachea and toward the esophagus to avoid food from "going down the wrong pipe" (see Figure 3.2). The larynx is also important in maintaining air pressure in the thoracic cavity during strenuous activities such as giving birth, lifting a heavy object, and elimination. During these activities, air is held in the lungs to provide extra muscular strength derived from the thorax. The vocal folds are held tightly together along their margins during these activities in order to stop the escape of air from the lungs. If you lift weights, you know the importance of good breath control to help you with your workout.

The Supralaryngeal System and Articulation

The supralaryngeal system is comprised of the **pharynx,** or throat, the oral cavity, the nasal cavity, and the articulators (see Figure 3.3). Collectively, these structures comprise what is known as the **vocal tract.** The length of the vocal tract from larynx to lips is about 17 cm (almost 7 inches) in the average adult male, and about 14 or 15 cm in the average adult female (Kent, 1997).

The pharynx directs airflow from the larynx to the oral and nasal cavities. It connects to the esophagus, which lies posteriorly to the larynx. The pharynx can be divided into three major sections. In ascending order from the larynx, they are (1) the *laryngopharynx,* the portion of the pharynx adjoining the larynx; (2) the *oropharynx,* adjacent to the posterior portion of the oral cavity; and (3) the *nasopharynx,* adjacent to the posterior portion of the nasal cavity. The **eustachian tubes,** important in equalizing changes in air pressure (when flying or diving in water), connect the nasopharynx with the middle ear systems on either side of the head.

The *nasal cavity* begins at the nostrils, or **nares,** and continues to the nasopharynx, posteriorly. Directly inferior to the nasal cavity (separated by the palate) is the oral cavity. The *oral cavity,* or mouth, begins at the lips and continues posteriorly to the oropharynx. The oral and nasal cavities join at the pharynx (see Figure 3.3).

During phonation (vocal fold vibration), air bursts or pulses escape from the glottis when subglottal pressure becomes sufficient to push the folds apart. These pulses are modulated by the opening and closing of the vocal folds. The air bursts collide with a column of air residing in the vocal tract. This collision sends acoustic vibrations at the speed of sound through the vocal tract to the lips (Daniloff, Shuckers, & Feth, 1980).

During production of voiceless phonemes, the vocal folds do not modulate the airstream because the vocal folds are abducted. Instead, acoustic vibrations are created when air, streaming from the lungs, is impeded by a constriction formed by the speech organs in the oral cavity. As the flow of air is forced through the constriction, a turbulent airstream is generated. The turbulence generates acoustic vibrations, which then travel toward the lips along with the airstream.

As the airstream from the lungs (and the accompanying acoustic vibrations) is directed to the oral and nasal cavities, the vibrations are modified by the speech organs to produce the individual phonemes of a language. This process is called **articulation.** The term articulation means "to join together." Articulation of speech, therefore, involves the joining together of the speech organs for the production of phonemes.

The major articulators of the vocal tract are located in the oral cavity. It is these structures that are directly responsible for the production of speech sounds. A detailed description of these organs and their role in the production of speech follows. While reading the descriptions of the articulators in the next few paragraphs, you may find it helpful to refer to Figures 3.3 and 3.4.

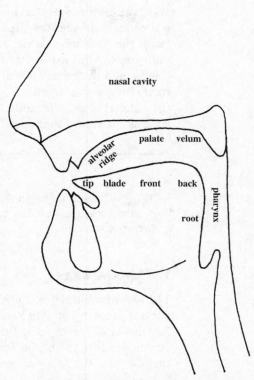

FIGURE 3.4 The landmarks of the tongue in relation to the other structures in the vocal tract.

The Lips

The purpose of the lips is to open and close in the production of several English speech sounds. The upper lip is supported by the **maxilla,** or upper jaw, and the lower lip is supported by the mandible. In production of English phonemes, the lower lip is more mobile because the mandible is quite active in speech production. The phonemes associated with the lips are called **labial** sounds. Phonemes produced with both lips are called **bilabial.** During production of speech, the lips may become rounded, as in the word "who," or unrounded as in the word "see."

Examples of labial (bilabial) sounds are the initial phonemes in the words "pear," "boy," "meet," and "witch." Notice that the formation of the phoneme /w/ is slightly different from the other three labial phonemes.

EXERCISE 3.2

Say the words "witch" and "pear" and pay attention to your lips in the formation of /w/ and /p/. What is the difference in the way the lips come together in the formation of these sounds?

The Teeth

The role of the teeth in the production of speech is more important than one might imagine. The top front teeth, the **central incisors,** and the lower lip are used in combination to produce the phonemes /f/ and /v/ as in the words "fat" and "vat." Phonemes that involve the articulation of the lower lip and the teeth are called **labiodental** (lips and teeth). The top and bottom central incisors (with the assistance of the tongue) are important in production of the initial phonemes in the words "think" and "that." Phonemes that are produced by the tongue and the teeth are called **dental** or **interdental**. In addition to being directly involved in the production of several phonemes, the teeth (most notably the *molars*) also help guide the tongue in production of other speech sounds, such as the initial sounds in "top," "sit," "ship," and "zebra."

EXERCISE 3.3

The phonemes that begin the words "think" and "that" both have a "th" sound, yet they are considered to be two separate phonemes. What is the difference in their production?

The Alveolar Ridge

The **alveolar ridge** (or *gum ridge* of the maxilla) is the bony ridge containing the sockets of the teeth. It is located directly posterior to the upper central incisors. Say the word "team." The tip of your tongue touches the anterior alveolar ridge as you produce the initial /t/ phoneme. Other examples of **alveolar** phonemes include /d/, /l/, /n/, /s/, and /z/.

The Palate

The **hard palate** (or simply, palate) is the bony structure located just posterior to the alveolar ridge. You can feel the palate by sliding the tip of your tongue from the alveolar ridge toward the back of the mouth. The palate, often referred to as the roof of the mouth, separates the oral cavity from the nasal cavity. Individuals born with a *cleft palate* may have an incomplete closure of the hard or soft palate that allows air to escape from the oral cavity directly into the nasal cavity. Sounds produced in conjunction with the palate (and tongue) are called **palatal.** Examples of palatal sounds include the sounds at the beginning of the words "<u>sh</u>ip" and "<u>y</u>ou."

The Velum

The **velum,** another name for the soft palate, is a muscular structure located directly posterior to the hard palate. (Some of you may be able to touch the soft palate with your tongue tip.) **Velar** sounds are those produced by articulation of the soft palate with the back of the tongue. Examples include the initial sounds in the words "kite" and "goat" and "ng" in the word "king."

The **uvula** is the rounded, tablike, fleshy structure located at the posterior tip of the velum. Although the uvula is not used in production of speech sounds in English, it is used in other languages, such as French and Arabic.

Because the velum is muscular, it is capable of movement. The velum acts as a switching mechanism that directs the flow of air coming from the lungs and larynx. When the velum is raised, it contacts the back wall of the pharynx, closing off the nasopharynx from the oropharynx. This process is called **velopharyngeal closure.** Closure of the velopharyngeal port prevents air from entering the nasal cavity. On the other hand, when the velum is lowered, air flows into both the oral and nasal cavities.

Phonemes produced with a raised (closed) velum are called **oral phonemes;** the airstream is directed solely into the oral cavity. Phonemes produced while the mouth is closed and the velum is lowered are called **nasal phonemes** because the breath stream flows into the nasal cavity as well. In English, there are only three nasal phonemes: /m/, /n/, and /ŋ/. The symbol /ŋ/ represents "ng" as in the words "sing" and "hunger." All of the other phonemes in English are oral.

The Glottis

The *glottis* is the place of production for the English phoneme /h/. This phoneme is considered a **glottal** sound because it is produced when the airstream from the lungs is forced through the opening between the vocal folds. Because the vocal folds do not vibrate during the production of /h/, it is considered to be voiceless.

The Tongue

The tongue is the major articulator in the production of speech. It is composed of muscle and is a quite active and mobile structure. The tongue is supported by the mandible and the hyoid bone through muscular attachments. The tongue also has muscular attachments to several other structures, including the epiglottis, the palate, and the pharynx.

Sounds produced with the tongue are called **lingual** sounds. The tongue is the primary articulator for all of the English vowels. In addition, the tongue articulates with the lips, teeth, alveolar ridge, palate, and velum in production of the consonants. The **root** of the tongue arises from the anterior wall of the pharynx and is attached to the mandible (see Figure 3.4). As a result, tongue movement is very much related to movements of the lower jaw.

In addition to the root, the tongue has several other geographical landmarks (see Figure 3.4). These landmarks include the **tip** of the tongue (also known as the **apex**) and the **blade,** which lies immediately posterior to the tip. The **body** of the tongue is found just posterior to the blade. The body is comprised of two portions, the **front** and the **back.** The front of the tongue generally lies inferior to the hard palate, and the back lies inferior to the velum. The entire tongue body is sometimes referred to as the tongue **dorsum.** (The term *dorsum* is also used to refer specifically to just the back of the tongue.) The landmarks are useful in describing the portion of the tongue involved in production of the various English phonemes. For instance, the /t/ phoneme is produced by placing the apex or blade of the tongue against the alveolar ridge, and the phoneme /g/ is produced by articulation of the back of the tongue and the soft palate.

EXERCISE 3.4

Provide the name of the articulator referenced by each of the following adjectives.

1. velar   _____
2. alveolar   _____
3. lingual   _____
4. labial   _____

5. palatal   _____
6. glottal   _____
7. dental   _____

Review Exercises

A. Matching

   Match each of the laryngeal cartilages at the right with its correct description.

   _____ 1. shaped like a class ring   a. epiglottis
   _____ 2. forms the Adam's apple   b. cricoid
   _____ 3. situated atop the cricoid   c. thyroid
   _____ 4. prevents food from entering the larynx d. arytenoids

B. Fill in the blank.

   1. The basic rate of vocal fold vibration is called _____.
   2. The _____ is another name for the lower jaw.
   3. a. The anatomical term *anterior* means _____.
       b. The anatomical term *inferior* means _____.
       c. The anatomical term *superior* means _____.
       d. The anatomical term *posterior* means _____.
   4. The _____ is a major muscle that separates the chest cavity from the abdomen.
   5. _____ pressure is the air pressure *below* the vocal folds.
   6. Inherent voice pitch is also known as _____ pitch.
   7. The _____ connect both middle ears with the nasopharynx.
   8. The _____ is the portion of the tongue just posterior to the tip. The tip is also known as the _____.
   9. The tongue dorsum is composed of the _____ and the _____.

C. Match the anatomical term at the right to the structures referenced.

   1. The pharynx is _____ to the esophagus.   a. anterior
   2. The lips are _____ to the teeth.   b. posterior
   3. The dorsum of the tongue is _____ to the tip.   c. superior
   4. The uvula is _____ to the velum.   d. inferior
   5. The nasal cavity is _____ to the oral cavity.
   6. The tongue is _____ to the palate.
   7. The larynx is _____ to the trachea.
   8. The arytenoid cartilages are _____ to the thyroid cartilage.
   9. The alveolar ridge is _____ to the hard palate.
   10. The laryngopharynx is _____ to the oropharynx.

D. True or False

T	F	1.	The phoneme /s/ is an alveolar sound.
T	F	2.	Vibration of the vocal folds is termed *articulation*.
T	F	3.	The tongue is involved in production of *labiodental* phonemes.
T	F	4.	The hyoid bone does not attach to any other bone.
T	F	5.	The upper lip is supported by the *maxilla*.
T	F	6.	When speaking, the period of time devoted to inhalation and exhalation is fairly equal.
T	F	7.	The root of the tongue attaches to the mandible.
T	F	8.	When the vocal folds are together, they are said to be *adducted*.
T	F	9.	The oral and nasal cavities join at the larynx.
T	F	10.	The diaphragm contracts and lowers during the process of inhalation.

Study Questions

1. Describe the process of inhalation and exhalation. Which anatomical structures are involved in these processes?
2. What is the *Bernoulli effect*? What is its importance in the production of speech?
3. Define the following terms:
    a. *glottis*
    b. *abduction/adduction*
    c. *hyoid bone*
    d. *uvula*
4. Which structures comprise the vocal tract?
5. What is the difference between a voiced and voiceless sound?
6. What is the *pharynx*, and what are its three major components?
7. What is the *larynx*, and what are its major cartilaginous components?
8. What is *phonation*? Which anatomical structures are involved in phonation?
9. What is *articulation*?
10. Identify and describe each of the geographical landmarks of the tongue.
11. What is the difference between an oral sound and a nasal sound?
12. Why does an adult male have a different habitual pitch than an adult female?

Online Resources

Hall, Daniel, University of Toronto. (nd). Interactive vocal tract. Retrieved from:
www.chass.utoronto.ca/~danhall/phonetics/sammy.html
(interactive visual display of the vocal tract for all English phonemes)

National Center for Voice and Speech. (2005). Tutorials. Retrieved from:
www.ncvs.org/ncvs/tutorials/voiceprod/tutorial/index.html
(tutorials on a number of topics related to voice and speech; pay particular attention to the tutorials related to *laryngeal anatomy* (Chapter 1), *breathing* (Chapter 3), and *vocal fold oscillation* (Chapter 4).

UCLA Phonetics Lab Demo Page. (nd). Retrieved from:
www.linguistics.ucla.edu/faciliti/demos/vocalfolds/vocalfolds.htm
(video of vocal fold vibration)

University of Iowa Phonetics Flash Animation Project: fənɛtɪks: the sounds of spoken English. (2001–2005). Retrieved from:
www.uiowa.edu/~acadtech/phonetics/#
(schematic diagram of the articulators for speech; *follow the anatomy link*)

University of Michigan Medical School. (nd). Three-dimensional rotatable model of the larynx. Retrieved from:
http://anatomy.med.umich.edu/qtvr/qtvr_larynx.html

CHAPTER

4

Vowels

Learning Objectives

After reading this chapter you will be able to:

1. Describe the relationship between the vowel quadrilateral and the articulatory description of the English vowels in terms of tongue height and tongue advancement.
2. Describe the effects of tongue position on resonance of the vocal tract during vowel production.
3. Define the major parameters of speech acoustics: *time, intensity,* and *frequency,* and describe how they are represented on a spectrogram.
4. Identify the acoustic characteristics of speech associated with vowel production.
5. Transcribe all of the English vowels and diphthongs in spoken utterances, using the appropriate IPA symbols.

Beginning with this chapter, the focus will be on phonetic transcription. Chapter 4 will emphasize the vowel sounds, and Chapter 5 will introduce the consonants. In these two chapters, each phoneme of English will be discussed in terms of the phonetic symbol used in transcription practice, the manner in which each phoneme is articulated, and its associated acoustic characteristics.

As stated in Chapter 1, learning phonetics is much like learning a new language. In order for you to feel comfortable with the use of the IPA, ample opportunity will be given for practice. The importance of practice cannot be emphasized enough in the study of phonetic transcription. Therefore, in addition to the printed exercises in this text, you will also have the opportunity to transcribe speech while listening to the instructor and other speakers, either in class or with the optional audio CDs.

What Is a Vowel?

Vowels are phonemes that are produced without any appreciable constriction or blockage of air flow in the vocal tract. As you know, English has many more vowel sounds than those represented by the five Roman alphabet letters, a, e, i, o, and u. Table 4.1 lists all of the vowel phonemes in English along with the way in which they are classified.

The tongue is the primary articulator in the production of vowels. Because the tongue has muscular attachments to the mandible, changes in jaw position also are

TABLE 4.1   The Fourteen Vowels of English (diphthongs not included)

Vowel Phoneme	Key Word	Tongue Height	Tongue Advancement	Tense/ Lax	Lip Rounding
/i/	*key*	high	front	tense	unrounded
/ɪ/	*win*	high	front	lax	unrounded
/e/	*reb<u>a</u>te*	high-mid	front	tense	unrounded
/ɛ/	*red*	low-mid	front	lax	unrounded
/æ/	*had*	low	front	lax	unrounded
/u/	*moon*	high	back	tense	rounded
/ʊ/	*wood*	high	back	lax	rounded
/o/	*<u>o</u>kay*	high-mid	back	tense	rounded
/ɔ/	*law*	low-mid	back	tense	rounded
/ɑ/	*cod*	low	back	tense	unrounded
/ə/	*<u>a</u>bout*	mid	central	lax	unrounded
/ʌ/	*bud*	low-mid	back-central	lax	unrounded
/ɚ/	*butt<u>er</u>*	mid	central	lax	rounded
/ɝ/	*bird*	mid	central	tense	rounded

linked directly to vowel production. As the tongue changes position for production of the individual vowels, the size and shape of the pharynx also change correspondingly. The airstream passes through the oral cavity with virtually no obstruction by the tongue or other major articulators. If the tongue did create a constriction in the vocal tract, a consonant phoneme would be produced. How then are vowels produced if no obstruction occurs in the vocal tract? To answer this question, say the following five words aloud. Pay particular attention to the position of your tongue as you produce the vowel (the middle element) in each word.

b<u>ea</u>d, b<u>i</u>d, b<u>ay</u>ed, b<u>e</u>d, b<u>a</u>d

Now say the words again and leave off the consonant phonemes /b/ and /d/ so that you are saying only the vowel. Once again, pay attention to the position of the tongue. What did you observe? Hopefully, you noted that as you said these words in order, the position of your tongue continually lowered. Specifically, it was the body of the tongue that lowered during the production of these vowels. Also, you may have noted that your jaw lowered at the same time.

Vowel phonemes are categorized in relation to the position of the body of the tongue in the mouth during their production. Specifically, vowels are characterized by height and advancement of the tongue body. **Tongue height** refers to how high (or low) in the oral cavity the tongue is when producing a particular vowel. **Tongue advancement** relates to how far forward (or backward) in the mouth the tongue is when producing a particular vowel. All of the vowels in English can be described by using these two dimensions of tongue position in the oral cavity.

To better understand the idea of tongue height and advancement, it is convenient to think of the oral cavity as the space schematically represented in Figure 4.1. This figure is called the **vowel quadrilateral** due to its characteristic shape. All of the vowels in English are plotted on this two-dimensional figure to represent tongue advancement and height. Examination of Figure 4.1 shows that tongue height can be divided into three dimensions: high, mid, and

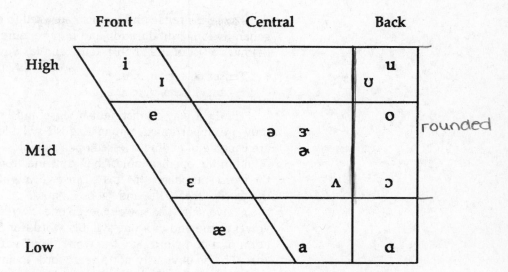

FIGURE 4.1 The vowel quadrilateral.

low. Tongue advancement also is divided into three dimensions: front, central, and back. It is these dimensions that will be discussed as each of the vowels are introduced in the following sections. Keep in mind that the vowel quadrilateral is only an approximation of tongue positions for the production of vowels.

A secondary characteristic of vowels involves lip rounding, that is, whether the lips are **rounded** or **unrounded** (retracted) in their production. For example, compare the vowel sounds in the following two words: "moon" and "mean." Notice that the first vowel is produced with the lips rounded, whereas the lips are unrounded in association with the second vowel. In English, most vowels produced in the back of the mouth are rounded; the front vowels are all unrounded. Other languages, such as German and French, have rounded front vowels. A summary of the rounded and unrounded vowels of English follows:

Unrounded: /i, ɪ, e, ɛ, æ, ɑ, ə, ʌ/
Rounded: /u, ʊ, o, ɔ, ɚ, ɝ/

Every vowel in English has a unique articulatory position based on the combination of tongue height, tongue advancement, and lip rounding.

PRELIMINARY EXERCISE 1–
ROUNDED AND UNROUNDED VOWELS

Using Table 4.1 as your guide, indicate whether the following one-syllable words have a rounded or an unrounded vowel (vowel graphemes are in **bold letters**). Write either R (rounded) or U (unrounded) in the blanks.

_____ 1. l**ea**n   _____ 6. thr**ow**

_____ 2. h**oo**k   _____ 7. b**a**ck

_____ 3. r**oa**d   _____ 8. th**e**n

_____ 4. m**i**nt   _____ 9. w**ai**t

_____ 5. ch**ew**   _____ 10. sh**ou**ld

The terms **tense** and **lax** also are used to classify vowels. Tense vowels are generally longer in duration and require more muscular effort than lax vowels. Below is a list of the English tense and lax vowels:

Tense: /i, e, u, o, ɔ, ɑ, ɝ/
Lax: /ɪ, ɛ, æ, ʊ, ə, ʌ, ɚ/

The best way to distinguish tense and lax vowels is to examine the way they are apportioned among English syllables when speaking. Tense vowels are capable of ending stressed open syllables. Examples of tense vowels can be found in the open syllables "he" /hi/ and "too" /tu/ and in the first syllable of the word "purchase" /pɝtʃəs/. Tense vowels also occur in closed syllables, as in the words "feet" /fit/ and "goose" /gus/.

Conversely, lax vowels never end a stressed open syllable. Placing a lax vowel at the end of a one-syllable word, for instance, would result in the creation of a non-word. Say the word "him" without the final /m/, for example, /hɪ/. This is obviously not a real word. Examples of lax vowels can be found in the words "had" /hæd/ and "look" /lʊk/ (closed syllables) and in the first syllable of the word "aloud" /əlaʊd/ (an *unstressed* open syllable).

PRELIMINARY EXERCISE 2–TENSE AND LAX VOWELS

Using Table 4.1 as your guide, indicate whether the following one-syllable words have a tense or a lax vowel (vowel graphemes are in **bold letters**). Write either T (tense) or L (lax) in the blanks.

_____ 1. s**ee**k	_____ 3. s**i**nge	_____ 5. h**o**t	_____ 7. m**a**p
_____ 2. p**u**sh	_____ 4. h**ea**d	_____ 6. h**oo**t	_____ 8. cl**e**rk

---

Most English vowels are **monophthongs** ("one sound"), because they have one primary articulatory position in the vocal tract. Vowel sounds that have two distinct articulatory positions are called **diphthongs** ("two sounds"). Diphthongs are actually two vowels that comprise one phoneme. Table 4.2 lists the English diphthongs.

During articulation of a diphthong, the tongue is placed in the appropriate position for production of the first element. The tongue then moves to the second element in a continuous gliding motion. The first element of a diphthong is referred to as the **onglide** portion, and the second element is referred to as the **offglide.** The tongue rises in the oral cavity when moving from the onglide to the offglide for all

TABLE 4.2　The English Diphthongs

Diphthong	Key Word
/aɪ/	*buy* bye
/aʊ/	*cow*
/ɔɪ/	*toy*
/eɪ/	*hate*
/oʊ/	*coat*

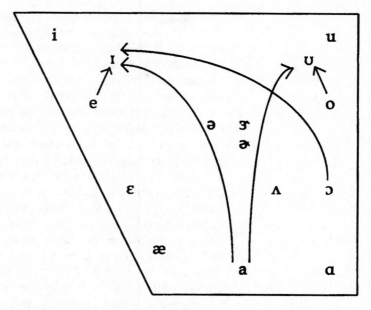

FIGURE 4.2   Onglide and offglide positions for the diphthongs /eɪ/, /oʊ/, /aɪ/, /ɔɪ/, and /aʊ/ (in reference to the traditional vowel quadrilateral).

of the English diphthongs. Therefore, the offglide is always produced at a higher position in the oral cavity than the onglide (see Figure 4.2). Note that all English offglides consist of only two vowels, either /ɪ/ (a front vowel) or /ʊ/ (a back vowel).

Because all English vowels are oral sounds, the velum is generally raised to prevent air from being directed into the nasal cavity during their production. In some instances, vowels may take on a nasal quality due to the phonemic environment of a word. This process is called **nasalization.** Generally, vowels tend to be nasalized when they precede or follow a nasal consonant. For example, the vowel /ɪ/ would be nasalized in articulation of the word "rim" [rɪ̃m]. (The *tilde* over the /ɪ/ indicates nasalization.) Because /m/ is a nasal consonant, the preceding vowel would become nasalized due to the fact that the velum remains lowered throughout the production of the word. Say the word aloud and you will be able to observe the nasalization of the vowel. Nasalized vowels are typical of some dialects of English and, in some cases, also may be characteristic of a speech disorder.

The Vocal Tract and Resonance

Every phoneme in a language has a unique sound quality associated with it due to a unique vocal tract shape and accompanying vibratory pattern, or **resonance.** Resonance deals with the vibratory properties of *any* vibrating body (including the vocal tract, a guitar, a harmonica, or a tuning fork). All objects have natural frequencies of vibration, or resonances. Consider blowing across the top of a bottle. When you blow across the opening, a particular tone is produced due to the inherent vibratory properties of the air mass in the bottle. Imagine adding some water to the bottle. Now what happens when you blow across the top? The tone that is produced will sound higher in pitch because the mass of air is less than before.

During the process of articulation, the tongue and other articulators constantly change their positions to produce different sounds as acoustic vibrations from the larynx (or from a vocal tract constriction) flow through the vocal tract on their way to the lips. As the articulators move from one position to the next, the natural frequencies of vibration (or resonances) of the vocal tract change accordingly. These resonance changes are the direct result of modifications in the air mass in the vocal tract brought about by the ever-changing shape of the tongue, pharynx, lips, and jaw during production of speech. (This process is similar to changing the water level in the bottle.) Recall in our earlier discussion of the production of the vowels in the words *bead, bid, bayed, bed,* and *bad* that the tongue and lower jaw assume different positions for each vowel. Because the oral structures (including the shape of the pharynx) change during the production of each individual vowel, there is a corresponding change in the natural frequencies of vibration (resonances) of the vocal tract. These changes in resonance not only give each separate vowel a unique acoustic characteristic or *quality,* they also provide acoustic cues to listeners so that each vowel can be recognized individually. **Quality** can be defined as the perceptual character of a sound based on its acoustic resonance patterns. **Timbre** is a synonym often used for sound quality.

Figure 4.3 shows spectrograms of the words "heed" /hid/ and "who'd" /hud/ (a minimal pair). A **spectrogram** is a graphic representation of the three major parameters that describe the acoustic characteristic of any sound, including speech sounds. These three parameters are *time, frequency,* and *intensity.* The measurement of **time** in acoustics simply refers to the duration of any particular sound. Time is usually recorded in milliseconds (msec.) but also may be recorded in seconds. (There are 1000 msec. in one second.) On a spectrogram, time is denoted on the *abscissa,* or x-axis.

The **frequency** of a sound can be defined as the number of cycles a vibrating body completes in one second. Recall that in males, the vocal folds open and close approximately 125 times per second. Therefore, the frequency of vibration of the average male larynx is 125 cycles per second, or 125 Hz. Similarly, the tines of a 500 Hz tuning fork vibrate back and forth 500 times per second. The term *Hz* (shorthand for *Hertz,* and named after Heinrich Hertz, a famous German physicist) is more commonly used

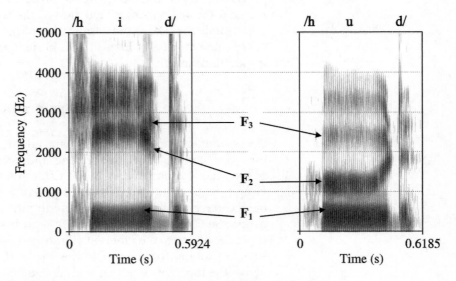

FIGURE 4.3 Spectrograms of the words /hid/ and /hud/.

to represent the frequency characteristic of a sound (as opposed to the term *cycles per second*). Frequency information (in Hz) is displayed on the *ordinate,* or y-axis on a spectrogram. Acoustically, each phoneme of a language has unique frequency information associated with it, due to not only the movement of the vocal folds (fundamental frequency), but also due to the resonances of the vocal tract linked to that phoneme. Frequency is perceived in terms of **pitch.** Frequency and pitch are directly related; this means that as the frequency of a sound increases, so does its perceived pitch.

Intensity is more difficult to define than frequency. It is best to start with an example. Lightly clap your hands together. Now clap them more forcefully. In both cases, you created a disturbance (movement) of air molecules on and surrounding your hands. The disturbance of air molecules was less when you lightly brought your hands together than when you clapped more forcefully. That is, the disturbance created a greater movement of air molecules when you clapped harder. The greater the movement of air molecules, the greater the energy expended, and the greater the intensity generated. *Intensity* refers to the amplitude (magnitude) of energy associated with a particular sound. The greater the energy associated with a particular auditory event, the greater its intensity. For example, as a whisper escapes the lips, a disturbance of the air molecules will result, creating a sound wave that will reach the listener's ear. The amplitude of the wave related to this disturbance in the air molecules would be appreciably less than the amplitude of a sound wave consistent with yelling. Typically, intensity is recorded in *decibels* (dB); however, other units of measurement also may be used (e.g., watts/meter^2). Please note that the term dB is both singular *and* plural. If a sound measures 25 decibels, the correct notation is 25 dB, *not* 25 dBs. Also, the decibel scale is logarithmic, not linear. On a spectrogram, sounds of greater intensity (in dB) appear darker than sounds of lesser intensity. Intensity is perceived in terms of **loudness.** Similar to frequency/pitch, there is a direct relationship between intensity and loudness; as the intensity of a sound increases, so does its loudness.

In terms of the intensity of all English phonemes, the vowels and diphthongs are greater in intensity than the consonants. This is mainly because of the greater amplitude of acoustic energy associated with the resonance of the vocal tract during their production, when compared to consonants. The least intense vowel, /i/, is greater in intensity than /r/, the consonant with the greatest intensity. Vowels generally will appear darker than the consonants on a spectrogram.

Next to vowels, the liquids and nasals have the greatest intensity, followed by the affricates. The fricatives and the stops are the least intense of all phonemes in English, with the voiceless fricatives (except for /ʃ/) being the least intense. The phoneme with the greatest acoustic energy, the vowel /ɔ/, is approximately 680 times more powerful than the voiceless fricative /θ/, the phoneme with the least acoustic energy (Fletcher, 1953). The difference in decibels between these two phonemes is approximately 28 dB. Keep in mind that these are average intensity values; the intensity of individual phonemes in connected speech varies considerably from speaker to speaker and from conversation to conversation. For instance, the intensity of connected speech varies depending on whether we are whispering (45 dB), speaking at a conversational level (65 dB), or talking loudly (85 dB) (Fletcher, 1953). The spectrograms in Figure 4.3 hopefully will help clarify the concepts of time, frequency, and intensity, and also will point out the acoustic specifications of the two words displayed in the figure.

Each of the spectrograms in Figure 4.3 is labeled phonetically at the top so that you can identify each phoneme with its corresponding acoustic representation. As you can see, time is indicated on the x-axis. The time it took the speaker to produce these two words is approximately 600 msec. (.6 seconds). Note that the vowels /i/ and /u/ are greater in intensity (darker shading) and longer in duration than the consonants /h/ and /d/. Look at the spectrograms in order to verify this fact. With respect to duration, vowels are generally longer than consonants in any particular syllable. Because vowels are longer than consonants, they comprise the largest part of any individual syllable. The actual length of any vowel or consonant phoneme varies in relation to the following: (1) whether the phoneme occurs in a stressed syllable; (2) the phonemic context (the other vowels and consonants that surround a particular phoneme in a word); and (3) the importance of the meaning of a word in an utterance that contains the phoneme.

Frequency is indicated on the y-axis. You can see that the phonemes /h/ and /d/ have frequency patterns that cover a wide range of frequencies. This can be seen by examining the *vertical* shadings that extend over a range of almost 5000 Hz from the bottom to the top of each spectrogram.

It is easy to identify vowels on a spectrogram, not only due to their greater duration (when compared to the consonants), but also due to the dark *horizontal* bars indicated in each spectrogram. These dark bars are known as **formants.** Formants are resonant frequencies of the vocal tract. Each vowel has a unique set of formant frequencies (or resonances that occur throughout the vocal tract) due to the specific positioning of the articulators necessary in production of each vowel. It is obvious from examining these two spectrograms that the formant patterns associated with these two vowels is quite different because the shape of the vocal tract during their production is also quite different. The vowel /i/ is produced further forward in the oral cavity (i.e., a "front" vowel), whereas the vowel /u/ is produced further back in the oral cavity (i.e., a "back" vowel).

The resonances of the vocal tract associated with vowel production contain primarily low-frequency energy (although higher than the fundamental frequency of the voice). The frequency array, or energy pattern, associated with a particular phoneme is called its **spectrum.** Therefore, vowels are considered to have low-frequency spectra and are perceived as being low in spectral pitch. Consonants, on the other hand, may be either low or high in spectral pitch. The frequency specification of consonants will be discussed further in Chapter 5.

The first three formants in Figure 4.3 are numbered from F_1 to F_3, starting with the formant that is the lowest in frequency. Generally, the higher-frequency formants are less intense than the lower-frequency formants. Examine the shading of the three formants of the vowel /u/ in /hud/. You will see that the shading (intensity) of F_3 is considerably lighter when compared to the shading of F_1 and F_2. There does not appear to be a difference in intensity between the three marked formants for the vowel /i/ in /hid/. This is only because the formants were artificially darkened so that they would show up better in print.

Now, compare the second formant *frequency* of each vowel. Note how much higher in frequency the F_2 of /i/ is when compared to /u/. Careful inspection of Figure 4.3 shows that the second formant of /i/ is greater than 2000 Hz, whereas the second formant of /u/ is closer to 1000 Hz. Generally, front vowels (such as /i/) have higher second formants than do the back vowels (such as /u/). Keep in mind that vowels do have more than three formants. See if you can identify F_4 for the vowels in both words in Figure 4.3. For the purpose of speech perception, listeners only need to perceive the

TABLE 4.3 F_1 and F_2 Values for Adult Male Speakers. Values are Given in Hz. Data from Peterson and Barney (1952)

					Vowels					
	/i/	/ɪ/	/ɛ/	/æ/	/ɑ/	/ɔ/	/ʊ/	/u/	/ʌ/	/ɝ/
F_1	270	390	530	660	730	570	440	300	640	490
F_2	2290	1990	1840	1720	1090	840	1020	870	1190	1350

lower formants, specifically F_1, F_2, and F_3, in order to be able to recognize and distinguish all of the vowels in English (that is, to be able to tell them apart). Table 4.3 gives average values for the first two formants of 10 English vowels spoken by adult males (data from Peterson & Barney, 1952). In Figure 4.4, the formant values from Table 4.3 are plotted with F_1 on the ordinate and F_2 on the abscissa.

As you examine Figure 4.4, you will notice that it closely resembles Figure 4.1, the vowel quadrilateral. In reality, the vowel quadrilateral is based more so on the F_1 and F_2 patterns of vowels than the exact placement of the articulators in the oral cavity as each vowel is spoken. In essence, the vowel quadrilateral is more of a schematic diagram representing where the various vowels are actually produced in the

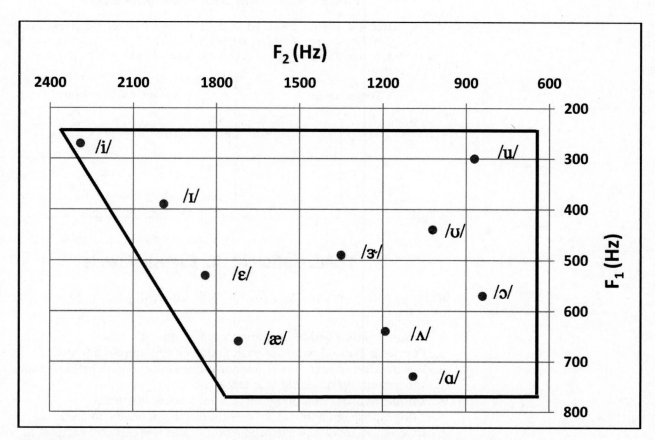

FIGURE 4.4 Plot of average male F_1 and F_2 values (in Hz) for 10 American English vowels.

oral cavity. Recall that in the vowel quadrilateral, tongue height is displayed on the ordinate and tongue advancement is displayed on the abscissa. Given the similarity of Figures 4.1 and 4.4, it appears there must be some relationship between tongue height, tongue advancement, and the formant values associated with each vowel. In fact, there are two rules that relate F_1 and F_2 to tongue height and tongue advancement, respectively:

1. F_1 is *inversely related to tongue height.* That is, the higher the tongue is elevated during vowel production, the lower the value of F_1. For example, the average F_1 of /i/ (a high vowel) is 270 Hz, whereas the average F_1 of /æ/ (a low vowel) is 660 Hz.
2. F_2 is *directly related to tongue advancement.* The more fronted the tongue placement during vowel production, the higher the value of F_2. For example, the average F_2 for the front vowel /i/ is 2290 Hz, whereas the average F_2 for the back vowel /u/ is 870 Hz.

Make sure you compare tongue placement for the vowels represented in the quadrilateral (Figures 4.1 and 4.4) with the F_1 and F_2 rules, as well as the formant values given in Table 4.3 to make sure you understand the relationship between place of articulation for vowels and the corresponding change in vocal tract resonance as indicated by the varying formant patterns.

PRELIMINARY EXERCISE 3–FORMANT RULES

Using Table 4.3 as your guide, write the formant values in the blanks for the vowels given. How do these values relate to the F_1 and F_2 rules given above? You may want to refer to the vowel quadrilateral (Figure 4.1) in helping you to answer this question.

Tongue Height		*Tongue Advancement*	
F_1	F_1	F_2	F_2
_____ /i/	_____ /u/	_____ /i/ ⟶	_____ /u/
_____ /ɪ/	_____ /ʊ/	_____ /ɪ/ ⟶	_____ /ʊ/
_____ /ɛ/	_____ /ɔ/	_____ /ɛ/ ⟶	_____ /ɔ/
_____ /æ/	_____ /ɑ/	_____ /æ/ ⟶	_____ /ɑ/

Transcription of the English Vowels

In the following sections, the vowels of English will be introduced using the following format:

1. **Pronunciation Guide** for the phonemes being discussed
2. **Phonetic Symbol Name** of each phoneme (Pullum & Ladusaw, 1986)
3. **Description** of each vowel on four dimensions: tongue height, tongue advancement, lip rounding, and tense/lax
4. **Sample Words** containing the phoneme being discussed
5. **Allographs** commonly used to represent the phoneme in spelling
6. **Discussion** involving the production of the vowel, and examples of some dialectal variants

7. **Acoustic Information** relative to production of the English vowels and diphthongs
8. **Exercises**

The Front Vowels
Pronunciation Guide

/i/	as in "keep"	/kip/
/ɪ/	as in "hit"	/hɪt/
/e/	as in "reb<u>a</u>te"	/ribet/
/eɪ/	as in "state"	/steɪt/ (allophone of /e/)
/ɛ/	as in "led"	/lɛd/
/æ/	as in "mat"	/mæt/

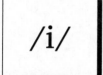

Lower-Case i
Description

Height:	high
Advancement:	front
Lip rounding:	unrounded
Tense/lax:	tense

Sample Words

fleet	we	eke	t<u>ea</u>cher
<u>TV</u>	eaves	creek	cr<u>e</u>dence
<u>Ea</u>ster	yeast	reach	piece
seeks	<u>e</u>dict	r<u>ecei</u>pt	p<u>i</u>laf

Allographs

Grapheme	Example	Grapheme	Example
i	mosquito	ee	keel
e	she	ey	key
ei	seizure	ie	relieve
ea	reach	oe	amoeba

Discussion   The vowel /i/ is produced by raising the body of the tongue to a high front position in the oral cavity. During production of /i/ (as well as for the other front vowels), the tongue is raised in the vicinity of the hard palate (Figure 4.5). If you examine the vowel quadrilateral (Figure 4.1), you will see that the vowel /i/ is the highest and most fronted of all vowels. Because it represents an extreme point or corner of the vowel quadrilateral, it is referred to as one of the **point vowels.** The other point vowels in English include the front vowel /æ/ and the back vowels /u/ and /ɑ/. The lips are unrounded in production of /i/. In addition, /i/ is considered to be tense, because it is capable of ending a one-syllable word (open monosyllable), for example, "key" /ki/ and "pea" /pi/.

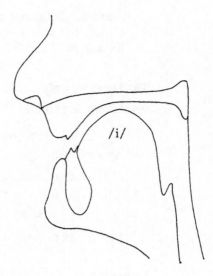

FIGURE 4.5 /i/ articulation.

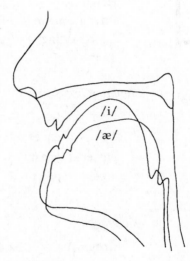

FIGURE 4.6 /i/ and /æ/ articulation.

The mandible is raised during production of /i/, because the tongue is in a high position. In fact, the jaw is in a somewhat closed position. Also, the oropharynx enlarges during production of /i/ because the tongue body and root move superiorly and anteriorly away from the pharynx. As the tongue lowers in production of the front vowels (from /i/ to /æ/), the jaw lowers, and the size of the oropharynx decreases (as the tongue moves closer to the pharyngeal area). See Figure 4.6 for a comparison of the tongue, jaw, and pharyngeal positions for the two front vowels /i/ and /æ/. Since each front vowel has distinct tongue, jaw, and pharyngeal articulatory positions, they each have distinct vocal tract resonances.

Acoustic Information Figure 4.7 shows spectrograms of the words "heed," "hid," "hayed," "head," and "had." Each word contains one of the five front vowels in the same phonetic context, i.e., /h_d/. Inspection of the spectrograms

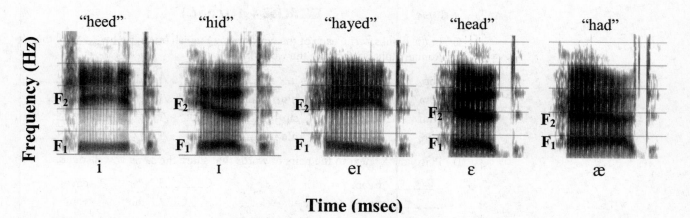

FIGURE 4.7 Spectrograms of the five front vowels in /h_d/ context.

helps demonstrate the F_1 and F_2 formant rules discussed previously. Note the general *increase* in the frequency of the first formant for each of the vowels as the tongue lowers from production of /i/ in "heed" to /æ/ in "had." The change in F_1 is most evident when directly comparing the vowels in "heed" and "had." Now compare F_2 in the words "heed" and "had." Note the fact that F_2 *lowers* in frequency as the tongue lowers in production from "heed" to "had." This is due to the fact that the tongue systematically moves from front to back as the tongue lowers in production of the front vowels (see Figures 4.1 and 4.4). Obviously, then, each front vowel has a distinct resonance pattern linked to changes in vocal tract shape consistent with each vowel's articulation.

Note: In this exercise and several others in this chapter, *consonant* IPA symbols are used. The IPA consonant symbols to be used are the same as their Roman alphabet counterparts. These consonant phoneme symbols are /b, d, f, g, h, k, l, m, n, p, r, s, t, v, w, z/. For example: "ease" /iz/; "dean" /din/.

EXERCISE 4.1—THE VOWEL /i/

A. Circle the words that contain the /i/ phoneme.

paper	train	Cleveland	seaside
please	picture	trip	trail
tribal	machine	labor	trees
settle	screen	Toledo	lip
nice	foreign	Levi	jeans

B. Circle the phonetic transcriptions that represent English words.

/ist/	/flip/	/min/	/hid/
/iv/	/hig/	/lim/	/wins/
/rift/	/if/	/trit/	/lik/

Continues

EXERCISE 4.1 (*cont.*)

C. In the blanks, write each of the words using English orthography (i.e., use the Roman alphabet to write the words).

/lip/	_____	/it/	_____	/brizd/	_____
/pip/	_____	/hip/	_____	/spik/	_____
/mit/	_____	/sip/	_____	/klin/	_____
/rid/	_____	/did/	_____	/krist/	_____

D. Place an "X" next to the pairs of words that share the same vowel sound.

_____	dream	drip	_____	east	eaves
_____	seek	wheel	_____	chief	vein
_____	same	land	_____	base	lease
_____	creek	steam	_____	need	pain
_____	bean	heed	_____	creed	cream

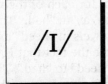

Small Capital ɪ
Description

Height:	high (lower than /i/)
Advancement:	front
Lip rounding:	unrounded
Tense/lax:	lax

Sample Words

flit	wh<u>i</u>ttle	<u>i</u>nside	dr<u>ea</u>ry
b<u>u</u>siness	king	s<u>i</u>ster	steer
l<u>i</u>sten	p<u>i</u>stol	<u>i</u>ntend	prince
reall<u>y</u>	stink	choos<u>y</u>	kitt<u>y</u>

Allographs

Grapheme	Example	Grapheme	Example
i	with, ring	e	England, pretty
y	gym	ea(r)	fear
ui	guilt	ee(r)	deer
u	business	i(r)	mirror
-y	baby	ei(r)	weird
ee	been	ie(r)	pierce
o	women	e(re)	here
ie	sieve		

Discussion   The body of the tongue is only slightly lower in production of /ɪ/ when compared to /i/ (Figure 4.8). This is why it is also classified as a high vowel. The jaw is in a fairly closed position during production of /ɪ/, and the lips are unrounded. One distinction between /i/ and /ɪ/ is that /ɪ/ is lax. Placing /ɪ/ in the

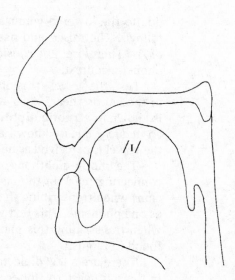

FIGURE 4.8 /ɪ/ articulation.

final position of a monosyllable would result in a nonsense word, that is, /bɪ/ or /wɪ/. The phoneme /ɪ/ does occur in closed syllables such as in "l̠isten" and "ɪ̠ndent."

The vowel /ɪ/ has some peculiarities in phonetic transcription. In final, unstressed syllables that end in "y," in words like "crazy," "gloomy," and "quantity," it has been debated by phoneticians and linguists as to whether the phoneme /i/ or /ɪ/ should be used in the transcription of the final sound (i.e., /kreɪzɪ/ or /kreɪzi/). In reality, what is heard by listeners is a phoneme that tends to be shorter in duration than the vowel /i/ found in stressed syllables (as in "heed"), but longer than /ɪ/ (as in "hid"). Also, the vowel in final, unstressed syllables tends to be retracted, that is, produced farther back in the oral cavity than the traditional place of articulation for /i/ (but not as low as /ɪ/) (Ball & Müller, 2005). Yavaş (2006) states that /i/ and /ɪ/ occur in *free variation* (see Chapter 2) in the final unstressed position of words for some speakers. In addition, both Yavaş (2006) and Ladefoged (2001) suggest that the use of /i/ and /ɪ/ in final, unstressed syllables may be associated with regional dialect. Although phoneticians and linguists differ in opinion as to which phoneme is the correct choice in transcribing the final sound in words like "crazy" or "gloomy," what is clear is that the correct sound can be thought of as an allophone of either /i/ or /ɪ/. Some sources (Singh & Singh, 2006; Shriberg & Kent, 2003) recommend the use of /ɪ/, while others (Ladefoged, 2001; Ball & Müller, 2005) recommend the use of /i/ in transcription of this sound.

In this text, when transcribing the final "y" in final, unstressed syllables, the sound will be treated as an allophone of /ɪ/. Keep in mind that some individuals will treat this sound as an allophone of /i/ in this particular phonetic context. As pointed out in Chapter 1, the phonetic symbol you adopt in this context is not as important as your consistency and understanding of the underlying rationale for your selection of that symbol. Also remember that although we will be using the phonemic symbol /ɪ/ in this particular case, the symbol is representing an *allophone* of /ɪ/.

Another peculiarity with /ɪ/ involves words that contain the letter string "ing," such as in the words "running," "finger," and "ink." Their actual transcriptions are /rʌnɪŋ/, /fɪŋgɚ/, and /ɪŋk/. Notice the use of the phoneme /ɪ/ and not /i/ in these words. In this phonetic context, /ɪ/ is raised from its usual position (but not so high that it is produced as /i/). /ɪ/ also becomes nasalized due to the lowered velum associated with the nasal consonant "ng" /ŋ/ that follows. The raised and nasalized /ɪ/ in these words is actually an allophone of /ɪ/. Therefore, it is considered more accurate to use /ɪ/ instead of /i/ in this phonetic context.

Last, the vowel /ɪ/ is often found in combination with the consonant /r/ as in the words "hear" /hɪr/ and "ear" /ɪr/. In this case, /ɪ/ + /r/ become what is known as a **rhotic diphthong** or **r-colored vowel.** R-colored vowels possess an *auditory quality* known as **rhotacization.** Rhotacization simply means that the vowel is perceived as having an "r" quality or "r-coloring" associated with it.

The rhotic diphthong, /ɪr/, also may be transcribed as /ɪɚ/ or /ɪɚ͜/. The connecting mark in the last example is used by some phoneticians and clinicians when transcribing the diphthong to signify the production of two sounds as one phoneme. This text will adopt the use of /ɪr/, as opposed to /ɪɚ/ or /ɪɚ͜/ when transcribing this phoneme. /ɪr/ is only one of several r-colored vowels found in English.

There are a few dialectal variants involving the phoneme /ɪ/. For instance, in the southeastern United States, some people pronounce the r-colored vowel /ɪr/ with /i/, as in "here" /hir/ or "ear" /ir/ (Hartman, 1985). /ɪ/ is also found to occur before /l/ in some southern pronunciations, as in "really" /rɪlɪ/ and "meal" /mɪl/. Both in African American English and in southern American dialect, words such as "many," "pen," and "cents" might be pronounced as /mɪnɪ/, /pɪn/, and /sɪnts/, respectively.

EXERCISE 4.2—THE VOWEL /ɪ/

A. Contrast the vowels in the following pairs of words (minimal pairs) by saying them aloud.

/i/	/ɪ/		/i/	/ɪ/
reed	rid		keel	kill
heed	hid		deal	dill
deep	dip		ceased	cyst
seat	sit		bean	been
sleek	slick		feet	fit

B. Circle the words that contain the /ɪ/ phoneme.

peace	friend	enthrall	bitter
mythical	silver	woman	tryst
click	ingest	build	fear
thread	pink	bowling	tried
pride	clear	sporty	synchronize

C. Circle the phonetic transcriptions that represent English words.

/vɪl/	/sɪst/	/fɪld/	/wɪns/
/izɪ/	/klip/	/spid/	/hik/
/hɪr/	/ɪl/	/sɪg/	/pɪgɪ/

Continues

EXERCISE 4.2 (*cont.*)

D. In the blanks, write each of the words using English orthography.

/stip/ _____   /pɪk/ _____

/pliz/ _____   /kɪst/ _____

/mɪt/ _____   /bik/ _____

/dɪd/ _____   /pɪp/ _____

/fɪr/ _____   /mɪstɪ/ _____

/rilɪ/ _____   /ɪndɪd/ _____

E. Place an "X" next to the pairs of words that share the same vowel sound.

_____ feel   teach   _____ win   king

_____ lip   thread   _____ mint   inch

_____ been   drink   _____ deed   flea

_____ vent   list   _____ dish   ill

_____ tied   pig   _____ kick   mill

F. Indicate with an "X" the words that contain the r-colored vowel /ɪr/.

1. _____ flirt   5. _____ smeared   9. _____ stirred

2. _____ peerless   6. _____ worried   10. _____ stared

3. _____ bird   7. _____ steered   11. _____ earring

4. _____ shrill   8. _____ harder   12. _____ cursor

/e/
/eɪ/

Lower-Case e
Description

Height:	high-mid
Advancement:	front
Lip rounding:	unrounded
Tense/lax:	tense

Sample Words   The following set of words all take /e/ in their transcriptions because the syllables that contain the vowel do not receive primary stress.

chaOtic	UNdulate
GYrate	layETTE
PHOnate	DECade
MANdate	ROtate

The following words all take the allophone /eɪ/ because the syllables are either stressed or at the end of a word.

aWAY	(also ends the word)	conTAgious
touPEE	(also ends the word)	STATed
creATE		BAby
TAble		BRAID

Allographs

Grapheme	Example	Grapheme	Example
ea	great	ei	veil
a..e	hate	ay	stray
au	gauge	ey	grey
ai	faint		

Discussion   The /e/ vowel is produced with the body of the tongue slightly higher than the exact middle of the mouth, therefore it is referred to as a *high-mid vowel* (see Figure 4.9). /e/ also is unrounded. Like the vowel /i/, it is tense and can be found in the word "bay." An allophone of /e/, written as /eɪ/, occurs in stressed syllables and at the ends of words (regardless of stress). This allophone of /e/ is actually a diphthong and occurs in these particular phonetic contexts as a result of vowel lengthening.

The diphthongal allophone is comprised of the onglide /e/ plus the offglide /ɪ/. In producing /eɪ/, the tongue and vocal tract assume the initial position for the /e/ vowel. The tongue then continues to glide to the high, front position for /ɪ/ (see Figure 4.2). As mentioned, the diphthongal form, /eɪ/, is usually produced in stressed syllables and at the end of words (regardless of stress) when the vowel is lengthened; the shorter monophthong /e/ generally occurs in unstressed syllables. Strictly speaking, phonemic (broad) transcription would dictate the use of /e/ when transcribing the diphthongal variant /eɪ/. However, many individuals prefer to indicate the use of the diphthong when it occurs, even though technically, use of the symbol /eɪ/ would result in an *allophonic* transcription. In this text, the diphthong /eɪ/ will be used in transcription when this particular allophone occurs in stressed syllables and at the ends of words (even though this breaks with the true definition of phonemic transcription). Check with your instructor to determine which method is preferred.

The use of /eɪ/ may also vary with regional pronunciation. For example, some southern speakers in the United States use the diphthong /eɪ/ in words such as "fresh" /freɪʃ/ and "leg" /leɪg/.

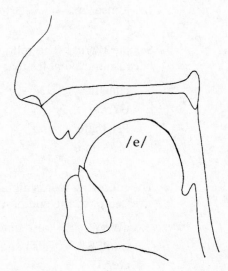

FIGURE 4.9   /e/ articulation.

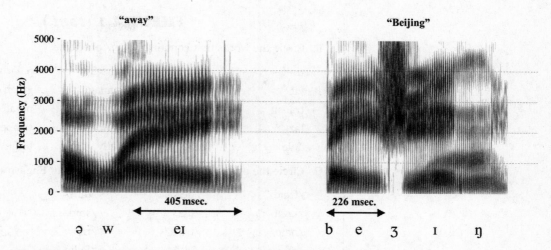

FIGURE 4.10 Spectrograms of the words "away" and "Beijing."

Acoustic Information   Figure 4.10 demonstrates the effect of syllabic stress on the duration of the diphthong /eɪ/ and the vowel /e/ in the words "away" and "Beijing," respectively. Both words have second syllable stress. The vowel in the first syllable of "Beijing" would be transcribed with /e/ because the syllable is unstressed. The second syllable in "away" contains the diphthong /eɪ/ because it is a stressed syllable. Note the difference in the duration of these two vowels as indicated by the length of the horizontal arrows in Figure 4.10. The duration of /eɪ/ is 405 msec., whereas the duration of /e/ is only 226 msec. It is clear that stressed vowels are lengthened when compared to unstressed vowels. The diphthong in "away" is also lengthened due to the fact that it is in the final position of the word.

Figure 4.10 indicates that the F_2 of the onglide of /eɪ/ begins at approximately 1000 Hz and rises to an offglide frequency greater than 2000 Hz. Also, consistent with the F_1 rule, note how the frequency of F_1 decreases over the length of the diphthong as the tongue rises from /e/ to /ɪ/.

EXERCISE 4.3—THE VOWEL /e/ – /eɪ/

A. Contrast the vowels in the following minimal pairs.

/eɪ/	/ɪ/	/eɪ/	/i/
grade	grid	tame	team
tape	tip	grain	green
drape	drip	trait	treat
take	tick	sale	seal
late	lit	Grace	grease
tale	till	wade	weed
faze	fizz	raid	reed

Continues

EXERCISE 4.3 (*cont.*)

B. Circle the words that contain the /eɪ/ phoneme.

trail	rage	wheel	palatial
vice	razor	manage	green
transit	machine	whale	potato
lazy	bread	football	temperate
dale	tackle	daily	bright

C. Circle the phonetic transcriptions that represent English words.

/freɪd/	/deɪs/	/dɪnt/	/deɪlɪ/
/kreɪt/	/bɪz/	/spid/	/deɪm/
/neɪp/	/trɪps/	/treɪ/	/frɪl/
/pɪln/	/blid/	/feɪlm/	/streɪp/

D. In the blanks, write each of the words using English orthography.

/bleɪz/	_____	/pleɪket/	_____
/pleɪd/	_____	/rimeɪn/	_____
/beɪn/	_____	/ɪnmet/	_____
/iveɪd/	_____	/ribet/	_____
/krɪmp/	_____	/steɪnd/	_____
/rikt/	_____	/deɪzɪ/	_____

E. Indicate whether the syllable that contains /eɪ/ is either open or closed by writing O or C in the blank.

_____ crayon		_____ unmade	
_____ prepay		_____ stay	
_____ baking		_____ tailor	
_____ masonry		_____ betrayed	

F. Place an "X" next to the pairs of words that share the same vowel sound.

_____ braid	hid		_____ state	rain	
_____ feed	hate		_____ fist	flea	
_____ lane	aim		_____ cringe	hid	
_____ fill	kissed		_____ deal	will	
_____ treat	sling		_____ wheel	meat	

G. Indicate whether you should use /e/ or /eɪ/ when transcribing the following words.

_____ neighbor		_____ Crayola	
_____ crate		_____ basin	
_____ donate		_____ stay	
_____ hooray		_____ prostrate	
_____ saber		_____ incubate	

/ɛ/

Epsilon
Description

Height:	low-mid
Advancement:	front
Lip rounding:	unrounded
Tense/lax:	lax

Sample Words

met	etch	bury	intend
steady	where	terror	tender
pretend	repent	heather	elephant
relish	stencil	marry	pleasures

Allographs

Grapheme	*Example*	*Grapheme*	*Example*
e	let	ai	said
ei	heifer	ai(r)	flair
ea	meant	ei(r)	their
a	many	ea(r)	bear
ie	friend	u(r)	bury
ue	guest	a(re)	bare
eo	Leonard	e(re)	where

Discussion   The /ɛ/ vowel is commonly referred to as "epsilon," an IPA symbol borrowed from the Greek alphabet. It is categorized as a low-mid, front vowel (see Figure 4.11). Examination of the vowel quadrilateral indicates the tongue body is located midway between the mid and low positions in the mouth for its production. Epsilon is an unrounded and lax vowel. (Placing /ɛ/ at the end of a monosyllabic word creates a nonsense word, e.g., /tɛ/ or /wɛ/.) The vowel /ɛ/

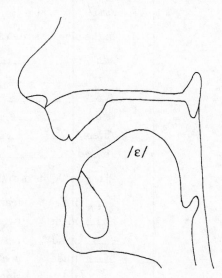

FIGURE 4.11   /ɛ/ articulation.

often occurs before the consonant /r/ in words such as "hair" /hɛr/ and "fair" /fɛr/. /ɛr/ is another example of an r-colored vowel (rhotic diphthong). This phoneme is transcribed by some individuals as /ɛɚ/ or /ɛ͜ɚ/. In the northeastern and southeastern United States, /ɛr/ may be pronounced as /er/ as in "hair" /hɛr/ and "fair" /fɛr/ (Hartman, 1985). Also, some speakers in the Great Lakes region substitute /ɛ/ for /ɪ/ in words such as "pillow" /pɛloʊ/ and "milk" /mɛlk/ (Hartman, 1985).

EXERCISE 4.4—THE VOWEL /ɛ/

A. Contrast the vowels in the following minimal pairs by saying them aloud.

/ɛ/	/ɪ/		/ɛ/	/eɪ/
red	rid		wed	wade
dead	did		tread	trade
head	hid		shed	shade
etch	itch		met	mate
bell	bill		bread	braid
bear	beer		every	Avery
fair	fear		bell	bale

B. Circle the words that contain the /ɛ/ phoneme.

pimple	trip	ensure	tryst
syrup	caring	women	contend
pencil	butter	build	pretzel
thing	thread	prepare	tried
jeep	pistol	unscented	remember

C. Circle the phonetic transcriptions that represent English words.

/mɛri/	/hint/	/split/	/istɛr/
/slɛpt/	/fɛr/	/ɪrk/	/meɪd/
/sɪsɪ/	/kleɪ/	/wɛl/	/krip/

D. In the blanks, write each of the words using English orthography.

/reɪk/	_____	/stɛr/	_____
/fɪz/	_____	/treɪl/	_____
/smɛl/	_____	/pritɛnd/	_____
/sid/	_____	/hɛvi/	_____
/kreɪn/	_____	/friz/	_____
/breɪzd/	_____	/blɛst/	_____

E. Place an "X" next to the pairs of words that share the same vowel sound.

_____ fill	fear		_____ step	edge
_____ made	cage		_____ bread	breathe
_____ wind	best		_____ flit	red
_____ trade	peel		_____ sill	kit
_____ rid	sing		_____ care	meant

Continues

EXERCISE 4.4 *(cont.)*

F. Indicate whether the words below end with an open (O) or closed (C) syllable (write C or O in the blanks).

_____ 1. trail   _____ 6. spree

_____ 2. repay   _____ 7. arouse

_____ 3. strike   _____ 8. rough

_____ 4. plea   _____ 9. undo

_____ 5. late   _____ 10. chow

G. Indicate with an "X" the words that contain the r-colored vowel /ɛr/.

_____ 1. share   _____ 6. careful

_____ 2. early   _____ 7. sparrow

_____ 3. dearly   _____ 8. third

_____ 4. compare   _____ 9. corridor

_____ 5. fluoride   _____ 10. certain

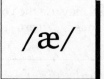

Ash

Description

Height:	low
Advancement:	front
Lip rounding:	unrounded
Tense/lax:	lax

Sample Words

trash	jazz	smacked	language
thank	stand	asterisk	Capricorn
manage	batter	aster	blasphemy
Alabama	tamper	fantastic	trespass

Allographs

Grapheme	**Example**
a	back
a(ng)	hang
a(nk)	tank
au	laugh
ai	plaid

Discussion   The vowel /æ/, referred to as "ash," is the lowest of the five front vowels. (The vowel /a/, found in some eastern American dialects, is slightly lower.) It is also one of the four point vowels. In reference to the front vowels, the mandible and tongue are in their lowest position for /æ/ (see Figure 4.6). The size of the oropharynx is small for /æ/ because the tongue body is in an inferior and posterior position (see Figures 4.6 and 4.12). Like all of the other front vowels, /æ/ is unrounded. Also, /æ/ is lax; no monosyllables end with this sound. The one peculiarity of "ash" is its use in words in which it precedes the nasal /ŋ/, as in "rank" /ræŋk/ and

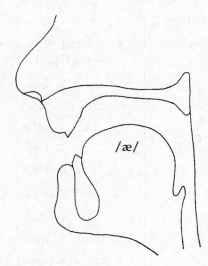

FIGURE 4.12   /æ/ articulation.

"bang" /bæŋ/. You might be tempted to use the vowel /eɪ/ in these words. Keep in mind that this vowel is an allophone of /æ/ in this particular context; its perception is affected by nasalization due to the nasal consonant that follows.

In the eastern and southern United States, speakers may use the vowel /æ/ in words such as "marry," "Harry," and "carry," that is, /mærɪ/, /hærɪ/, and /kærɪ/.

EXERCISE 4.5—THE VOWEL /æ/

A. Contrast the vowels in the following pairs of words by saying them aloud.

/ɛ/	/æ/	/eɪ/	/æ/
led	lad	bade	bad
tend	tanned	haze	has
den	Dan	shale	shall
Ben	ban	mate	mat
bed	bad	lane	language
Kent	can't	bane	bank
spend	spanned	Dane	dank

B. Circle the words that contain the /æ/ phoneme.

straddle	practice	lapse	revamp
pale	panther	repast	straight
Lester	pacific	pacify	farmer
baseball	hanged	chances	cards
jazz	pistol	tamed	bombastic

C. Circle the phonetic transcriptions that represent English words.

/klæd/	/prid/	/strɪv/	/wæd/
/slæpt/	/bɪrd/	/bæz/	/trækt/
/web/	/steɪp/	/sprɪg/	/læzɪ/

Continues

EXERCISE 4.5 (*cont.*)

D. In the blanks, write each of the words using English orthography.

/klæn/ _____   /spɪr/ _____

/sprɪnt/ _____   /hɛrɪ/ _____

/rɛk/ _____   /pækt/ _____

/teɪstɪ/ _____   /dræg/ _____

/præns/ _____   /bɛrɪ/ _____

/læft/ _____   /tinz/ _____

E. Place an "X" next to the pairs of words that share the same vowel sound.

_____ badge   rage   _____ hair   bend

_____ seed   shade   _____ lick   beer

_____ cab   blonde   _____ beak   bless

_____ tray   whale   _____ trap   bake

_____ crank   shag   _____ lapse   crag

Complete Assignment 4-1.

The Back Vowels

Pronunciation Guide

/u/	as in "toot"	/tut/
/ʊ/	as in "look"	/lʊk/
/o/	as in "<u>o</u>bese"	/obis/
/oʊ/	as in "vote"	/voʊt/	(allophone of /o/)
/ɔ/	as in "dawn"	/dɔn/
/ɑ/	as in "not"	/nɑt/

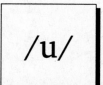

Lower-Case u
Description

Height:	high
Advancement:	back
Lip rounding:	rounded
Tense/lax:	tense

Sample Words

chew	ewe	unc<u>ou</u>th	strewn
f<u>u</u>tile	truth	spew	loot
Tr<u>u</u>man	cr<u>ue</u>l	cucumber	t<u>u</u>lip
clue	st<u>u</u>pid	t<u>u</u>na	s<u>u</u>per

Allographs

Grapheme	*Example*	*Grapheme*	*Example*
u	Pluto	wo	two
ue	true	oe	shoe
u..e	tune	o	to
ui	suit	ew	stew
ou	through	ieu	lieu
oo	moon	eu	maneuver
o..e	move	ioux	Sioux

Discussion   If you compare the placement of /u/ with the placement of /i/ in the vowel quadrilateral, you will see that these two vowels are mirror images of one another, that is, they are the two highest vowels in English. (See the spectrograms in Figure 4.3 for an acoustic comparison of /i/ and /u/.) Actually, all of the back vowels are approximate mirror images of their front vowel counterparts in terms of height. Because of the extremely high back tongue body position, /u/ is considered to be another point, or corner, vowel in English (see Figure 4.13). /u/ is a rounded vowel. As previously stated, although all of the front vowels are unrounded, most of the English back vowels are rounded. The vowel /u/ is a tense vowel; it is found at the end of the one-syllable words "through," "you," and "true."

In raising the tongue to such a high position for /u/, the tongue root is forced to be somewhat advanced, widening the pharynx. As the tongue lowers in production of the back vowels from /u/ to /ɑ/, the pharynx narrows accordingly, due to the retreating movement of the tongue root, posteriorly. Figure 4.14 displays the different tongue, jaw, lip, and pharyngeal positions for /u/ and /ɑ/.

There is one peculiarity associated with the phoneme /u/ and its transcription. Notice that in words like "you," "few," and "music," /u/ is actually preceded by the consonant phoneme /j/ (/ju/, /fju/, and /mjuzɪk/). (The /j/ phoneme is the

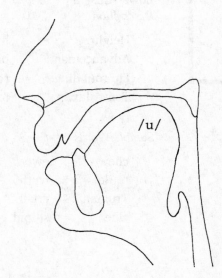

FIGURE 4.13   /u/ articulation.

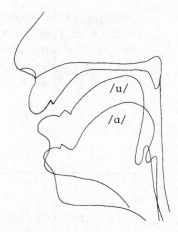

FIGURE 4.14 /u/ and /ɑ/ articulation.

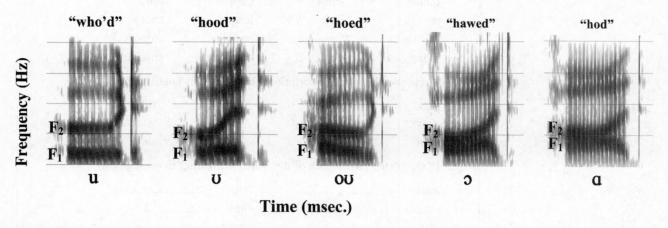

FIGURE 4.15 Spectrograms of the five back vowels in /h_d/context.

palatal "y" sound.) Without the /j/ phoneme, these words would sound like "oo," "foo," and "moosic." Some phonetics texts do treat the phoneme sequence /ju/ as a diphthong. In this text, however, we will treat /j/ + /u/ as separate phonemes. As you examine the allographs of /u/ above, you will see several varied spellings for this phoneme.

Acoustic Information   Figure 4.15 shows spectrograms of the five back vowels in /h_d/ context. Examine the acoustic characteristics of the five vowels, paying attention to changes in the formant patterns as the tongue lowers in production of the five back vowels. As predicted by the F_1 rule, as the tongue lowers in production from /u/ to /ɑ/, the frequency of F_1 rises. The second formant frequency is quite similar at the onset of each of the five vowels. This is because the back vowels are fairly consistent in terms of tongue advancement; they do not change as much in the front/back dimension as do the front vowels. Note, however, that the second formant rises throughout the production of each of the vowels. This is because each vowel begins with the tongue toward the back of the oral cavity (in the velar region) for production of the vowel. Then the tongue moves forward toward the alveolar ridge for production of /d/ at the end of each word. This dynamic change in the frequency of the formant from vowel to following consonant is known as a **formant transition.** The formant transition helps demonstrate how changes in tongue position alter the resonance of the vocal tract. Also, the formant transition is an acoustic cue that identifies the place of articulation (where the consonant is produced in the oral cavity) of the post-vocalic consonant (/d/ in this case). Formant transitions also occur between pre-vocalic consonants and vowels.

EXERCISE 4.6—THE VOWEL /u/

A. Circle the words that contain the /u/ phoneme.

ghoul	oboe	crew	plural
butter	stuck	Lucifer	must
should	luck	lusty	shook
fuchsia	look	molding	stupor
loosely	glue	blouse	choose

B. Circle the phonetic transcriptions that represent English words.

/ust/	/krud/	/prus/	/tul/
/suv/	/tug/	/pus/	/wund/
/pul/	/rup/	/lus/	/slug/

C. In the blanks, write each of the words using English orthography.

/spun/ _____	/sup/ _____
/tun/ _____	/lud/ _____
/rut/ _____	/stru/ _____
/mud/ _____	/flu/ _____
/klu/ _____	/grum/ _____
/ruf/ _____	/snut/ _____

D. Indicate with an "X" the pairs of words that share the same vowel phoneme.

____ 1.	could	showed	____ 6.	brood	hood
____ 2.	suit	loon	____ 7.	stood	could
____ 3.	lute	book	____ 8.	hoops	poor
____ 4.	crew	scoot	____ 9.	feud	moose
____ 5.	push	foot	____ 10.	muse	cook

E. Indicate with an "X" the words that have the phoneme sequence /j/ + /u/, as in "you."

____ 1. oozing		____ 6. fuming
____ 2. cute		____ 7. Pluto
____ 3. huge		____ 8. useful
____ 4. ruined		____ 9. viewing
____ 5. sloop		____ 10. spooky

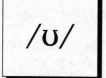

/ʊ/

Upsilon

Description

Height:	high (lower than /u/)
Advancement:	back
Lip rounding:	rounded
Tense/lax:	lax

Sample Words

could	s<u>u</u>gar	pushed	bull
should	would	c<u>u</u>shion	lure*
obsc<u>u</u>re*	uns<u>u</u>re*	took	hood
wolf	full	stood	put

*/ʊ/ in these words may be pronounced differently, depending on a speaker's dialect.

Allographs

Grapheme	**Example**
u	push
ou	could
u(r)	sec<u>u</u>re
oo	book
o	wolf

Discussion The vowel /ʊ/ is produced with the tongue body only slightly lower in the oral cavity than for /u/ (see Figure 4.16). Therefore, it also is termed high. Like /u/, the vowel /ʊ/ is rounded; unlike /u/, it is lax. You will never see open syllables ending with this phoneme, as in /bʊ/ or /tʊ/. This vowel, in combination with the consonant /r/, forms the r-colored vowel /ʊr/ (also transcribed as /ʊɚ/ or /ʊɚ/). The combination of /ʊ/ + /r/ may be used in the pronunciation of the words "tour" /tʊr/ and "lure" /lʊr/ by some individuals. Others may

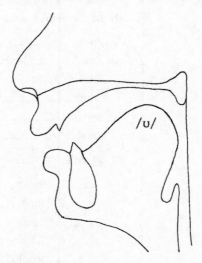

FIGURE 4.16 /ʊ/ articulation.

pronounce these words as if they rhymed with "core," that is, /tɔr/ and /lɔr/ (see the vowel /ɔ/ on page 82). Notice that there are many fewer allographs associated with /ʊ/ than for the vowel /u/.

When the allograph "oo" is followed by /l/ (as in pool, cool, fool, and tool), the resulting pronunciation may be either /ʊ/ or /u/, depending on a speaker's dialect. Examine the following possible pronunciations of these words:

| *pool* | /pʊl/ | or | /pul/ | | *fool* | /fʊl/ | or | /ful/ |
| *cool* | /kʊl/ | or | /kul/ | | *tool* | /tʊl/ | or | /tul/ |

Some eastern speakers use the vowel /ʊ/ in words such as "room" /rʊm/ and "broom" /brʊm/.

EXERCISE 4.7—THE VOWEL /ʊ/

A. Contrast the vowels in the following words.

/u/	/ʊ/	/u/	/ʊ/
who'd	hood	food	foot
cooed	could	shoed	should
Luke	look	stewed	stood

B. Circle the words that contain the /ʊ/ phoneme.

hole	wooden	snooze	stunned
shut	punched	luscious	spook
hood	couldn't	pulled	shook
flushed	mistook	beauty	person
rudely	cooker	brood	stood

C. Circle the phonetic transcriptions that represent English words.

/buk/	/stʊ/	/rul/	/sul/
/lʊv/	/lum/	/rʊk/	/frut/
/trups/	/stʊr/	/buts/	/slʊg/

D. In the blanks, write each of the words using English orthography.

/pʊs/	_____	/tʊr/	_____
/tru/	_____	/hʊk/	_____
/stʊd/	_____	/lum/	_____
/dum/	_____	/fluk/	_____
/gru/	_____	/prun/	_____
/gʊd/	_____	/krʊk/	_____

E. Place an "X" next to the pairs of words that share the same vowel sound.

_____ 1.	loot	foot	_____ 6.	what	look
_____ 2.	tune	mute	_____ 7.	nook	stood
_____ 3.	coupe	soon	_____ 8.	rust	rook
_____ 4.	flood	cute	_____ 9.	goof	cruise
_____ 5.	would	soot	_____ 10.	mutt	look

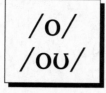

Lower-Case o

Description

Height:	high-mid
Advancement:	back
Lip rounding:	rounded
Tense/lax:	tense

Sample Words The following words all take the allophone /o/ in their transcription because the syllables that contain the vowel are not stressed.

boDAcious	RIboflavin
CroAtian	floTILla
broCADE	proHIBit
ptoMAINE	roTAtion

The following words all take the allophone /oʊ/ because the syllables are either stressed (including monosyllables), or are at the end of a word.

cone	flow
bowl	whole
PRObate	toad
STOic	SLOWer
BLOATed	reMOTE
beLOW (also end of word)	BELLow (end of word)

Be sure to compare and contrast the words "below" and "bellow." The second syllable in "below" is stressed and the second syllable in "bellow" is not. However, both words are transcribed with /oʊ/ because this sound ends both words. In either case, the final phoneme is correspondingly lengthened.

Allographs

Grapheme	Example	Grapheme	Example
o	open	oe	foe
o..e	rose	oh	oh
oa	road	ou	soul
ow	bowl	eau	beau
ew	sew	au	cafe au lait

Discussion The body of the tongue is in the high-middle portion of the oral cavity during production of /o/ (see Figure 4.17). In many ways this phoneme is similar to the front allophones /e/ and /eɪ/. That is, the diphthong /oʊ/ occurs in stressed syllables and at the ends of words (regardless of stress), and the monophthong /o/ occurs in unstressed syllables. Therefore, /oʊ/ and /o/ are allophones of the same phoneme. The production of the diphthong begins with the tongue in position for the onglide /o/, in the mid-back portion of the mouth. The tongue then glides to a higher position for production of the offglide /ʊ/ (see Figure 4.2). *Phonemic* (broad) transcription would technically dictate the use of /o/

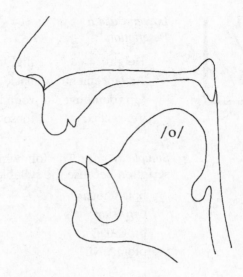

FIGURE 4.17   /o/ articulation.

when transcribing the allophone /oʊ/. In this text, however, the diphthong /oʊ/ will be used when transcribing this particular allophone when it occurs in stressed syllables and at the ends of words. Check with your instructor to determine which method is preferred.

Acoustic Information   Figure 4.18 illustrates the effect of syllabic stress not only on the duration of the diphthong /oʊ/ and the monophthong /o/, but also on the length of the entire syllables in which they are located. Figure 4.18 shows spectrograms of the words "probate" and "protest." Note that each word begins with the same phonetic string, that is, /pro(ʊ)/. The first syllable is stressed in the word "PRObate" /ˈproʊbeɪt/ and the second syllable is stressed in the word "proTEST" /proˈtɛst/. Note the difference in the duration of these two syllables as indicated by the length of the horizontal arrows in Figure 4.18. The duration of /proʊ/ in the word "probate" (approximately 292 msec.) is almost double the length of the

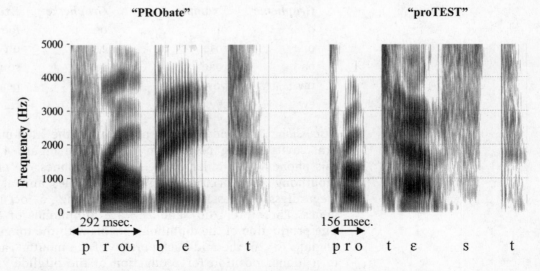

FIGURE 4.18   Spectrograms of the words "probate" and "protest."

syllable /pro/ in "pro̱test" (approximately 156 msec.). Although it is not immediately obvious from the spectrograms in Figure 4.18, the diphthong also is lengthened in the stressed syllable /proʊ/ compared to the vowel in the unstressed syllable /pro/. The actual duration of /oʊ/ in "pro̱bate" is approximately 129 msec. whereas the duration of /o/ in "pro̱test" is approximately 76 msec. In either case, the vowel comprises almost 50% of the syllable.

EXERCISE 4.8—THE VOWEL /o/ – /oʊ/

A. Contrast the vowels in the following minimal pairs.

/oʊ/	/u/	/oʊ/	/ʊ/
grow	grew	coke	cook
slope	sloop	broke	brook
cope	coop	code	could
lobe	lube	hoed	hood
grope	group	showed	should
stowed	stewed	croak	crook

B. Circle the words that contain the /oʊ/ phoneme.

mope	aloof	root	toll
noose	slowed	pond	push
soda	lost	loaded	lasso
nosy	book	sugar	remote
dole	spoke	doily	wholly

C. Circle the phonetic transcriptions that represent English words.

/toʊ/	/boʊn/	/stup/	/prʊb/
/bʊt/	/floʊd/	/boʊd/	/krud/
/stub/	/stud/	/flʊk/	/woʊnt/

D. In the blanks, write each of the words using English orthography.

/moʊld/ _____	/tupeɪ/ _____
/kupt/ _____	/bruzd/ _____
/boʊnɪ/ _____	/bændeɪd/ _____
/ivoʊk/ _____	/kʊkɪ/ _____
/stoʊd/ _____	/koʊɛd/ _____
/doʊpɪ/ _____	/rizum/ _____

E. Indicate whether you should use /o/ or /oʊ/ when transcribing the following words.

_____ Romania	_____ snowman	_____ bowling
_____ corroded	_____ location	_____ though
_____ stolen	_____ jello	_____ notation
_____ magnolia	_____ coagulate	_____ potential

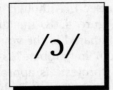

Open o
Description

Height:	low-mid
Advancement:	back
Lip rounding:	rounded
Tense/lax:	tense

Sample Words

prawn	thought	vault	wrong
awl	ought	autumn	haul
all	sought	off	gone
cord	frog	hoard	soar

Note: Some speakers may use the phoneme /ɑ/ in the production of some of these words.

Allographs

Grapheme	Example	Grapheme	Example
ou	wrought	o	log
au	laud	a	call
aw	lawn	oa	broad

Discussion　The /ɔ/ vowel is often referred to as "open o." This rounded vowel is produced with the tongue slightly lower in the oral cavity than /o/, in the low-mid position (see Figure 4.19). In addition, it is a tense vowel, and it is found in some individuals' pronunciations of the words "saw," "haul," "caught," and "awl." This vowel is difficult for many students to recognize since it is not produced by all speakers of American English; its use varies considerably with regional dialect. In many regions of the United States, the vowel has merged with /ɑ/ (discussed in the next section) so that both vowels are produced as /ɑ/. This topic will be discussed in greater detail in Chapter 8.

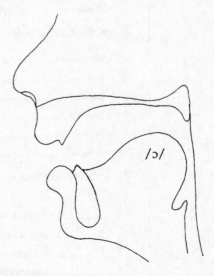

FIGURE 4.19　/ɔ/ articulation.

In words such as "corn," "bored," and "fort," it is the r-colored vowel /ɔr/ (also transcribed as /ɔɚ/ or /ɔɚ̯/) that is used in their transcriptions—that is, /kɔrn/, /bɔrd/, and /fɔrt/. Also, some individuals will pronounce the words "lure" and "tour" as /lɔr/ and /tɔr/, respectively. Some individuals will use /ɔr/ in the production of the word "sure," that is, /ʃɔr/.

EXERCISE 4.9—THE VOWEL /ɔ/

A. Circle the phonetic transcriptions that represent possible pronunciations of English words.

/bɔt/	/drʊm/	/stɔn/	/brɔn/
/koʊt/	/grɔn/	/tɔk/	/pʊl/
/lups/	/fɔrt/	/flum/	/ɔrn/

B. In the blanks, write each of the words using English orthography.

/spɔrt/ _____   /sprɔl/ _____

/kʊd/ _____   /stʊd/ _____

/proʊb/ _____   /frɔt/ _____

/pruv/ _____   /kɔrps/ _____

/stɔrd/ _____   /hʊkt/ _____

/ɔfʊl/ _____   /doʊnet/ _____

C. Indicate with an "X" the words that contain the r-colored vowel /ɔr/.

1. _____ farm   4. _____ storm   7. _____ lured

2. _____ third   5. _____ worm   8. _____ worth

3. _____ horrid   6. _____ thorn   9. _____ spar

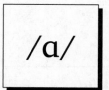

Script a
Description

Height:	low
Advancement:	back
Lip rounding:	unrounded
Tense/lax:	tense

Sample Words

r**o**tten	**o**strich	p**o**sse	cause
f**a**ther	ap**a**rt	l**a**tte	watch
bond	stop	car	pr**o**blem
plod	bronze	Hans	smart

Note: Some speakers may use the phoneme /ɔ/ in production of some of these sample words.

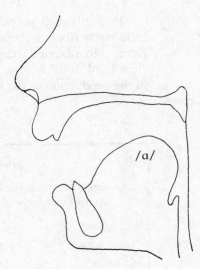

/ɑ/

FIGURE 4.20   /ɑ/ articulation.

Allographs

Grapheme	Example	Grapheme	Example
a	shawl	ea(r)	heart
o	rob	e(r)	sergeant
a(r)	mart		

Discussion   /ɑ/ is a point vowel due to the tongue's extremely low, back articulatory position in the oral cavity during its production (see Figure 4.20). It is the only unrounded back vowel in English. /ɑ/ is also tense. Due to dialectal variation in pronunciation, some individuals use this vowel instead of /ɔ/, especially in pronunciation of words such as "saw," "haul," "caught," and "awl." The /ɑ/ vowel is most commonly used in combination with /r/ to form the r-colored vowel /ɑr/ (also transcribed as /ɑɚ/ or /ɑ͡ɚ/) as in the words "bark" /bɑrk/ and "art" /ɑrt/.

EXERCISE 4.10—THE VOWEL /ɑ/

A. Contrast the vowels in the following words.

/oʊ/	/ɑ/ (or) /ɔ/ (depending on dialect)
boat	bought
bowl	ball
coat	caught
load	laud
sewed	sawed
loan	lawn

Continues

EXERCISE 4.10 (*cont.*)

B. Circle the phonetic transcriptions that represent possible pronunciations of English words.

/wond/	/tɔb/	/harm/	/blab/
/koʊd/	/sɔt/	/blad/	/armɪ/
/frɔd/	/pʊnt/	/ad/	/kad/

C. In the blanks, write each of the words using English orthography.

/frast/ _____	/zɑr/ _____
/lʊkt/ _____	/prund/ _____
/bɔrd/ _____	/blɔnd/ _____
/kroʊm/ _____	/ansɛt/ _____
/want/ _____	/krɔdæd/ _____
/starvd/ _____	/ardvark/ _____

D. Indicate with an "X" the words that contain the r-colored vowel /ar/.

1. _____ war
2. _____ cleared
3. _____ quartz
4. _____ flare
5. _____ starred
6. _____ dirt
7. _____ orchard
8. _____ March
9. _____ poorly
10. _____ smarter
11. _____ carbon
12. _____ spore

Complete Assignment 4-2.

The Central Vowels

Pronunciation Guide

/ə/	as in "alone"	/əloʊn/	(unstressed)
/ʌ/	as in "but"	/bʌt/	(stressed)
/ɚ/	as in "perhaps"	/pɚhæps/	(unstressed)
/ɝ/	as in "heard"	/hɝd/	(stressed)

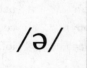

Schwa
Description

Height:	mid
Advancement:	central
Lip rounding:	unrounded
Tense/lax:	lax

Sample Words

astound	paraded	plantation	command
rearrange	tangent	spumoni	relevant
roasted	salami	mountain	carousel
ransom	ketchup	tuna	undone

Note: /ə/ occurs in unstressed syllables in all of these words.

Allographs

Grapheme	Example	Grapheme	Example
u	<u>u</u>ntrue	ou	jealous
o	c<u>o</u>logne	i	merrily
a	machine	oi	porpoise
ai	villain	e	happen
ia	parliament	eo	surgeon
io	nation		

Discussion   /ə/ is commonly known as "schwa." Schwa is produced with the tongue body in the most central portion of the mouth cavity. The entire vocal tract is in its most neutral configuration during production of /ə/. It is difficult to discuss this vowel without discussing another vowel concurrently, namely /ʌ/, referred to as *turned v* or "wedge." These vowels are used to represent allophones of the same sound, even though most phoneticians and clinicians treat them as two separate vowel phonemes. (There *is* actually a slight difference in their place of production in the oral cavity.) The basic distinction between these vowels is that schwa *occurs only in unstressed syllables* and turned v *occurs only in stressed syllables*. The distribution of these vowels is similar to /e/ and /eɪ/ and /o/ and /oʊ/, in reference to their occurrence in stressed and unstressed syllables:

Stressed	Unstressed
eɪ	e
oʊ	o
ʌ	ə

Schwa is unrounded because the lips do not protrude in its production. It is also a lax vowel.

EXERCISE 4.11–THE VOWEL /ə/

A. Circle the words that contain the /ə/ phoneme.

rowing	decision	control	untamed	laundry
lasagna	injure	glamor	opera	petunia
wooded	poorly	motion	puppy	cockroach
Laverne	ruled	holding	fuchsia	lotion

B. Circle the phonetic transcriptions that represent English words.

/sətɪn/	/zəbrɑ/	/əbeɪt/	/əluf/
/drɑmə/	/ləpʊr/	/bəlun/	/rədæn/
/səpoʊz/	/rəpik/	/brəzɪl/	/əndu/

Continues

EXERCISE 4.11 (*cont.*)

C. In the blanks, write each of the words using English orthography.

/pɪnət/ _____   /kənteɪn/ _____

/əkrɔs/ _____   /lɛmən/ _____

/vəlɔr/ _____   /bətɑn/ _____

/səpɔrt/ _____   /əwɔrd/ _____

/kɔfɪn/ _____   /eɪprəl/ _____

/plətun/ _____   /kəsɛt/ _____

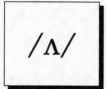

/ʌ/

Turned V
"Wedge"
Description

Height:	low-mid
Advancement:	back-central
Lip rounding:	unrounded
Tense/lax:	lax

Sample Words

rub	button	Monday	mustard
trouble	luncheon	luckily	scrumptious
flood	undone	rushing	public
abundance	stumble	redundant	wonderful

Note: /ʌ/ occurs in only the stressed syllables of these words.

Allographs

Grapheme	Example	Grapheme	Example
u	crumb	oe	does
o	done	ou	double
oo	flood		

Discussion Turned v is found in monosyllabic words and stressed syllables. It is produced slightly lower and farther back in the oral cavity than /ə/ (see Figure 4.21). Like /ə/, /ʌ/ is unrounded and lax. Although /ʌ/ can occur in one-syllable words, it does not usually occur in open syllables in English. One exception might be in the production of the word "the," which usually does not receive stress in conversational English.

Students often confuse /ʌ/ with the vowel /ʊ/. Compare the minimal pairs in Exercise 4.12A that contrast these two phonemes.

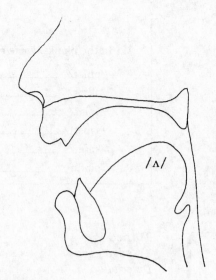

FIGURE 4.21   /ʌ/ articulation.

EXERCISE 4.12—THE VOWEL /ʌ/

A. Contrast the vowel /ʌ/ in the following minimal pairs.

/ʌ/	/ʊ/	/ʌ/	/u/	/ʌ/	/ɑ, ɔ/
cud	could	rub	rube	hut	hot
shuck	shook	done	dune	mum	mom
tuck	took	bust	boost	hug	hog
buck	book	dumb	doom	bust	bossed
stud	stood	rum	room	rub	rob
putt	put	spun	spoon	gun	gone
luck	look	glum	gloom	rubbed	robbed

B. Circle the words that contain the /ʌ/ phoneme.

awful	blunder	laundry	Hoover
custard	laborious	Sunday	lawyer
pushy	cushion	hundred	trumpet
cologne	abundant	plural	shouldn't
charades	mundane	wander	conducive

Continues

EXERCISE 4.12 (*cont.*)

C. Examine the English words in the first column and the transcriptions in the second column. Place an "X" next to the transcription if it is wrong.

Examples:

book	/bʊk/	_____
subbed	/sʊbd/	_____

1.	hooked	/hʌkt/	_____
2.	bond	/bʊnd/	_____
3.	bluff	/blʌf/	_____
4.	hood	/hud/	_____
5.	cluck	/klʌk/	_____
6.	rookie	/rʌkɪ/	_____
7.	mistook	/mɪstʊk/	_____
8.	lucky	/lʌkɪ/	_____
9.	rubbing	/rʊbɪŋ/	_____
10.	crooked	/krɔkəd/	_____

D. Circle the phonetic transcriptions that represent English words.

/klʊstɪ/	/əpʊft/	/dʊkɪ/	/sʌntæn/
/rizən/	/krɑmd/	/pʊlɪ/	/vɪstʌ/
/mʌstɪ/	/əndʌn/	/plʌmət/	/plæzə/

E. In the blanks, write each of the words using English orthography.

/pɛrəs/	_____	/robʌst/	_____
/hʌnɪ/	_____	/sʌdən/	_____
/əlɑt/	_____	/kəbus/	_____
/kənvɪns/	_____	/tʌndrə/	_____
/gɑrdəd/	_____	/kəlæps/	_____
/flʌbd/	_____	/bəfun/	_____

F. Indicate whether /ʌ/ or /ə/ should be used in transcribing the following words by circling the appropriate symbol.

lumber	/ʌ/	/ə/		suspend	/ʌ/	/ə/
abort	/ʌ/	/ə/		suppose	/ʌ/	/ə/
shaken	/ʌ/	/ə/		induct	/ʌ/	/ə/
contain	/ʌ/	/ə/		serpent	/ʌ/	/ə/
thunder	/ʌ/	/ə/		rusty	/ʌ/	/ə/

G. Indicate with an "X" the following pairs of words that share the same vowel phoneme.

_____	1. nuts	could		_____	6. crook	fund
_____	2. foot	stoop		_____	7. blood	crust
_____	3. done	rubbed		_____	8. runs	floods
_____	4. crumb	rust		_____	9. loom	food
_____	5. cook	should		_____	10. rush	look

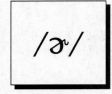

Right-Hook Schwa
"Schwar"
Description

Height:	mid
Advancement:	central
Lip rounding:	rounded
Tense/lax:	lax

Sample Words

pertain	luxury	cursor*	percussion
surround	treasure	flirtatious	mattered
runner	under	countered	Herbert*
ergonomic	ferocious	Saturday	harbor

*****Note:** /ɚ/ occurs only in the unstressed syllables in the sample words above. (The words "Herbert" and "cursor" have stress on the first syllable and would be transcribed with /ɝ/, for example, /hɝbɚt/ and /kɝsɚ/.)

Allographs

Grapheme	Example	Grapheme	Example
or	labor	er	winner
ar	lunar	ir	flirtatious
ur	urbane	yr	martyr

Discussion   /ɚ/ is sometimes referred to as "schwar" because the phonetic symbol visually resembles schwa, but in addition possesses rhotacization (r-coloring). /ɚ/ is not easily defined by referring only to the four categories used previously to describe the other English vowels, that is, height, advancement, lip rounding, and tenseness. Production of /ɚ/ involves additional tongue movement and is formed by constricting the pharynx and increasing the space in the oral cavity in front of the tongue by either: (1) raising the tongue tip and curling it posteriorly toward the alveolar ridge, or (2) lowering the tongue tip while bunching the tongue body in the region of the palate (*Handbook of the International Phonetic Association,* 1999; Ladefoged, 2001; MacKay, 1987). In either case, the associated "r" quality is due to a constriction in the pharynx brought about by retraction of the portion of the tongue below the epiglottis (Ladefoged, 2001).

Inspection of the IPA chart (Figure 2.1) reveals that schwar is missing from the vowel quadrilateral. At one time, the recommended IPA notation for this vowel was in the form of a rhotic diphthong, i.e., /əɹ/ or /əʴ/, indicating the rhotacization of the vowel (Pullum & Ladusaw, 1996). Currently, the IPA recommends the use of /ə/ plus /ʴ/, the diacritic for *rhoticity* (known as the "right-hook"), as the proper notation for transcribing this rhotacized mid-central vowel, i.e., /ə/ + /ʴ/ = /ɚ/. You will find the rhoticity diacritic /ʴ/ located in the IPA chart in the last row of the first column of the diacritics section (Figure 2.1). Interestingly, the *Handbook of the International Phonetic Association* (1999) also recommends the use of the rhoticity diacritic in transcribing other rhotic diphthongs, e.g., "far" /fɑʴ/.

Like schwa, /ɚ/ is produced only in unstressed syllables. Therefore, it is lax. One distinguishing feature of /ɚ/ is that it is produced with lip rounding.

The degree of lip rounding varies from speaker to speaker. (Some phoneticians argue that this vowel is unrounded.) The tense vowel, /ɝ/, is found only in stressed syllables (see the next section). We now can add these two phonemes to the table of stressed and unstressed vowel allophones:

Stressed	*Unstressed*
eɪ	e
oʊ	o
ʌ	ə
ɝ	ɚ

Note: Words such as "ring" and "raisin" begin with the phoneme /r/, *not* with the phoneme /ɚ/. That is, /rɪŋ/ and /reɪzɪn/ *not* /ɚɪŋ/ and /ɚeɪzɪn/. Similarly, the words, "unread" and "berate" should be transcribed as /ənrɛd/ and /bireɪt/, *not* /ənɚɛd/ and /biɚeɪt/.

EXERCISE 4.13—THE VOWEL /ɚ/

A. Contrast the underlined sounds in the words below.

/ɚ/	/r/	/r/-colored vowels
slumb<u>er</u>	<u>d</u>ress	quee<u>r</u>
p<u>er</u>use	<u>r</u>ibbon	me<u>re</u>
ov<u>er</u>	c<u>r</u>eam	sna<u>re</u>
stup<u>or</u>	th<u>r</u>ead	chai<u>r</u>
walk<u>er</u>	<u>fr</u>ost	sto<u>re</u>d
must<u>ard</u>	a<u>r</u>ound	floo<u>r</u>

B. Circle the words that contain the /ɚ/ phoneme.

clover	rebel	barley	dearly
fearless	endear	perjure	fester
carbon	torment	harbor	electric
tremor	written	poorly	breezy
laundered	perhaps	torpedo	surprise

C. Circle the phonetic transcriptions that represent English words.

/kɑnvɚt/	/pɚteɪn/	/pɚsɛnt/	/lɛpɚd/
/rabɚ/	/tɚoʊd/	/drimɚ/	/fɚəst/
/sɚvɛs/	/ɚɛdi/	/ʌnfɛr/	/hɪndɚ/

D. In the blanks, write each of the words using English orthography.

/drɛsɚ/ _____	/kəntɔrt/ _____
/kæmrə/ _____	/pɚɑnə/ _____
/rʌbɚ/ _____	/pɚu/ _____
/marbəl/ _____	/sɪmɚ/ _____
/tɚeɪn/ _____	/kɛrosin/ _____
/flʌstɚd/ _____	/əweɪtəd/ _____

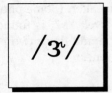

Right-Hook Reversed Epsilon
Description

Height:	mid
Advancement:	central
Lip rounding:	rounded
Tense/lax:	tense

Sample Words

curse	third	Thursday	murder*
deter	surgeon	worry	reverse
rehearse	purple	thirsty	nursery
furnace	service	percolate	aversion

***Note:** The word "murder" would be transcribed as /mɝdɚ/.

Allographs

Grapheme	Example	Grapheme	Example
or	word	ir	shirt
ear	learn	ur	curt
er	perk	yr	Myrtle

Discussion   /ɝ/ occurs only in stressed syllables. It is produced in a manner similar to /ɚ/ with the lips rounded, although the degree of rounding varies among speakers (see Figure 4.22). (Like schwar, this vowel is considered un-rounded by some phoneticians.) /ɝ/ is the only central vowel that is considered to be tense. It is found at the end of the one-syllable words "her," "stir," and "fur," and for some speakers "sure." Keep in mind that /ɝ/ occurs in only the stressed syllables of the sample words provided above.

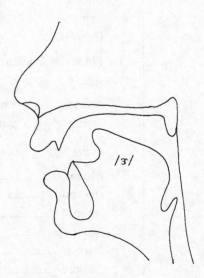

FIGURE 4.22   /ɝ/ articulation.

Similar to the symbol for schwar /ɚ/, /ɜ˞/ is not located in the vowel quadrilateral. Instead the symbol is a combination of *reversed epsilon* /ɜ/ plus the right-hook diacritic /˞/, hence its name, "right-hook reversed epsilon." Reversed epsilon /ɜ/ is a non-rhotacized, mid-central vowel, part of the IPA chart, but not generally used by speakers of American English. However, in British English it is the vowel commonly found in words such as "word" and "curtains" (i.e., /wɜd/ and /kɜtənz/). Try saying these two words without r-coloring when trying to produce reversed epsilon.

Right-hook reversed epsilon /ɜ˞/ is often confused with the rhotic diphthongs, previously introduced in this chapter. Especially confusing are /ɜ˞/ versus /ɪr/ and /ɛr/. Examine the following word combinations, paying close attention to the distinction between /ɜ˞/ and the rhotic diphthongs. Each of the words in the left column contain a different rhotic diphthong. All of the words in the right column contain /ɜ˞/. Say each word pair (i.e., fear-fur; hair-her, etc.) listening to the differences between the rhotic diphthongs and /ɜ˞/. Also, be sure to look at Exercise 4.14A.

		/ɜ˞/			/ɜ˞/
/ɪr/	fear	___ fur	/ɪr/	beer	___ burr
/ɛr/	hair	___ her	/ɛr/	spare	___ spur
/ɑr/	star	___ stir	/ɑr/	shark	___ shirk
/ɔr/	court	___ curt	/ɔr/	ward	___ word
/ʊr/	tour	___ tur(n)	/ʊr/	lure	___ lear(n)

In some dialects of English, notably Southern and Eastern American English, the central rhotic vowels /ɜ˞/ and /ɚ/ may be produced as /ɜ/ and /ə/, respectively. The result is the production of /ɜ/ in words that normally require /ɜ˞/, and the production of /ə/ in words that normally require /ɚ/, e.g., "girl" /gɜl/ and "tiger" /taɪgə/. This will be discussed in more detail in Chapter 8.

EXERCISE 4.14—THE VOWEL /ɜ˞/

A. Contrast the vowel /ɜ˞/ with the rhotic diphthongs in the following minimal contrasts.

/ɜ˞/	/ɑr/	/ɔr/	/ɪr/	/ɛr/
stir	star	store	steer	stare
purr	par	pore	peer	pair
fur	far	for	fear	fair
burr	bar	bore	beer	bare
myrrh	mar	more	mere	mare

B. Circle the words that contain the /ɜ˞/ phoneme.

forward	muster	warship	steered	morale
disturbed	pretend	wordy	distort	persistent
terrible	turban	January	conserve	choir
conversion	arid	stirrup	barren	fearless

Continues

EXERCISE 4.14 (*cont.*)

C. Circle the phonetic transcriptions that represent English words.

/kʌstəd/   /lɝdɪ/   /kərɪr/   /vɝsəz/

/pɝsən/   /hɝdəd/   /fɝmɚ/   /dɝsənt/

/plædɝ/   /fɔrən/   /ɝbɔrt/   /kɝsɚ/

D. In the blanks, write each of the words using English orthography.

/smɝkt/ _____   /kənvɝt/ _____

/ovɝt/ _____   /wɪspɚ/ _____

/kɛrət/ _____   /bɝbən/ _____

/sʌbɚb/ _____   /skwɝts/ _____

/supɝb/ _____   /səhɛrə/ _____

E. Indicate whether /ɝ/ or /ɚ/ should be used in transcribing the following words by circling the appropriate symbol.

erasure	/ɝ/	/ɚ/	ermine	/ɝ/	/ɚ/
surprise	/ɝ/	/ɚ/	color	/ɝ/	/ɚ/
furnace	/ɝ/	/ɚ/	infer	/ɝ/	/ɚ/
curtail	/ɝ/	/ɚ/	terror	/ɝ/	/ɚ/
immerse	/ɝ/	/ɚ/	duster	/ɝ/	/ɚ/

F. Indicate with an "X" the pairs of words that share the same vowel phoneme.

_____ 1. herd   cheered   _____ 6. hair   queer

_____ 2. cord   word   _____ 7. birch   lurk

_____ 3. lured   stored   _____ 8. hoard   lord

_____ 4. ark   smart   _____ 9. pear   heard

_____ 5. fears   cheer   _____10. term   peered

G. For the following, indicate whether the word contains a rhotic diphthong or /ɝ/ (in any syllable) by placing the correct symbol in the blank.

Examples:

<u>/ɪr/</u>   cheer   <u>/ɝ/</u>   stir

_____ 1. mirth   _____ 11. appearance

_____ 2. flared   _____ 12. Carol

_____ 3. cirrus   _____ 13. furtive

_____ 4. serenade   _____ 14. larynx

_____ 5. Merlin   _____ 15. experience

_____ 6. cherub   _____ 16. disturbing

_____ 7. portion   _____ 17. clearance

_____ 8. farming   _____ 18. nervous

_____ 9. sparrow   _____ 19. furious

_____ 10. nervous   _____ 20. clairvoyant

Complete Assignment 4-3.

More on Diphthongs

The diphthongs /eɪ/ and /oʊ/ were discussed earlier as allophones of /e/ and /o/, respectively. In English, there are three additional diphthong phonemes that do not exist in a monophthongal form. That is, they do not vary in relation to phonetic context. These three diphthongs are /aɪ/ as in "kite," /aʊ/ as in "loud," and /ɔɪ/ as in "void."

There is considerable variation in the symbols use to transcribe these three diphthongs. This is due to the fact that the exact articulation of these phonemes varies by dialect and by phonetic context. Similar to /eɪ/ and /oʊ/, these diphthongs should be thought of as having two distinctive articulations. That is, there is a gliding of the tongue from the first articulatory position (the onglide) to the second position (the offglide); the exact starting and ending position varies from speaker to speaker. The one commonality among all of the diphthongs (including /eɪ/ and /oʊ/) is the fact that the tongue always glides from a lower to a higher position in the oral cavity (see Figure 4.2). The symbols chosen for this text to represent the three diphthongs are the ones most often adopted by most phonetics texts. They also represent a fairly close approximation of the actual articulation of these sounds.

Acoustic Information   The spectrogram of the diphthongs /ɔɪ/, /aɪ/, and /aʊ/ can be seen in Figure 4.23. Note that F_2 rises between the onglide and the offglide in production of the words "boy" and "buy." This is predictable from the F_2 rule because the tongue moves forward in the oral cavity as the tongue glides from /ɔ/ to /ɪ/ in "boy" and from /a/ to /ɪ/ in "buy" (see Figure 4.23). The F_2 of the diphthong /aʊ/ in "bough" behaves somewhat differently due to the fact that the offglide is a back vowel. As the tongue moves toward the back of the oral cavity as it changes position from /a/ to /ʊ/, there is a corresponding decrease in the frequency of F_2 as would be predicted by the F_2 rule.

For all three diphthongs, there is not much separation in frequency between F_1 and F_2 from the beginning of the word throughout the onglide. However, F_1 in /aɪ/ and /aʊ/ begins at a higher frequency than that seen in /ɔɪ/. The F_1 rule can explain this difference because /ɔ/, the onset of /ɔɪ/, is produced higher in the oral cavity than the onset /a/ in the diphthongs /aɪ/ and /aʊ/.

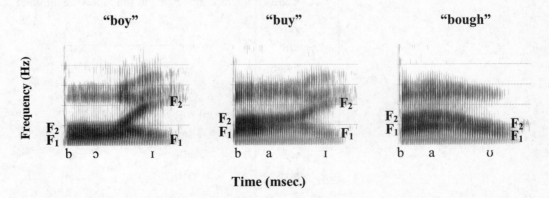

FIGURE 4.23 Spectrograms of the diphthongs /ɔɪ/, /aɪ/, and /aʊ/ in the words "boy," "buy," and "bough."

Pronunciation Guide

/aɪ/	as in "buy"	/baɪ/
/aʊ/	as in "bough"	/baʊ/
/ɔɪ/	as in "boy"	/bɔɪ/

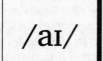

Sample Words

lye	ice
fiber	light
thyme	tie
buy	feisty

Allographs

Grapheme	Example	Grapheme	Example
i..e	write	uy	buy
i	sigh	ie	tried
ai	aisle	ei	height
ae	maestro	ey	eye
y	my	ay	aye

Discussion The tongue body begins in the low central or low back portion of the mouth (depending on dialect) in the production of the onglide /a/ and moves to the high front position for the offglide /ɪ/. The initial phoneme in this diphthong represents a vowel monophthong not commonly used by all speakers in the United States. It does exist in the speech patterns of individuals from Boston and other areas of the eastern United States in pronunciation of words such as "park" /pak/ or "car" /ka/. Some speakers in the East and South produce this diphthong as the monophthong /a/ as in the words "might" /mat/ and "ice" /as/.

EXERCISE 4.15—THE DIPHTHONG /aɪ/

A. Contrast the diphthong /aɪ/ in the following minimal pairs.

/aɪ/	/ɪ/	/eɪ/
kite	kit	Kate
height	hit	hate
sight	sit	sate
wind (verb)	wind (noun)	waned
lime	limb	lame
style	still	stale
tyke	tick	take

Continues

EXERCISE 4.15 (*cont.*)

B. Circle the words that contain the /aɪ/ phoneme.

power	spacious	machine	replaced
slice	delicious	Formica	traded
contrite	spider	maybe	piped
lever	Cairo	cider	supplied
rivalry	razor	piano	spigot

C. Circle the phonetic transcriptions that represent English words.

/fraɪdeɪ/	/braɪmɚ/	/taɪfraɪn/	/rəvaɪz/
/məbaɪ/	/naɪlɔn/	/prədaɪt/	/traɪdɛnt/
/traɪd/	/laɪɚ/	/haɪəst/	/straɪpt/

D. In the blanks, write each of the words using English orthography.

/səpraɪz/ _____   /klaɪmæks/ _____

/kəlaɪd/ _____   /preɪlin/ _____

/treɪlɚ/ _____   /baɪsɛps/ _____

/praɪmet/ _____   /waɪɚd/ _____

/vaɪrəs/ _____   /taɪred/ _____

/deɪlaɪt/ _____   /daɪmənd/ _____

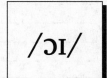

Sample Words

toy	join	ah<u>oy</u>	flamb<u>oy</u>ant
expl<u>oit</u>	b<u>oi</u>sterous	f<u>oi</u>ble	c<u>oi</u>ned

Allographs

Grapheme	**Example**
oy	soy
oi	foil

Discussion   The tongue body begins in the low-mid back position of the mouth (for /ɔ/) and glides to a high front position (for /ɪ/). When initiating this diphthong, the lips are rounded. As the tongue glides upward in the oral cavity toward the offglide portion, the lips become unrounded. In the East and South, some speakers will produce this diphthong as the monophthong /ɔ/, as in "oil" /ɔl/ and "soil" /sɔl/.

EXERCISE 4.16—THE DIPHTHONG /ɔɪ/

A. Contrast the diphthong /ɔɪ/ in the following minimal pairs.

/ɔɪ/	/aɪ/	/eɪ/
Boyd	bide	bade
soy	sigh	say
coil	Kyle	kale
hoist	heist	haste
loin	line	lane
boys	buys	bays
poise	pies	pays

B. Circle the words that contain the /ɔɪ/ phoneme.

repay	hoisted	voiceless	reward
loiter	crowded	fiery	tiled
straight	feisty	coy	cloying
crime	broiler	stoic	destroy
goiter	razor	avoid	supplied

C. Circle the phonetic transcriptions that represent English words.

/kwaɪət/	/sprɔɪdɪn/	/dɔɪəz/	/plɔɪdənt/
/mɝdɚ/	/blaɪndlɪ/	/ənstraɪt/	/taɪpsɛt/
/pɔɪzən/	/vɔɪdəd/	/rikɔɪld/	/taɪwɑn/

D. In the blanks, write each of the words using English orthography.

/ɔɪlɪ/	_____	/ændrɔɪd/ _____
/maɪstroʊ/	_____	/laɪvlɪ/ _____
/taɪfɔɪd/	_____	/ɪnvɔɪs/ _____
/parbɔɪl/	_____	/ɔɪstɚ/ _____
/haɪndsaɪt/	_____	/haɪɔɪd/ _____
/baɪaʊt/	_____	/deɪlaɪt/ _____

/aʊ/

Sample Words

loud	sour
clown	trousers
around	powder
flower	roused

Allographs

Grapheme	Example
ou	house
ow	cow

Discussion   The tongue begins in the low back position of the mouth for the onglide /a/ and glides upward to the high back position for the production of the offglide /ʊ/. When initiating this diphthong, the lips are unrounded. As the glide progresses toward the offglide, the lips become rounded.

EXERCISE 4.17—THE DIPHTHONG /aʊ/

A. Contrast the diphthong /aʊ/ in the following minimal pairs.

/aʊ/	/oʊ/	/aɪ/	/ɔɪ/
bough	bow	buy	boy
sow	sew	sigh	soy
cowl	coal	Kyle	coil
row (quarrel)	row	rye	Roy
towel	toll	tile	toil
fowls	foals	files	foils

B. Circle the words that contain the /aʊ/ phoneme.

toilet	dowdy	frown	bounty
mousy	allowed	loaded	probate
beauty	explode	soils	proud
astound	toil	chowder	crowbar
hello	toad	chastise	scrolled

C. Circle the phonetic transcriptions that represent English words.

/taɪɚd/	/laʊzi/	/aɪvri/	/hoʊmbɔɪ/
/rɪbaʊ/	/blaʊkɚ/	/rɔɪdɪ/	/kaʊtaʊ/
/waʊntɪd/	/roʊgbi/	/pauzɚ/	/auɚli/

D. In the blanks, write each of the words using English orthography.

/bɔɪfrɛnd/ _____	/roʊboʊt/ _____
/klɑndaɪk/ _____	/pispaɪp/ _____
/daʊntaʊn/ _____	/sɚaʊnd/ _____
/sloʊɚ/ _____	/doʊnʌt/ _____
/faʊndəd/ _____	/klaɪənt/ _____
/vaɪzɚ/ _____	/braʊzɚ/ _____

Complete Assignment 4-4.

Review Exercises

A. Describe each of the following vowels by providing their tongue height, tongue advancement, lip rounding, and tense/lax characteristics.

	Height	Advancement	Rounded	Tense/Lax
i	high	front	no	tense
ʊ	_____	_____	_____	_____
ɝ	_____	_____	_____	_____
ə	_____	_____	_____	_____
o	_____	_____	_____	_____
u	_____	_____	_____	_____
ɛ	_____	_____	_____	_____
ɚ	_____	_____	_____	_____
ʌ	_____	_____	_____	_____
e	_____	_____	_____	_____
ɪ	_____	_____	_____	_____
ɑ	_____	_____	_____	_____
ɔ	_____	_____	_____	_____
æ	_____	_____	_____	_____

B. For the following items, fill in the blank with the appropriate vowels from the description given. Then write the word in English orthography.

Example:

/mi̱t/	high, front, tense vowel	__meat__
1. /b__d/	low, front	_____
2. /s__n/	low-mid, back-central	_____
3. /sl__pt/	low-mid, front	_____
4. /s__p/	high, back, tense	_____
5. /k__rd/	low-mid, back	_____
6. /f__t/	high, back, lax	_____
7. /f__z/	high, front, lax	_____
8. /p__rk/	low, back	_____
9. /w__d/	mid-central, tense	_____
10. /kr__z/	high-mid, back	_____

C. For each of the the following two-syllable words, indicate whether each vowel is tense (T) or lax (L).

Example:

lasso	L	T

1. Sunday	_____	_____	4. confused	_____	_____
2. bashful	_____	_____	5. fender	_____	_____
3. laundry	_____	_____	6. concern	_____	_____

7. regroup   _____   _____   9. layette   _____   _____
8. obese   _____   _____   10. abrupt   _____   _____

D. For the following two-syllable words, indicate whether each vowel is rounded (R) or unrounded (U).

   Example:

   lasso   <u>U</u>   <u>R</u>

   1. foolish   _____   _____   6. Pluto   _____   _____
   2. curfew   _____   _____   7. person   _____   _____
   3. decade   _____   _____   8. pursuit   _____   _____
   4. collate   _____   _____   9. rugby   _____   _____
   5. football   _____   _____   10. lower   _____   _____

E. Transcription Practice—Front Vowels

   Use the correct IPA symbol(s) (i, ɪ, e, eɪ, ɛ, æ) for each of the front vowels in the following words.

   ____ 1. straight   ___ ___ 11. empty
   ____ 2. bees   ___ ___ 12. rabies
CD #1 ____ 3. bread   ___ ___ 13. instead
Track 20 ____ 4. can   ___ ___ 14. stampede
   ____ 5. filled   ___ ___ 15. vacate
   ____ 6. bring   ___ ___ 16. pleasing
   ____ 7. lapse   ___ ___ 17. transit
   ____ 8. sang   ___ ___ 18. beer can
   ____ 9. fair   ___ ___ 19. implant
   ____ 10. mean   ___ ___ 20. barely

F. Transcription Practice—Back Vowels

   Use the correct IPA symbol(s) (u, ʊ, o, oʊ, ɔ, ɑ) for each of the back vowels in the following words.

   ____ 1. moat
   ____ 2. push   ___ ___ 11. awful
CD #1 ____ 3. laud   ___ ___ 12. Clorox
Track 21 ____ 4. locks   ___ ___ 13. loco
   ____ 5. crude   ___ ___ 14. oboe
   ____ 6. chose   ___ ___ 15. taco
   ____ 7. raw   ___ ___ 16. monarch
   ____ 8. lure   ___ ___ 17. popcorn
   ____ 9. sword   ___ ___ 18. truthful
   ____ 10. card   ___ ___ 19. costume
                              ___ ___ 20. crouton

G. Transcription Practice—Central Vowels

Use the correct IPA symbol(s) (ə, ʌ, ɚ, ɝ) for each of the central vowels in the following words.

CD #1
Track 22

_____ _____ 1. certain   _____ _____ 11. purpose
_____ _____ 2. rusted   _____ _____ 12. sudden
_____ _____ 3. perturb   _____ _____ 13. luster
_____ _____ 4. assert   _____ _____ 14. purchase
_____ _____ 5. upper   _____ _____ 15. sherbet
_____ _____ 6. merger   _____ _____ 16. mother
_____ _____ 7. clutter   _____ _____ 17. converge
_____ _____ 8. verbal   _____ _____ 18. herder
_____ _____ 9. traverse   _____ _____ 19. worded
_____ _____ 10. learner   _____ _____ 20. mustard

H. Diphthong Practice

Some of the following words have the wrong diphthong/vowel symbol in their transcriptions.
If there is an error, write the correct symbol in the blank.

1. word   /wɝd/   _____   16. maestro   /maɪstroʊ/   _____
2. lard   /lɔrd/   _____   17. flour   /floʊɚ/   _____
3. carp   /kɝp/   _____   18. pouring   /pɔrɪŋ/   _____
4. war   /wɑr/   _____   19. liar   /laɪɚ/   _____
5. mere   /mɪr/   _____   20. appear   /əpɛr/   _____
6. wide   /weɪd/   _____   21. tighter   /taɪtɝ/   _____
7. curd   /kʊrd/   _____   22. parrot   /pɝət/   _____
8. stay   /steɪ/   _____   23. corner   /kɔrnɚ/   _____
9. pray   /praɪ/   _____   24. oyster   /ɔɪstɛr/   _____
10. crow   /kraʊ/   _____   25. squarely /skwɛrlɪ/   _____
11. coin   /kɔɪn/   _____   26. silence   /sɪləns/   _____
12. pride   /praɪd/   _____   27. smarter   /smɔrtɚ/   _____
13. firm   /fɪrm/   _____   28. avoid   /əvaɪd/   _____
14. tour   /tʊr/   _____   29. prowess   /proəs/   _____
15. fair   /fɛr/   _____   30. license   /leɪsəns/   _____

I. Using /ɝ/ and the rhotic diphthongs listed below, create as many meaningful English words as possible for each of the following items.

/ɪr, ʊr, ɔr, ɑr, ɛr, ɝ/

Example:

b ____   beer, boor, bore, bar, bear, burr _____

1. p ____   _____
2. r ____   _____
3. d ____ t   _____
4. w ____ d   _____
5. k ____ d   _____

J. Using the vowels listed below, create as many meaningful English words as possible for each of the following items.

/i, ɪ, eɪ, ɛ, æ, u, ʊ, oʊ, ɔ, ɑ, ɝ, ʌ/

Example:

	—— z	ease, is, as, ooze, owes, awes, Oz
1.	—— d	_____
2.	—— n	_____
3.	l —— st	_____
4.	sk —— n	_____
5.	st —— d	_____
6.	b —— rd	_____
7.	t —— nt	_____
8.	s —— t	_____
9.	r —— t	_____
10.	r —— bd	_____
11.	sp —— t	_____
12.	w —— d	_____

K. Write each of the following transcribed words in English orthography.

1. /kʌstəmz/ _____
2. /əbaʊnd/ _____
3. /twɔrd/ _____
4. /slɛndɚ/ _____
5. /kɛrfri/ _____
6. /veɪkənt/ _____
7. /bʌntəd/ _____
8. /klaʊdɪ/ _____
9. /steɪplɚ/ _____
10. /kəntɔrt/ _____
11. /saɪrənz/ _____
12. /klɔɪstɚd/ _____
13. /ohaɪoʊ/ _____
14. /reɪdɪoʊ/ _____
15. /kɚoʊsɪv/ _____
16. /plətɑnək/ _____
17. /rɛzənet/ _____
18. /daɪgrɛs/ _____
19. /saɪfənd/ _____
20. /ɑrkənsɔ/ _____
21. /wʌndɚful/ _____
22. /kæləndɚ/ _____

23. /rimɔrsfʊl/ _____
24. /stupɛndəs/ _____
25. /læksətɪv/ _____
26. /sɪnsɪrlɪ/ _____
27. /kɑləndɚ/ _____
28. /rezənɛts/ _____
29. /bɛrəton/ _____
30. /disɛmbɚ/ _____
31. /mɛksɪkoʊ/ _____
32. /kwægmaɪɚ/ _____
33. /ɔrdɚlɪ/ _____
34. /hɝbəsaɪd/ _____
35. /rəpʌlsɪv/ _____
36. /kɛrəktɚ/ _____
37. /sæsəfræs/ _____
38. /zaɪləfon/ _____
39. /kwɔrtɚbæk/ _____
40. /ɛmbɛrəst/ _____

L. Transcription Practice—Front, Back, and Central Vowels

Use the correct IPA symbol(s) for each of the vowels in the following words.

CD #1
Track 23

____ ____ 1. epic
____ ____ 2. faster
____ ____ 3. wonder
____ ____ 4. octet
____ ____ 5. woolen
____ ____ 6. depot
____ ____ 7. soldier
____ ____ 8. itchy
____ ____ 9. worship
____ ____ 10. palace
____ ____ 11. barely
____ ____ 12. nation
____ ____ 13. genius
____ ____ 14. cupboard
____ ____ 15. cartoon
____ ____ 16. nasty
____ ____ 17. fearless
____ ____ 18. number
____ ____ 19. sanction
____ ____ 20. ocean

____ ____ 21. inkling
____ ____ 22. Fairbanks
____ ____ 23. car pool
____ ____ 24. machine
____ ____ 25. Athens
____ ____ 26. autumn
____ ____ 27. rebus
____ ____ 28. torment
____ ____ 29. utter
____ ____ 30. bushel
____ ____ 31. corner
____ ____ 32. quandary
____ ____ 33. aster
____ ____ 34. phone booth
____ ____ 35. turban
____ ____ 36. key case
____ ____ 37. boarder
____ ____ 38. blaring
____ ____ 39. strangle
____ ____ 40. awesome

M. Transcribe the vowels in the following words.

CD #1
Track 24

_____ _____ 1. broiler
_____ _____ 2. mousetrap
_____ _____ 3. boardwalk
_____ _____ 4. closure
_____ _____ 5. nylons
_____ _____ 6. steroid
_____ _____ 7. starstruck
_____ _____ 8. regime
_____ _____ 9. bashful
_____ _____ 10. perjure
_____ _____ 11. spearmint
_____ _____ 12. lightbulb
_____ _____ 13. destroy
_____ _____ 14. banquet
_____ _____ 15. eyesore

_____ _____ 16. gender
_____ _____ 17. China
_____ _____ 18. jaundiced
_____ _____ 19. turquoise
_____ _____ 20. invoice
_____ _____ 21. financed
_____ _____ 22. merchant
_____ _____ 23. proclaim
_____ _____ 24. probate
_____ _____ 25. July
_____ _____ 26. martian
_____ _____ 27. future
_____ _____ 28. prospect
_____ _____ 29. product
_____ _____ 30. tofu

N. Compare each pair of vowels. Then, indicate how F_1 and F_2 would vary as the tongue changes in production from the first vowel to the second vowel. Write either "rises" or "lowers" in the blanks.

Example:

/i/ /ɪ/ F_1 _____rises_____

1. /u/ /ɑ/ F_1 _____
2. /ɛ/ /i/ F_1 _____
3. /o/ /e/ F_2 _____
4. /ɪ/ /ʊ/ F_2 _____
5. /æ/ /u/ F_1 _____ F_2 _____

Study Questions

1. What is the vowel quadrilateral and what is its importance in the study of phonetics?
2. Which vowels in English are tense? Which ones are lax? How does your understanding of syllables help in understanding the use of tense and lax vowels in English?
3. How are vowels produced in the vocal tract?
4. Which vowels in English are rounded? Which ones are unrounded?
5. What is a point vowel? List the English point vowels.
6. Why isn't the final sound in the word "lucky" transcribed with /i/?
7. Define the terms onglide and offglide.
8. Which vowels in English are affected by syllable stress?
9. What is the difference between a monophthong and a diphthong?
10. What is the relationship between tongue movement and pharyngeal shape during vowel production?
11. What is a formant?

12. What is a spectrogram? What three parameters of speech acoustics are plotted on a spectrogram?

13. What affect does tongue position have on F_1 and F_2?

14. What is the difference between *frequency/pitch* and *intensity/loudness*?

Online Resources

University of Iowa Phonetics Flash Animation Project: fənɛtɪks: the sounds of spoken English (2001–2005). Retrieved from:
www.uiowa.edu/~acadtech/phonetics/#
(video and animation of English, German, and Spanish vowel/diphthong production)

University of Victoria Department of Linguistics: Linguistics IPA Lab (nd). *Public IPA Chart.* Retrieved from:
http://web.uvic.ca/ling/resources/ipa/charts/IPAlab/IPAlab.htm
(interactive IPA chart with pronunciations of all IPA vowel symbols)

Assignment 4-1
Front Vowels

Name _____

Transcribe the front vowels in the following words.

CD #1
Track 25

_____ 1. cramp

_____ 2. stared

_____ 3. each

_____ 4. spleen

_____ 5. skim

_____ 6. bless

_____ 7. mist

_____ 8. trapped

_____ 9. fears

_____ 10. axe

_____ _____ 11. impasse

_____ _____ 12. hearsay

_____ _____ 13. eclipse

_____ _____ 14. cheesecake

_____ _____ 15. skinflint

_____ _____ 16. banish

_____ _____ 17. Sinbad

_____ _____ 18. herring

_____ _____ 19. reindeer

_____ _____ 20. kinship

_____ _____ 21. Band-Aid

_____ _____ 22. headband

_____ _____ 23. keychain

_____ _____ 24. cheery

_____ _____ 25. barely

_____ _____ 26. pin head

_____ _____ 27. revamp

_____ _____ 28. cherry

_____ _____ 29. invest

_____ _____ 30. chin strap

_____ _____ 31. welfare

_____ _____ 32. immense

_____ _____ 33. farewell

_____ _____ 34. baby

_____ _____ 35. filly

_____ _____ 36. bareback

_____ _____ 37. staircase

_____ _____ 38. bereft

_____ _____ 39. playpen

_____ _____ 40. eggplant

Assignment 4-2
Front and Back Vowels

Name _____

Transcribe the front and back vowels in the following words.

CD #1
Track 26

____ ____ 1. feud
____ ____ 2. bull
____ ____ 3. spore
____ ____ 4. rocks
____ ____ 5. strew
____ ____ 6. rook
____ ____ 7. lost
____ ____ 8. bog
____ ____ 9. oats
____ ____ 10. crone
____ ____ 11. carpool
____ ____ 12. wrongful
____ ____ 13. pseudo
____ ____ 14. oxbow
____ ____ 15. doorknob
____ ____ 16. careful
____ ____ 17. bookshelf
____ ____ 18. bootleg
____ ____ 19. bamboo
____ ____ 20. barnyard

____ ____ 21. arrow
____ ____ 22. borax
____ ____ 23. faux pas
____ ____ 24. forceps
____ ____ 25. footstool
____ ____ 26. boorish
____ ____ 27. Fargo
____ ____ 28. ballroom
____ ____ 29. romance
____ ____ 30. offshoot
____ ____ 31. meatballs
____ ____ 32. jaw bone
____ ____ 33. awning
____ ____ 34. inkblot
____ ____ 35. romaine
____ ____ 36. armhole
____ ____ 37. hardware
____ ____ 38. previewed
____ ____ 39. artful
____ ____ 40. airborne

Assignment 4-3
Name _____
Front, Back, and Central Vowels

Transcribe the front, back, and central vowels in the following words.

CD #1
Track 27

____ ____ 1. bedbug
____ ____ 2. revered
____ ____ 3. yogurt
____ ____ 4. yuppie
____ ____ 5. virtue
____ ____ 6. uproar
____ ____ 7. tortoise
____ ____ 8. performed
____ ____ 9. tether
____ ____ 10. terror
____ ____ 11. suburb
____ ____ 12. soldier
____ ____ 13. quasar
____ ____ 14. circus
____ ____ 15. gumdrop
____ ____ 16. ogre
____ ____ 17. gorgeous
____ ____ 18. mirthful
____ ____ 19. luggage
____ ____ 20. frontier
____ ____ 21. placard
____ ____ 22. opposed
____ ____ 23. hurrah
____ ____ 24. ferment
____ ____ 25. drunkard

____ ____ 26. govern
____ ____ 27. pewter
____ ____ 28. bonus
____ ____ 29. arrest
____ ____ 30. pungent
____ ____ 31. Thursday
____ ____ 32. parcel
____ ____ 33. goulash
____ ____ 34. cupcake
____ ____ 35. gleeful
____ ____ 36. morale
____ ____ 37. golfer
____ ____ 38. footage
____ ____ 39. exhaust
____ ____ 40. drama
____ ____ 41. conceit
____ ____ 42. teardrop
____ ____ 43. slogan
____ ____ 44. secrete
____ ____ 45. proclaim
____ ____ 46. dormant
____ ____ 47. bunker
____ ____ 48. acute
____ ____ 49. hundred
____ ____ 50. cedar

Assignment 4-4
Vowel/Diphthong Review

Name _____

Transcribe all of the vowels and diphthongs in the following words.

CD #1
Track 28

_____ _____ 1. corker
_____ _____ 2. irate
_____ _____ 3. absurd
_____ _____ 4. bagpipe
_____ _____ 5. Boise
_____ _____ 6. clubhouse
_____ _____ 7. bullfrog
_____ _____ 8. conjoin
_____ _____ 9. commute
_____ _____ 10. grotto
_____ _____ 11. errand
_____ _____ 12. fervor
_____ _____ 13. birthright
_____ _____ 14. jousting
_____ _____ 15. deltoid
_____ _____ 16. discount
_____ _____ 17. honor
_____ _____ 18. inform
_____ _____ 19. mastoid
_____ _____ 20. oblique
_____ _____ 21. outbreak
_____ _____ 22. goiter
_____ _____ 23. bloodshot
_____ _____ 24. parsnip
_____ _____ 25. downward

_____ _____ 26. bauxite
_____ _____ 27. crackdown
_____ _____ 28. perturb
_____ _____ 29. highbrow
_____ _____ 30. playwear
_____ _____ 31. poem
_____ _____ 32. ion
_____ _____ 33. proclaim
_____ _____ 34. beehive
_____ _____ 35. procure
_____ _____ 36. import
_____ _____ 37. punster
_____ _____ 38. carbide
_____ _____ 39. toystore
_____ _____ 40. outlaw
_____ _____ 41. unfair
_____ _____ 42. employed
_____ _____ 43. icebox
_____ _____ 44. x-ray
_____ _____ 45. furtive
_____ _____ 46. eyesore
_____ _____ 47. blowtorch
_____ _____ 48. ozone
_____ _____ 49. suburb
_____ _____ 50. voiceless

Consonants

What Is a Consonant?

Although this seems like a simple question, unfortunately the answer is not so simple. The term **consonant** can be defined in several ways. It is possible to define consonants in terms of the letters used to represent them or by the way they are formed by the articulators. Consonants also can be defined in terms of their particular role in the structure of syllables, or by their acoustic and physical properties. To best answer the question *What is a consonant?* we need to consider all of these issues.

We already know that there are many more consonant letters in the Roman alphabet than vowels. Likewise, there are more consonant than vowel phonemes. In Chapter 4, we learned that there are 14 vowel phonemes in English plus five diphthongs. In this chapter, 24 consonant phonemes will be introduced. As you are aware, the IPA symbols for the consonants are well represented by the letters of the Roman alphabet. There are only a few new symbols to learn in order to transcribe English consonants. In this respect, consonant transcription is easier to learn than vowel transcription. In addition to the 24 consonant phonemes, some of the more common allophonic variations of some of the consonants will be introduced.

Consonants Versus Vowels

In terms of production, vowels and consonants vary considerably. Unlike vowels, consonants are not produced solely by changes in tongue and lip positioning. Consonants are produced by vocal tract constrictions that modify the breath stream coming from the larynx. Consonant production generally involves the coming together of two articulators to modify the flow of air as it passes through the oral and/or nasal cavities. The tongue, the primary articulator in production of consonants, makes contact with other articulators to form most of the English consonants. In addition, there are several consonants that do not utilize the tongue in their production, for example, /h/, /b/, and /f/.

Another way in which vowels and consonants vary is in relation to where the sound generator (or sound source) is located during their production. The sound source for all of the vowels is at the level of the vocal folds. That is, for vowel production, the breath stream coming from the larynx is voiced (with the vocal folds vibrating). As you recall, changes in lip and tongue position cause alterations in the resonant frequencies of the vocal tract, giving each vowel its characteristic quality. Similar to the vowels, the **sonorant consonants,** or simply *sonorants,* are produced with resonance occurring throughout the entire vocal tract. This is why the sonorants are also sometimes referred to as **resonant consonants.** The sonorant consonants include the nasals, the liquids, and the glides, all of which are voiced. The sonorants are produced with little constriction in the vocal tract and with little turbulence in the airstream as it passes through the oral cavity. Refer to Table 5.1 for a classification of all the English consonants.

The sound source for several consonants, however, is not in the larynx. For some consonants, the sound source is the noise (or turbulence) created at the point of constriction in the oral cavity, formed by the articulators, as air flows through the supralaryngeal system. Consonants produced in this manner are called **obstruents** (because the airflow is obstructed during their articulation). Obstruents are sometimes referred to as **non-resonant consonants.** Obstruents include the stop, fricative, and affricate consonants. In the production of obstruents, resonance does not occur throughout the entire vocal tract, as it does for the vowels and the sonorants. Instead, resonance occurs primarily in the portion of the vocal tract anterior to the constriction formed by the articulators. For voiceless obstruent sounds, such as /s, f, t, and k/, the sound source is solely at the point of constriction in the vocal tract. However, for voiced obstruents, such as /z, v, d, and g/, the vibrating vocal folds do provide a second sound source, creating a modulation of the breath stream coming from the lungs.

TABLE 5.1   The Classification of English Consonant Phonemes

	Bilabial		Labiodental		Interdental		Alveolar		Palatal		Velar		Glottal
	vl	v	vl	v	vl	v	vl	v	vl	v	vl	v	vl
Obstruents													
Stops (Plosives)	p	b					t	d			k	g	ʔ
Fricatives			f	v	θ	ð	s	z	ʃ	ʒ			h
Affricates									tʃ	dʒ			
Sonorants													
Nasals		m						n				ŋ	
Approximants													
Glides		w								j		w	
Liquids								l		r			

vl = voiceless; v = voiced

In addition to the degree of vocal tract constriction involved in their production, vowels and consonants differ markedly in terms of their frequency specifications. As mentioned in Chapter 4, vowels are considered to have low-frequency spectra and are perceived as being low in spectral pitch. Similarly, the sonorants (nasals, glides, and liquids) also are characterized as having low-frequency spectra and, therefore, are perceived as low-pitched phonemes. The obstruents (especially the fricatives) have spectra higher in frequency than the vowels and resonant consonants and are perceived as having higher spectral pitch. This is due to the high frequency noise (turbulence) generally associated with obstruent production.

Whereas vowels can stand alone and create a meaningful utterance—for example, "oh," "a," and "I"—consonants do not have the ability to stand alone. Consonants are generally found at the beginning and/or the end of syllables. As such, they are often classified as to their position in relation to the vowel in each syllable. Consonants that occur before a vowel in any syllable are referred to as **prevocalic** and those that occur after a vowel are referred to as **postvocalic**. Consonants located between two vowels are termed **intervocalic**. See Table 5.2 for some examples of prevocalic, postvocalic, and intervocalic consonants.

TABLE 5.2 Examples of Prevocalic, Postvocalic, and Intervocalic Consonants (consonant graphemes are underlined)

Prevocalic	Postvocalic	Intervocalic
tee	eat	easy
hoe	ouch	anew
cow	Oz	okay
see	ail	away
ray	eyes	utter

PRELIMINARY EXERCISE 1–PREVOCALIC, INTERVOCALIC, AND POSTVOCALIC CONSONANTS

Match the appropriate term to each of the words below to indicate whether the underlined consonant is in the prevocalic, intervocalic, or postvocalic position.

a. prevocalic   b. intervocalic   c. postvocalic

_____ 1. seem
_____ 2. trade
_____ 3. away
_____ 4. cruise
_____ 5. oaf

_____ 6. oily
_____ 7. hotdog
_____ 8. hasten
_____ 9. open
_____ 10. football

As you learned in Chapter 2, vowels generally serve as the center or nucleus of a syllable. Vowels are considered to be the nucleus of a syllable because they are of greater intensity than consonants and are, therefore, the prominent aspect of a syllable. Because vowels can form the nucleus of a syllable, they are said to be **syllabic.** We will see later that in some instances a few consonants may become syllabic in some phonetic contexts. Consequently, they have the special ability to become the nucleus of a syllable as well.

Manner, Place, and Voicing

One last way in which consonants and vowels differ is the way in which consonant articulation is classified. Vowels are usually classified in terms of lip and tongue position. Consonants, on the other hand, are classified according to three different phonemic dimensions: manner of production, place of articulation, and voicing.

   Manner of production refers to *the way in which the airstream is modified* as it passes through the vocal tract. For instance, stops are produced when the articulators completely impede the airstream passing through the vocal tract. Fricatives, on the other hand, are produced by forcing air through a narrow channel formed by the articulators in the oral cavity. Stop and fricative consonants belong to separate manners of production. In addition to stops and fricatives, the other English manners of production include affricates, nasals, glides, and liquids. Examine Table 5.1 in order to see the distribution of the English consonants among the various manners of production.

PRELIMINARY EXERCISE 2–MANNER OF PRODUCTION

Referring to Table 5.1, match each of the following consonants to their manner of production.

_____ 1. /r/	a. stop
_____ 2. /d/	b. fricative
_____ 3. /w/	c. affricate
_____ 4. /f/	d. nasal
_____ 5. /n/	e. glide
_____ 6. /tʃ/	f. liquid

   To define **place of articulation** we must answer this question: *Where* in the vocal tract is the constriction located during the production of a particular consonant? In other words, to determine place of articulation, we need to know which speech organs are active in production of that consonant. From Chapter 3, you should be familiar with the various adjectives that refer to specific articulators located in the vocal tract. It is these adjectives that are used to refer to place of articulation. For example, if both lips are used to produce a phoneme, the place of production is *bilabial.* Likewise, if a phoneme is created by placing the tongue against the alveolar ridge, the place of articulation is considered to be *lingua-alveolar* or simply *alveolar.* (It is redundant to say lingua-alveolar because it is understood that the primary articulator is the tongue.) Table 5.3 reviews the various places of articulation most common to spoken English.

TABLE 5.3 Most Common Places of Articulation in English

Place of Articulation	Articulators Involved
Bilabial	upper and lower lips
Labiodental	lower lip and upper central incisors
Dental	tongue apex (or blade) and teeth
Alveolar	tongue apex (or blade) and alveolar ridge
Palatal	blade of tongue and hard palate
Velar	back of tongue and velum
Glottal	vocal folds
Lingual	tongue

The last dimension used in classifying consonants is **voicing.** Voicing refers to whether the vocal folds are vibrating during the production of a particular consonant. Several phonemes in English share the same manner of production and place of articulation, yet differ only in the voicing dimension (/s/ and /z/, for example). Phonemes that differ only in voicing are called **cognates.** Other examples of voiceless/voiced cognates include /k/ and /g/, /f/ and /v/, and /p/ and /b/. Keep in mind that word pairs differing only in the voicing dimension of one phoneme also are minimal pairs. For example, the word pairs "bit"/"pit" and "tuck"/"duck" are minimal pairs because they differ only in the voicing of the initial phoneme.

PRELIMINARY EXERCISE 3–VOICED/VOICELESS COGNATES

Place an "X" by each word pair having initial consonants that are voiced/voiceless cognates. You may need to refer to Table 5.1 for assistance.

_____	1. me, we	_____	6. shoot, suit
_____	2. seal, zeal	_____	7. flame, blame
_____	3. plan, clan	_____	8. dram, tram
_____	4. lice, rice	_____	9. yes, chess
_____	5. grain, crane	_____	10. vender, fender

Transcription of the English Consonants

In the following sections, the consonants of English will be introduced using the following format:

1. **Pronunciation Guide** for each consonant within each manner class, along with a detailed explanation of each manner.

2. **Acoustic Information** relative to the production of each manner of production.

3. **Phonetic Symbol Name** of each phoneme (Pullum & Ladusaw, 1986).

4. **Description** of each consonant on three dimensions: voicing, place of articulation, and manner. Voiced/voiceless cognates will be introduced together.

5. **Sample Words** and **Minimal Pairs** containing the phoneme(s) being discussed.

6. **Allographs** commonly used to represent the phoneme in spelling.

7. **Discussion** involving the production of each consonant.

8. **Practice Exercises** for the entire manner class—exercises will *not* be given for each separate phoneme, as with the vowels.

The Stop Consonants (Plosives)

Pronunciation Guide

/p/	as in "pan"	/pæn/	/b/	as in "ban"	/bæn/
/t/	as in "tune"	/tun/	/d/	as in "dune"	/dun/
/k/	as in "could"	/kʊd/	/g/	as in "good"	/gʊd/
/ɾ/	as in "better"	/bɛɾɚ/			
/ʔ/	as in "kitten"	/kɪʔn̩/			

Stop consonants (sometimes referred to as plosives) are produced by *completely* obstructing the airstream once it enters the oral cavity. This is why stops are part of the class of consonants termed obstruents. The obstruction in the vocal tract is more occluding for this manner of articulation than for any of the others. Stop production is marked not only by a closure in the oral cavity, but also by a closure of the velopharyngeal port. That is, the velum is raised to prevent the breath stream from entering the nasal cavity. The English stop consonants are produced by forming a closure in the oral cavity at one of three places of articulation: bilabial (both lips coming together), alveolar (the tip or blade of the tongue contacting the alveolar ridge), or velar (the back of the tongue contacting the velum).

The articulatory process in stop consonant production is very rapid. In fact, of all the phonemes in English, stops are among the shortest in duration. Although it is possible to prolong the production of a vowel (iiiiiiiiii), it is not possible to prolong the production of a stop consonant.

During the period of closure, **intraoral pressure** (air pressure within the oral cavity) increases due to the fact that the impeded airstream cannot escape the oral cavity. Once the constriction is released, the intraoral air pressure is relieved, resulting in the expulsion of an audible noise burst from the oral cavity (hence the name *plosive*). The burst of air is referred to as noise, since the airflow becomes turbulent when the stop is released.

One last thing to consider relating to the production of plosives is their sound source. Stops may have one or two sound sources, depending on whether they are voiced or not. In English there are three voiceless stops (/p, t, k/) and three voiced stops (/b, d, g/). The primary sound source for voiceless stop consonants is considered to be at the point of constriction in the vocal tract, formed by the articulators. More specifically, the source of sound is the turbulent airflow generated when the intraoral pressure is released. For this reason, the sound source for voiceless stops is considered to be a noise source. For voiced stops, the vocal folds vibrate in conjunction with the release of the stop in the oral cavity. Therefore, voiced stops have two separate sound sources: (1) the noise source produced at the constriction in the vocal tract, and (2) the vocal tone produced by the vibrating vocal folds.

Each stop consonant has a characteristic vocal tract shape due to the position of the articulators that form the stop constriction. Therefore, there is a separate, characteristic vocal tract resonance for the labial, alveolar, and velar places of production. Vocal fold vibration causes modifications in the vocal tract resonance during production of the voiced stops. The differences in the resonance of the larynx, pharynx, and oral cavity during production of the various stop consonants provide listeners the auditory cues necessary to distinguish their place of articulation.

Acoustic Information   Figure 5.1 shows spectrograms of the words "pay," "bay," "ape," and "Abe." The spectrograms are labeled phonetically to help you identify each of the phonemes in the words. During production of *voiceless* stops, a frictional noise burst follows the release of the stop, especially in the prevocalic position. This frictional noise is called **aspiration.** In spectrogram *a*, "pay," the stop /p/ begins with a hardly visible narrow spike of energy (stop release) followed by a long gray shaded band that runs vertically up to 8000 Hz on the y-axis. This vertical band is a display of the aspiration that follows the release of the voiceless stop /p/ (indicated with a white arrow). Notice that in spectrogram *b*, "bay," there is no such gap (aspiration) between the release of the

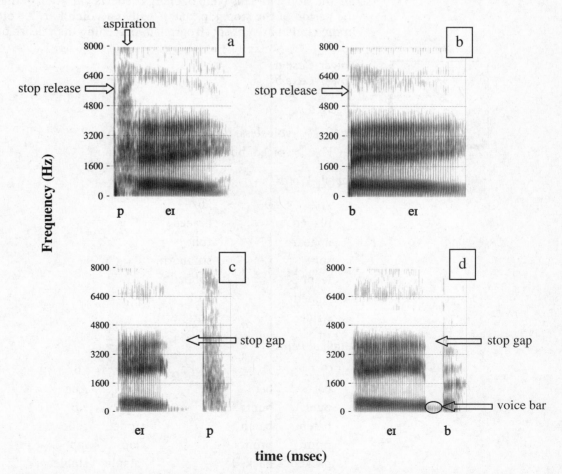

FIGURE 5.1   Spectrograms of the words (a) "pay," (b) "bay," (c) "ape," and (d) "Abe."

stop and the following vowel. This is because aspiration does not occur during production of voiced stops. It appears as though the vowel begins almost immediately following the release of the voiced stop /b/. Aspiration also may occur (depending on pronunciation) when a voiceless stop is in the coda position of a word. This can be observed with the release of /p/ in the word "ape" (spectrogram *c*). In spectrogram *d*, what looks like aspiration following the release of /b/ in the word "Abe" is actually a reflection of the way the speaker pronounced the word. The word was pronounced with the addition of schwa at the end of the word (i.e., /eɪbə/). If you look at the spectrogram, you will be able to visualize the formants of the /ə/ vowel.

In addition to aspiration, another defining characteristic of stop consonants as seen on a spectrogram is a **stop gap.** This gap, as seen on a spectrogram, *precedes the release* of a stop. A stop gap can be seen in spectrogram *c*, "ape," and spectrogram *d*, "Abe." The stop gap is a silent interval that reflects the actual time (in msec.) when oral pressure is building up in the oral cavity prior to the stop release. Notice that the stop gap preceding /p/ is longer in duration than the stop gap preceding /b/. Since intraoral pressure is greater for voiceless than for voiced stops, it takes more time to build up the necessary intraoral pressure to achieve greater pressure. Voiceless stops are perceived as being louder than voiced stops because of the greater acoustic energy being released during their production.

During production of *voiced* stops, a low-frequency energy band occurs during the stop gap. This band of energy reflects vibration of the vocal folds during the period of the stop gap, and is called a **voice bar.** A voice bar can be seen in the circled area of spectrogram *d*, preceding the release of the /b/ in "Abe."

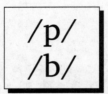

Lower-Case p
Lower-Case b

Description

/p/	voiceless, bilabial stop
/b/	voiced, bilabial stop

Sample Words

/p/	/b/
played	breeze
appear	rube
spite	stubborn
leapt	rubbed
ripped	club
stripe	abrade

Minimal Pairs

/p/	/b/		/p/	/b/
pet	bet		ape	Abe
punt	bunt		rip	rib
patch	batch		rope	robe
prim	brim		lap	lab
packed	backed		staple	stable
plead	bleed		ample	amble

Allographs

	/p/		/b/
Grapheme	*Example*	*Grapheme*	*Example*
p	pig	b	bear
pp	apple	bb	blubber

Discussion The airstream is impeded as both lips are brought together during production of the stops /p/ and /b/. Therefore, these two phonemes are classified as bilabial (see Figure 5.2). The jaws are in an almost closed position so that the lips can come together. The velopharyngeal port remains closed so that air does not flow into the nasal cavity. Recall that upon release, the burst of air for /p/ is more powerful than for /b/, because the amount of intraoral pressure is greater for voiceless phonemes. During production of /p/ or /b/, the tongue's position is determined by the following vowel. The use of the /p/ and /b/ phonemes in transcription is fairly straightforward (see the sample words above).

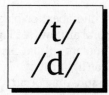

Lower-Case t
Lower-Case d

Description

/t/	voiceless, alveolar stop
/d/	voiced, alveolar stop

Sample Words

/t/	/d/
taste	dunce
stick	address
attack	pedestal
sate	door
tempest	edict
walk<u>ed</u>	mail<u>ed</u>

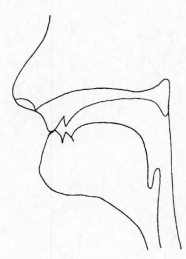

FIGURE 5.2 Bilabial articulation.

Minimal Pairs

/t/	/d/	/t/	/d/
talk	dock	pat	pad
to	do	trot	trod
touch	Dutch	state	stayed (staid)
troll	droll	straight	strayed
taffy	daffy	trait	trade
tram	dram	post	posed

Allographs

/t/		/d/	
Grapheme	**Example**	**Grapheme**	**Example**
t	toe	d	doe
ed	look<u>ed</u>	ed	wad<u>ed</u>

Discussion   To produce the alveolar stops /t/ and /d/, the apex, or blade, of the tongue makes contact with the alveolar ridge, impeding oral airflow (see Figure 5.3). The sides of the tongue are placed against the upper molars so that air does not escape from the sides of the tongue. In essence, a small airtight cavity is formed by the tongue and teeth so that an increase in intraoral pressure may occur.

The air burst associated with the release of the voiceless /t/ is greater than for the voiced /d/, due to greater intraoral pressure for the voiceless cognate. In certain phonetic contexts, the velopharyngeal port may open during release of /t/ or /d/, allowing release of air through the nasal cavity instead of through the oral cavity. In the words "mutton" and "sudden," for instance, the tongue may remain in contact with the alveolar ridge during the release of the consonant; the stop would then be released through the nasal cavity instead of through the oral cavity. This maneuver is accomplished by lowering the velum. The release of air through the nasal cavity is called **nasal plosion** for obvious reasons. Nasal plosion can be indicated in narrow transcription by using a raised "n" following the phoneme in question (e.g., "sudden" [sʌdⁿn̩]).

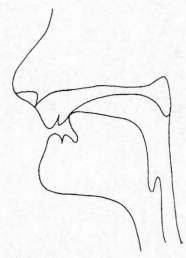

FIGURE 5.3   Alveolar articulation.

One other consideration regarding /t/ and /d/ is their use in transcribing the morpheme "-ed," used to represent the past tense ending in words. Notice that the words "bagged" /bægd/ and "reaped" /ript/ each end with a different phoneme. In the first case, "ed" is represented by /d/ and in the second case with /t/. Now, examine the following words and see if you can determine a pattern as to the use of /t/ and /d/ in representing the morpheme "-ed."

Example	*Final Phoneme*	*Example*	*Final Phoneme*
crowed	/d/	taped	/t/
teamed	/d/	hiked	/t/
hogged	/d/	lacked	/t/
carded (carted)	/d/	docked	/t/

Perhaps you noticed that if the phoneme preceding the "-ed" morpheme is voiced, the final phoneme also will be voiced, that is, /d/. Notice that a final /d/ also will be used if a tap precedes "-ed," as in the words "carded"/"carted" (see below). Conversely, if the phoneme preceding "-ed" is voiceless, then the voiceless /t/ will represent the morpheme "ed." Reexamine the words above to make sure you understand this concept.

Allophones of /t/ and /d/

Alveolar Tap /ɾ/

Glottal Stop /ʔ/

Sample Words

whittle	battle	coddle
Toto	cutie	ladder/latter

Sample Words

button	mountain	hat
fatten	Latin	atlas

Alveolar Tap An allophone of /t/ and /d/ often occurs in casual speech in words like "latter"/"ladder" and "Plato"/"play dough." Say these word pairs aloud to yourself and you will not see a difference in their production. For example, the pronunciation of the word "latter" is not truly a /t/, as in the pronunciation /lætɚ/, nor is it truly a /d/, as in /lædɚ/; the pronunciation is somewhere between the two. In this context, the (alveolar) **tap** /ɾ/ is the allophone used to represent the combination of /t/ and /d/ as in /læɾɚ/ or /pleɪɾoʊ/. Tap articulation involves a very rapid movement of the tongue tip against the alveolar ridge, creating a very brief stop consonant. The motion associated with a tapped stop consonant is more rapid than the "traditional" stop articulation of /t/ or /d/. The tap generally occurs in words with an intervocalic "t" or "d" digraph, in which the first syllable receives stress. Some examples include:

better	stutter	matted	battle
madder	huddle	coddle	riddle

The tap also is used in transcription when an intervocalic /t/ closes a stressed syllable. Examine the following words by saying them aloud:

fated	flirted	static	data

Notice that the /t/ becomes partially voiced, due to the voiced environment provided by the vowels preceding and following the consonant. Use of the tap in this instance is more accurate in transcription than using /t/ or /d/.

Glottal Stop   Another allophone of /t/, the **glottal stop** /ʔ/ appears quite often in American English. It generally occurs in syllable-final position. This stop is most readily noted in British English in the phrase, "Li'l bi' of tea" (Little bit of tea). The vocal folds are the articulators that both impede and release the flow of air in the production of this speech sound. Because the vocal folds do not vibrate during the production of the glottal stop, it is considered to be voiceless.

In American English, the glottal stop is found in some speakers' productions of words such as "kitten," "mountain," and "Dayton," where /t/ or /nt/ is followed by the /n/ phoneme. In saying these words, the /t/ is not released through the oral cavity. Instead, the release occurs at the level of the vocal folds. The reason for this is the tongue tip stays in place for both the /t/ and the following /n/ phonemes because they share the same (alveolar) place of articulation. Phonemes that share the same place of articulation are said to be **homorganic.** The transcription of the words "kitten," "mountain," and "Dayton" would be /kɪʔn̩/, /maʊnʔn̩/, and /deɪʔn̩/, respectively.

Notice the use of the symbol /n̩/ in the transcription of the words /kɪʔn̩/, /maʊnʔn̩/, and /deɪʔn̩/ above. The /n̩/ represents an entire syllable, that is, both the consonant and the vowel, because there is no fully articulated vowel in these words. In this context, /n̩/ has become a syllabic consonant. (Remember that vowels are considered to be syllabic because they are the nucleus of a syllable.) The syllabic marking indicates that /n̩/ has become the nucleus of the syllable and therefore also represents the vowel in the syllable.

Syllabic consonants (or simply syllabics) result most often when adjacent homorganic consonants occur in either the same word or in separate words in connected speech. Syllabics also can be found in conversational speech as in "cat 'n dog" /kæʔn̩dɑg/ and "sittin'" /sɪʔn̩/ (note the use of the glottal stop here). We will return to the topic of syllabics in the sections focusing on nasals and liquids later in the chapter.

The glottal stop also occurs between vowels in individual words such as "Hawaii" /həwaɪʔi/, and in connected speech between vowels in adjacent words, as in "pay Amos" /peɪʔeɪməs/. Some speakers replace syllable-final /t/ with a glottal stop. When this occurs, it almost sounds as though the speaker has deleted the /t/. Examples include "hat" /hæʔ/, "litmus" /lɪʔməs/, "Atlanta" /æʔlænə/, and "beatnik" /biʔnɪk/. In cases of disordered speech, it is important to listen carefully in order to determine if syllable-final /t/ is being deleted or if a glottal stop is being substituted.

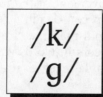

Lower-Case k
Lower-Case g

Description

/k/	voiceless, velar stop
/g/	voiced, velar stop

Sample Words

/k/	/g/
cotton	gold
wreck	rugged
opaque	Ghandi
queue	lager
squirts	aggressive

Minimal Pairs

/k/	/g/	/k/	/g/
crow	grow	luck	lug
cane	gain	back	bag
cut	gut	broke	brogue
cram	gram	shack	shag
kill	gill	pluck	plug
kale	gale	lacked	lagged

Allographs

	/k/		/g/
Grapheme	*Example*	*Grapheme*	*Example*
k	like	g	gone
ck	rock	gg	leggings
c	cat	gh	ghost
cc	occult	gu	guard
ch	chord		
cq	acquit		
cu	biscuit		
qu	liquor		

Discussion   The constriction in the oral cavity for production of /k/ and /g/ is considered to be velar because the stop is formed between the back of the tongue and the anterior portion of the velum (see Figure 5.4). As you would expect, there is greater intraoral pressure for the voiceless /k/ than for the voiced /g/. The release for both /k/ and /g/ is through the oral cavity. It is interesting to note the many allographs of the phoneme /k/. Of all the stop consonants, /k/ has the most variant spellings.

In some phonetic contexts, the back of the tongue may move slightly forward to articulate with the posterior portion of the palate during production of

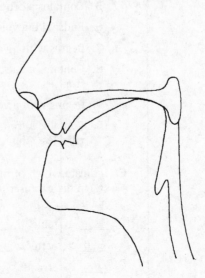

FIGURE 5.4 Velar articulation.

/k/ or /g/. To demonstrate, let us compare the production of the phoneme /k/ in two different phonetic contexts, that is, in the words "coop" and "keep." To produce the /k/ in /kup/, the back of the tongue would be close to the anterior portion of the velum because, in this context, it is followed by the back vowel /u/. To produce the /k/ in "keep," the tongue would be pulled forward, closer to the posterior portion of the palate, because /k/ is followed by the front vowel /i/. In anticipation of the forward place of articulation for /i/, the /k/ is produced more forward than normal. Keep in mind that a phoneme's identity often is altered by the other phonemes that precede or follow it.

EXERCISE 5.1–THE STOP CONSONANTS

A. Place an "X" by the words with a stop consonant in their transcriptions.

_____ 1. wish   _____ 6. runs   _____ 11. church   _____ 16. think

_____ 2. spring   _____ 7. whisper   _____ 12. tomb   _____ 17. rummage

_____ 3. loom   _____ 8. question   _____ 13. logical   _____ 18. realm

_____ 4. brush   _____ 9. system   _____ 14. jeans   _____ 19. guess

_____ 5. window   _____ 10. phase   _____ 15. Stephen   _____ 20. fox

B. For each item, select the word(s) that have the specified criterion *in their transcriptions*. (There may be more than one correct response for each question.)

man   about   perky   could   plaque   green

Example:

Contains a bilabial sound   man, about, perky, plaque

1. Contains a high front vowel   _____

2. Contains a voiceless alveolar stop   _____

3. Contains no stops   _____

4. Contains a velar stop   _____

5. Contains a central vowel   _____

6. Ends with a voiceless sound   _____

7. Begins with a voiced sound   _____

8. Contains a back vowel and a voiced
   stop   _____

9. Begins with a voiceless sound   _____

10. Contains a front vowel and a
    voiceless stop   _____

C. Indicate which of the following words have either a tap (T) or a glottal stop (G) in their transcriptions. Indicate which it would be by writing T or G in the blank.

_____ 1. table   _____ 4. listen   _____ 7. written   _____ 10. Lincoln

_____ 2. better   _____ 5. quittin'   _____ 8. beaten   _____ 11. pushin'

_____ 3. errand   _____ 6. uncle   _____ 9. walked   _____ 12. splatter

Continues

EXERCISE 5.1 (*cont.*)

____ 13. rotted ____ 15. bottle ____ 17. bitten ____ 19. rotten

____ 14. sweatin' ____ 16. talkin' ____ 18. wedded ____ 20. fodder

D. The words below all end with the "-ed" morpheme. Indicate in the blank whether the final phoneme should be transcribed as /t/ or /d/.

____ 1. wished ____ 6. danced ____ 11. sailed ____ 16. crabbed

____ 2. loaded ____ 7. wrapped ____ 12. leased ____ 17. placed

____ 3. endorsed ____ 8. hanged ____ 13. reached ____ 18. meshed

____ 4. endangered ____ 9. hoped ____ 14. toted ____ 19. burned

____ 5. robbed ____ 10. traded ____ 15. wrecked ____ 20. carved

E. Circle the real English words given below.

1. /kipət/ 5. /pɝkt/ 9. /pɝpət/ 13. /tʊki/

2. /təkɪd/ 6. /pækət/ 10. /pɪkɪ/ 14. /gækət/

3. /ədɛbt/ 7. /tɛpɪd/ 11. /ətæk/ 15. /dɛrbɪ/

4. /paʊrə/ 8. /taɪrə/ 12. /tɔrkot/ 16. /pipʔd/

F. In the blanks, write each of the words using English orthography.

1. /pɑrəɪ/ _____ 7. /gʌpɪ/ _____

2. /pʌkəd/ _____ 8. /pækɪŋ/ _____

3. /pəteɪɾoʊ/ _____ 9. /daɪpəd/ _____

4. /dɑktə/ _____ 10. /peɪpəɾbɔɪ/ _____

5. /tɑrgət/ _____ 11. /dækəɪ/ _____

6. /pʌpət/ _____ 12. /daɪətəd/ _____

G. For each item below, correct any vowel, diphthong, or stop consonant transcription errors by marking out the incorrect IPA symbol and placing the correct symbol above it. If no error is present, indicate by circling "no error."

Examples:

a. cap /kæp/ (no error)

b. tick /tɪ̶k/ ⁱ no error

1. direct /dəɛkt/ no error

2. tighter /taɪɾə/ no error

3. petted /pɛɾed/ no error

4. corker /kɔrkə/ no error

5. Carter /cɑrɾə/ no error

6. partake /pɔrteɪk/ no error

7. repeat /repit/ no error

Continues

EXERCISE 5.1 (*cont.*)

8. poet	/poʊət/	no error
9. oboe	/oʊboʊ/	no error
10. paper	/pɑpɚ/	no error

H. Word Analysis
Read the phonetic descriptions of the following words. Then write the appropriate IPA symbols and the English orthography on the two lines.

Example:

voiceless alveolar stop + low front lax   /tæg/
vowel + voiced velar stop   tag

1. voiceless velar stop + high front lax
    vowel + voiced alveolar stop

2. high front tense vowel + voiced velar
    stop + mid-central lax rounded vowel

3. voiceless alveolar stop + low-mid front
    vowel + voiceless bilabial stop + high
    front lax vowel + voiced alveolar stop

4. mid-central unrounded lax vowel +
    voiced bilabial stop + low-mid back-
    central unrounded lax vowel +
    voiceless alveolar stop

5. voiced alveolar stop + low back tense
    vowel + voiceless velar stop + voice-
    less alveolar stop

6. voiced velar stop + low-mid back tense
    vowel + voiced alveolar stop + high
    front lax vowel

I. Written Transcription Practice
Transcribe the following words. Remember to enclose your transcriptions with virgules.

1. cape		14. putt	
2. pared		15. coat	
3. dog		16. apart	
4. tied		17. guarded	
5. kept		18. boater	
6. debt		19. Bobby	
7. bake		20. barter	
8. pour		21. bigger	
9. bored		22. beaker	
10. pork		23. tuba	
11. peat		24. cabby	
12. taupe		25. peered	
13. took		26. backed	

Continues

EXERCISE 5.1 (*cont.*)

27. perky	_____	34. decked	_____
28. geared	_____	35. tired	_____
29. dagger	_____	36. bagboy	_____
30. giddy	_____	37. debate	_____
31. carpet	_____	38. torrid	_____
32. doctor	_____	39. parrot	_____
33. ticket	_____	40. dirty	_____

Complete Assignment 5-1.

The Nasal Consonants

Pronunciation Guide

/m/   as in "man"   /mæn/
/n/   as in "new"   /nu/
/ŋ/   as in "ring"   /rɪŋ/

The three *nasal* consonants /m, n, and ŋ/ are produced in a manner similar to the stop consonants. That is, the airstream is completely obstructed in the oral cavity during their production. Also, the obstruction occurs at the same three places of articulation as the stops, that is, bilabial, alveolar, and velar (see Figures 5.2, 5.3, and 5.4). However, this is where the similarity ends. Nasal consonants are sonorants, not obstruents. Nasal consonants are produced with the velum lowered so that the airstream and acoustic vibrations continually flow into the nasal cavity. The obstruction at the lips, alveolar ridge, or velum is maintained during the production of the nasal consonants as it is for stops. Therefore, there is no release of intraoral pressure from the oral cavity. The articulators simply block the flow of air out of the oral cavity so that the airstream may continually flow through the nasal cavity and out through the nares. If you sustain the production of /m/, and place your index finger under your nose (as if you were trying to stifle a sneeze), you can feel a lightly escaping airstream.

Another difference between stop and nasal consonants is the fact that all nasal consonants are voiced; they have no voiceless counterparts in English. Like vowels, the sound source for nasals is the vibration of the vocal folds. Recall that in some instances, nasal phonemes may become syllabic. In the word "written" /rɪʔn̩/, the syllabic /n̩/ marks both the consonant and the vowel in the second syllable.

Acoustic Information   Because airflow is directed through the nasal port during nasal consonant production, resonance occurs in the nasal cavity as well as in the oral cavity and pharynx. In production of nasal consonants, the oral cavity can be considered a sidebranch of the vocal tract. The size of the oral sidebranch decreases with the location of the constriction in the vocal tract from /m/ (bilabial) to /n/ (alveolar) to /ŋ/ (velar) (from anterior to posterior). Because the size of the oral cavity varies during production of the nasals, so does the resonance of the vocal tract during nasal consonant production. Due to the additional resonance provided by the nasal cavity, the nasal consonants have a sound quality quite different from the other phonemes in English.

Figure 5.5 shows spectrograms of the minimal pair "bay" and "may." The spectrograms allow you to contrast the differences in the production of a voiced

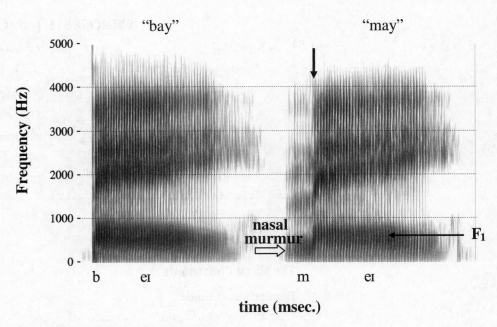

FIGURE 5.5   Spectrograms of "bay" and "may."

bilabial *nasal* and a voiced bilabial *stop*. Examine the spectrogram of the word "may." Notice that the spectrogram of /m/ looks somewhat like a vowel in that it has identifiable formants, unlike the spectrograms of stops. Recall that nasals are sonorants and in that respect they are similar to vowels. That is, sonorants are produced with resonance occurring throughout the entire vocal tract.

When the velum lowers in production of a nasal consonant and the tongue forms an obstruction in the oral cavity, acoustic energy radiates outward through the nasal cavity. This acoustic radiation is known as **nasal murmur.** Nasal murmur can be seen on a spectrogram below 500 Hz for /m/, /n/, and /ŋ/. The nasal murmur for /m/ in "may" is indicated in Figure 5.5 with a white arrow on the spectrogram. It is easy to locate due to the additional spectral energy in the lower frequencies. Note that the nasal murmur is lower in frequency than the F_1 of the vowel /eɪ/ in "may."

Compare the formants of /m/ and /eɪ/. What differences do you see? One obvious difference is the formants associated with /m/ are less intense (lighter shading) than the formant associated with /eɪ/. This is because when the velum lowers in production of a nasal phoneme, the vocal tract resonances become less intense due to absorption of sound energy in the nasal cavity. The reduction in the amplitude of energy (intensity) of a vibrating system is known as **damping.**

Damping only explains part of the reason why the nasal formants have less intensity when compared to vowel formants. Recall that during production of a nasal consonant, the oral cavity is constricted or closed off (at either the lips for /m/, alveolar ridge for /n/, or velum for /ŋ/). No sound escapes through the oral cavity; instead all sound is diverted to the nares. As the velum lowers, additional resonances are created in the vocal tract along with the creation of *negative* resonances or **antiresonances.** The antiresonances arise from changes in the resonance patterns of the *oral cavity* when it becomes a sidebranch of the vocal tract. These antiresonances cause *decreases* in the intensity of the formants of the nasal consonants.

Now compare the vowel /eɪ/ in the two words "bay" and "may." It should be obvious that the formants of /eɪ/ in "may" appear lighter than the formants of the same vowel in the word "bay." This is the result of *vowel nasalization* due to a lowered velum during its production. It is clear that the antiresonances of the vocal tract have caused a decrease not only in the intensity of the formants of the nasal consonant itself, but also in the formants of the vowel following it.

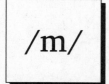

Lower-Case m
Description

/m/   voiced, bilabial nasal

Sample Words

/m/

mark	cramp
slam	dimpled
mend	alarming
maybe	amounted
drama	stomach
grump	mother

Minimal Pairs

/m/	/p/	/b/
mark	park	bark
roamed	roped	robed
messed	pest	best
crams	craps	crabs
sum	sup	sub
slam	slap	slab

Allographs

Grapheme	Example
m	cram
mm	hammer

Discussion   During production of /m/, the velum is lowered so that the airstream enters the nasal cavity. The lips are brought together in order to halt the airstream coming from the larynx (similar to the constriction for the phoneme /b/). Because /m/ is voiced, the vocal folds vibrate during its production. The oral resonating cavity for /m/ is the largest of the three nasals; it includes the entire oral cavity, extending from the lips to the oropharynx. The tongue is poised in position for the vowel following production of /m/. Figure 5.6 shows the articulation of the bilabial nasal /m/. Compare this figure with the articulation of a bilabial stop, as shown in Figure 5.2. Note the differing position of the velum in these two figures: It is lowered in Figure 5.6, and it is raised in Figure 5.2.

In some instances, /m/ may become syllabic in conversational speech, depending on the phonetic environment. For example, the word "happen" becomes /hæpm̩/, and the phrase "wrap them up" becomes "wrap 'em up" ræpm̩əp/. Note the occurrence of syllabic /m/ in these examples due to the homorganic /p/ preceding the bilabial /m/.

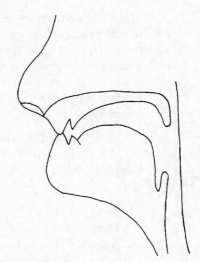

FIGURE 5.6   Bilabial nasal articulation.

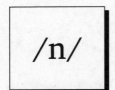

Lower-Case n

Description

/n/   voiced, alveolar nasal

Sample Words

/n/

note	runner
nail	Andover
Nile	nervous
loaned	answered
tunes	astound
snowball	mannerism

Minimal Pairs

/n/	/m/	/n/	/m/
nail	mail (male)	nine	mine
note	mote (moat)	Nate	mate
loan	loam	cunning	coming
grin	grim	warned	warmed
noon	moon	sunning	summing
roan	roam	dinner	dimmer

Allographs

Grapheme	Example
n	nice
nn	dinner

Discussion   The phoneme /n/ is produced in a manner similar to /m/, except for its place of articulation. For /n/, the tongue tip (or blade) contacts the alveolar ridge in order to impede the flow of air coming from the larynx. Because the place of articulation is posterior to that for /m/, the oral cavity is slightly smaller, causing a different resonance to be created in the vocal tract.

Transcription of this sound is fairly straightforward. However, when /n/ occurs at the end of a word, and the preceding consonant is an alveolar (homorganic) *obstruent,* such as /d, t, s, or ʔ/, the /n/ often becomes the nucleus of the syllable (syllabic). Some examples are given below with the homorganic consonant allograph underlined.

ri<u>dd</u>en	/rɪdn̩/	go<u>tt</u>en	/gɑʔn̩/
rea<u>s</u>on	/rizn̩/	cho<u>s</u>en	/tʃoʊzn̩/
le<u>ss</u>on	/lɛsn̩/	ea<u>t</u>en	/iʔn̩/

Note that for the word "ridden," the stop /d/ may be released through the nasal cavity as the velum is lowered in production of /n/ (nasal plosion).

Examine the following words. Although the preceding consonant (underlined) is not homorganic, many individuals still use the syllabic /n̩/ in transcription because the vowel between the consonants is almost nonexistent.

ri<u>bb</u>on	/rɪbn̩/
ha<u>pp</u>en	/hæpn̩/ (or /hæpm̩/)
mu<u>ff</u>in	/mʌfn̩/

One last word about the use, or actually nonuse, of /n/. Keep in mind that in words containing the letter string "ing," the phoneme /ŋ/ is used, not /n/ (see the section on /ŋ/ below).

Eng

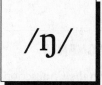

Description

/ŋ/   voiced, velar nasal

Sample Words

/ŋ/

ring	clank	stinky
wrangler	ankle	lingo
being	dangle	wrinkle
finger	larynx	wrangler

Allographs

Grapheme	**Example**
ng	sing
nk	link

Discussion   /ŋ/ is produced similarly to the other two nasal consonants in terms of voicing and velar opening. However, for /ŋ/, the point of constricted airflow in the oral cavity is the most posterior, between the back of the tongue and the anterior portion of the velum (or sometimes the posterior portion of the hard palate, in a manner similar to /k/ and /g/). The oral resonating cavity for /ŋ/ is the shortest of all (when compared to /m/ and /n/) given that the constriction in the vocal tract is adjacent to the pharynx.

/ŋ/ never begins a word in English; it is found only in the middle or at the end of a word. In relation to transcription, /ŋ/ poses some interesting dilemmas for beginning transcribers. Note the use of /ŋ/ with the following letter strings:

Letter String	Sample Word	Transcription
ink	kink	/kɪŋk/
ank	lanky	/læŋkɪ/
ynx	lynx	/lɪŋks/
inx	sphinx	/sfɪŋks/

It would not be possible to say these words using /n/ instead of /ŋ/ (try it for yourself). In some words, such as "English" and "finger," /ŋ/ is always followed by the voiced, velar stop /g/ in its pronunciation. However, there are other words in English, such as "longing" and "stinger," in which the production of /g/ is variable. Contrast the following two sets of words:

Word	Transcription	Word	Transcription		
linger	/lɪŋgɚ/	hanger	/hæŋgɚ/	or	/hæŋɚ/
ingot	/ɪŋgət/	singer	/sɪŋgɚ/	or	/sɪŋɚ/
anger	/æŋgɚ/	clanging	/klæŋgɪŋ/	or	/klæŋɪŋ/

Note that all of the words in the first set always have /g/ in their transcriptions, whereas the words in the second set may be pronounced with or without the /g/, depending on individual speaker differences and/or dialect. Similar to /m/ and /n/, /ŋ/ may become syllabic when it follows a homorganic velar obstruent such as /k/ or /g/ as in "bacon" /beɪkŋ̩/ or "wagon" /wægŋ̩/.

EXERCISE 5.2—THE NASAL CONSONANTS

A. Place an "X" by the words with a nasal phoneme in their transcription.

_____ 1. ring	_____ 6. jasmine	_____ 11. moan	_____ 16. ripen
_____ 2. bomb	_____ 7. crease	_____ 12. spanking	_____ 17. unfair
_____ 3. pet	_____ 8. inside	_____ 13. possible	_____ 18. monkey
_____ 4. stop	_____ 9. trait	_____ 14. trench	_____ 19. lure
_____ 5. tomb	_____ 10. loaner	_____ 15. lung	_____ 20. failure

B. Indicate with an "X" the words that have /ŋ/ in their transcription.

_____ 1. angle	_____ 8. singe	_____ 15. banging
_____ 2. angel	_____ 9. ginger	_____ 16. manx
_____ 3. brink	_____ 10. danger	_____ 17. ingest
_____ 4. mango	_____ 11. blinker	_____ 18. singer
_____ 5. Angie	_____ 12. hanger	_____ 19. hunger
_____ 6. single	_____ 13. ringing	_____ 20. jangle
_____ 7. conjure	_____ 14. mingle	_____ 21. congeal

Continues

EXERCISE 5.2 (*cont.*)

C. Circle the words in B that could have /ŋ/ followed by /g/ in their transcriptions. (Some words may be pronounced differently due to speaker dialect.)

D. Place an "X" next to the words that have /g/ in their transcriptions.

_____ 1. hinge	_____ 7. ring	_____ 13. tango
_____ 2. bangle	_____ 8. drank	_____ 14. flange
_____ 3. wings	_____ 9. onyx	_____ 15. engine
_____ 4. single	_____ 10. tingle	_____ 16. English
_____ 5. wrong	_____ 11. bungee	_____ 17. tongue
_____ 6. mangle	_____ 12. kangaroo	_____ 18. dangerous

E. Place an "X" next to the words that have /n/ in their transcriptions.

_____ 1. pharynx	_____ 7. engine	_____ 13. ginger
_____ 2. England	_____ 8. flank	_____ 14. blanket
_____ 3. bungee	_____ 9. tingle	_____ 15. tongue
_____ 4. length	_____ 10. lunge	_____ 16. danger
_____ 5. lungs	_____ 11. strength	_____ 17. vengeance
_____ 6. jungle	_____ 12. tango	_____ 18. ranges

F. For each item, select the word(s) that have the specified criterion *in their transcriptions.* (There may be more than one correct response for each question.)

good	mutton	curving	bank
napped	taken	carton	code

1. Contains an initial labial sound _____
2. Contains a voiced initial sound _____
3. Ends with a stop _____
4. Contains a central vowel _____
5. Ends with a voiceless sound _____
6. Contains a velar nasal _____
7. Contains a syllabic consonant _____
8. Contains no nasals _____
9. Contains a low front vowel and a labial consonant _____
10. Contains a velar consonant and a back vowel _____

G. Circle the words that represent real English words.

1. /kæmp/	5. /tɪŋgə/	9. /dænk/
2. /neɪm/	6. /nɪŋgɪd/	10. /bʌmpɪ/
3. /mɛlɪ/	7. /kræŋkɪ/	11. /pɪntoʊ/
4. /pint/	8. /kɔrn/	12. /pɑrmɔɪ/

Continues

EXERCISE 5.2 (*cont.*)

H. In the blanks, write each of the words using English orthography.

1. /næb/ _____
2. /kɑnd/ _____
3. /əmæs/ _____
4. /æŋgɚ/ _____
5. /mɔrnɪŋ/ _____
6. /bɛndɪŋ/ _____
7. /kændɪ/ _____
8. /əpɔɪnt/ _____
9. /kʊkɪŋ/ _____
10. /tumɚ/ _____
11. /taɪʔn̩/ _____
12. /maɪndəd/ _____

I. For each item below, correct any vowel, diphthong, nasal, or stop consonant transcription errors by marking out the incorrect IPA symbol and placing the correct symbol above it. If no error is present, so indicate by circling "no error."

1. camper   /kæmpɚ/   no error
2. adorn   /ədɔrn/   no error
3. duffer   /dəfɝ/   no error
4. bunting   /bʌntɪŋ/   no error
5. bingo   /bɪŋoʊ/   no error
6. pecking   /pɛckɪŋ/   no error
7. Dayton   /deɪʔən/   no error
8. batter   /bædɝ/   no error
9. baking   /bɑkɪŋ/   no error
10. doorknob   /dɔrknɑb/   no error

J. Word Analysis
Read the phonetic descriptions of the following words. Then write the appropriate IPA symbols and the English orthography on the two lines.

1. voiceless velar stop + low front vowel + alveolar nasal + voiced alveolar stop

   _____
   _____

2. voiced bilabial nasal + low-mid, back-central vowel + alveolar nasal + high front lax vowel

   _____
   _____

3. mid-central lax unrounded vowel + voiceless alveolar stop + high-mid front vowel + alveolar nasal

   _____
   _____

4. voiceless velar stop + low back vowel + velar nasal + voiced velar stop + high-mid back vowel

   _____
   _____

5. voiced bilabial stop + mid-central tense rounded vowel + voiceless bilabial stop + voiceless alveolar stop

   _____
   _____

Continues

EXERCISE 5.2 (*cont.*)

K. Transcription Practice
Transcribe the following words, using the IPA.

1. mink	_____	21. under	_____
2. pert	_____	22. tankard	_____
3. tan	_____	23. peanut	_____
4. king	_____	24. dandy	_____
5. done	_____	25. partake	_____
6. knead	_____	26. Monday	_____
7. bang	_____	27. nomad	_____
8. gnome	_____	28. bongo	_____
9. monk	_____	29. madam	_____
10. coin	_____	30. gander	_____
11. earn	_____	31. omit	_____
12. newt	_____	32. negate	_____
13. town	_____	33. tunic	_____
14. mood	_____	34. donkey	_____
15. knight	_____	35. command	_____
16. dumb	_____	36. mirror	_____
17. could	_____	37. countin'	_____
18. torn	_____	38. daring	_____
19. tongue	_____	39. empire	_____
20. gone	_____	40. coward	_____

Complete Assignment 5-2.

The Fricative Consonants

Pronunciation Guide

/f/	as in "form"	/fɔrm/		/v/	as in "van"	/væn/
/θ/	as in "thick"	/θɪk/		/ð/	as in "them"	/ðɛm/
/s/	as in "sip"	/sɪp/		/z/	as in "zoo"	/zu/
/ʃ/	as in "shell"	/ʃɛl/		/ʒ/	as in "rouge"	/ruʒ/
/h/	as in "ham"	/hæm/				

Fricatives are produced by forcing the breath stream (whether voiced or voiceless) through a narrow channel, or constriction, in the vocal tract. The articulators do not close completely during fricative production as they do in stop consonant production. They simply converge to form a slit to create the channel necessary for production of each fricative phoneme. There are five different places of articulation (points of constriction) in the vocal tract used for production of the nine English fricatives. These include the linguadental, labiodental, alveolar, palatal, and glottal places of articulation. Fricatives have voiced/voiceless cognate phonemes at each place of articulation. The only exception is the glottal fricative /h/, which is usually voiceless. Unlike stops and nasals, there are no bilabial or velar fricatives in English. However, these phonemes do exist in other languages. For instance, bilabial fricatives occur in Spanish and in Ewe, a West African language, and velar fricatives exist in German and Hebrew. Interestingly, bilabial and velar fricatives are sometimes produced by English-speaking adults and children as a result of a speech sound disorder.

Because the airstream from the lungs is being forced through a narrow channel, a turbulent, frictional noise is generated at the point of constriction. Fricatives, like stops, are considered to be obstruents, because their production involves an obstruction of the airstream in the vocal tract.

Voiceless fricatives, like voiceless stop consonants, are produced without the benefit of the vibrating vocal folds as the sound source. Therefore, the breath stream from the lungs must be forceful enough to create an audible turbulence at the point of constriction in the vocal tract. Similar to voiced stops, voiced fricatives have a second sound source—the vibrating vocal folds. In order to maintain voicing during their production, voiced fricatives have less airflow through the constriction in the oral cavity when compared to voiceless fricatives. Therefore, voiced fricatives are less intense than the voiceless fricatives; they are perceived as being softer than voiceless fricatives.

Acoustic Information   Figure 5.7 shows spectrograms of the words "Shaw," "saw," and "thaw." You will immediately see that the fricatives look nothing like the spectrograms of stops and nasals. Note that fricatives appear as wide bands of energy that cover a wide range of frequencies. These bands of energy visually depict the turbulence created by forcing the breath stream through a narrow channel in the oral cavity. The forcing of the breath stream through the constriction generally results in production of phonemes that have high-frequency spectra. The turbulent sound associated with fricatives sounds something like *white noise* because fricatives contain random energy that spans a wide range of frequencies. When compared to other consonants, fricatives are among the highest frequency phonemes.

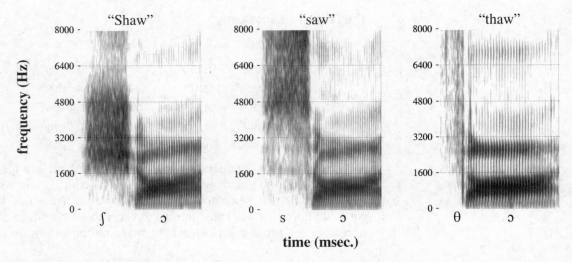

FIGURE 5.7 Spectrograms of the words "Shaw," "saw," and "thaw."

As you can see, the *primary* spectral energy for /ʃ/ (where the shading is the darkest) is between approximately 1600 and 5000 Hz. (It is evident that /ʃ/ does have additional resonance that extends up through 8000 Hz even though it is not as intense.) Now compare the primary resonant frequencies of /ʃ/ with /s/. You will see that /s/ has primary spectral energy at frequencies even higher than /ʃ/, that is, between 4000 and 8000 Hz (the frequency limit was set at 8000 Hz when creating the spectrograms). The frequency spectrum of the individual fricatives is dictated by the location of the constriction in the vocal tract during their production. The larger the cavity in front of the constriction, the lower the frequency spectrum of the fricative. Among all of the fricatives, /h/ has the largest cavity in front of the constriction, and consequently has the lowest frequency spectrum. Conversely, /f/ and /v/ have the smallest cavity in front of the constriction and therefore have the highest frequency spectra associated with them. Therefore, during production of fricatives, as the constriction formed by the tongue moves forward, the resonant frequencies of the frictional noise increase accordingly. It then follows that /s/ (alveolar place of production) would have higher frequency resonance than /ʃ/ (palatal place of production).

You can tell by looking at the spectrograms in Figure 5.7 that the noise associated with fricatives is significantly longer in duration than the brief noise bursts common in production of stop consonants. Unlike stops, the noise in fricatives is continuous. That is, it is possible to prolong the production of a fricative; it is not possible to prolong the production of a stop. Of all the obstruents, fricatives are the longest in duration. In addition, fricatives are longer than nasals.

The fricatives can be divided into two groups based on their intensity characteristics. The alveolar and palatal fricatives /s, z, ʃ, ʒ/ are the most intense of all the fricatives, and are known collectively as **sibilants.** The **non-sibilant** fricatives include /θ, ð, f, v, and h/. The sibilants are perceived as being louder than the non-sibilants. Therefore, they would appear darker on a spectrogram. The third spectrogram in Figure 5.7 is of the word "thaw." Notice how much less intense (lighter in shading) the non-sibilant /θ/ is when compared to the two sibilants /s/ and /ʃ/. In fact, /θ/ is the least intense of all the English phonemes.

As mentioned above, voiceless fricatives have greater airflow through the constriction during their production when compared to voiced fricatives. Therefore, voiceless fricatives also will appear darker on a spectrogram than voiced fricatives due to their greater intensity. Compare the two spectrograms of the words "leash" and "liege" in Figure 5.8. You can see by the darkness of the shading that /ʃ/ in "leash" is greater in intensity than /ʒ/ in "liege," especially in the higher frequencies.

When viewing a spectrogram, it is not difficult to distinguish voiced from unvoiced fricatives. This is because during production of voiced fricatives, it is possible to identify vertical striations throughout the period of noise. These striations correspond to the pulsing (opening and closing) of the vocal folds. Observe the spectrogram of the fricatives /ʃ/ and /ʒ/ in Figure 5.8. You should be able to see the vertical striations associated with the /ʒ/ in "liege;" no striations are evident for the /ʃ/ in "leash" since it is voiceless.

/f/
/v/

Lower-Case f
Lower-Case v

Description

/f/	voiceless, labiodental fricative
/v/	voiced, labiodental fricative

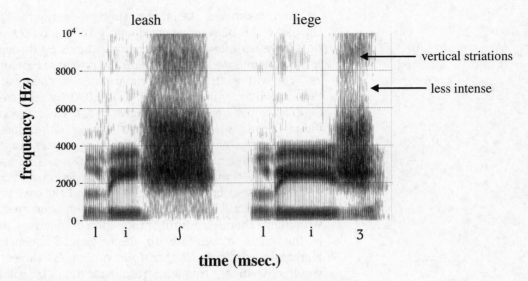

FIGURE 5.8   Spectrograms of the words "leash" and "liege."

Sample Words

/f/	/v/
free	veal
foam	love
phobia	calves
coffer	vane
rough	over
turf	vase

Minimal Pairs

/f/	/v/
fail	veil
fend	vend
fan	van
leaf	leave
first	versed
proof	prove

Allographs

/f/		/v/	
Grapheme	*Example*	*Grapheme*	*Example*
f	fix	v	vote
ff	muffin	f	of
gh	rough	ph	Stephen
ph	phone		

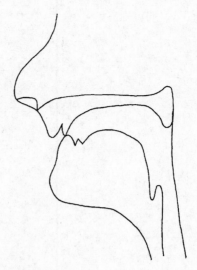

FIGURE 5.9 Labiodental articulation.

Discussion The point of constriction for /f/ and /v/ is formed by bringing the lower lip close to the edges of the upper central incisors (see Figure 5.9). The lower jaw must be raised near the upper jaw to accomplish this maneuver. The breath stream is forced through the narrow constriction formed by the lower lip and upper teeth.

The labiodental fricatives are quite easy to transcribe. The only allographs associated with /f/ that may cause trouble at first are "ph" and "gh." /v/ is generally used with words containing the letter "v" except in the rare case of "f" and "ph" (see allographs on page 142 for examples).

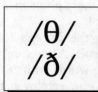

Theta
Eth

Description

/θ/ voiceless, interdental fricative
/ð/ voiced, interdental fricative

Sample Words

/θ/	/ð/	/θ/	/ð/
thermal	though	bath	bathe
thought	lathe	breath	breathe
froth	feather	thigh	thy
with	wither	ether	either

Note: "Either" and "ether" are minimal pairs, as are "thigh" and "thy."

Allographs

	/θ/		/ð/
Grapheme	**Example**	**Grapheme**	**Example**
th	thistle	th	although

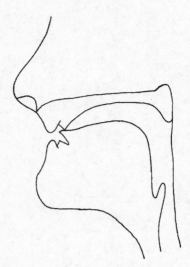

FIGURE 5.10   Interdental articulation.

Discussion   The interdental fricatives are named "theta" /θ/ (voiceless) and "eth" /ð/ (voiced). These phonemes are produced by forcing the breath stream through a constriction formed by the apex (or blade) of the tongue and the lower edge of the upper central incisors. The tongue is placed between the teeth for this articulation, hence the label *interdental*. Simultaneously, the sides of the tongue contact the upper molars to help direct the voiced or voiceless breath stream towards the constriction (see Figure 5.10).

A second way in which these phonemes may be produced is by forming a constriction between the apex of the tongue and the posterior portion of the upper central incisors. This particular articulation of these phonemes would be termed appropriately *dental,* as opposed to interdental.

/θ/ and /ð/ are both represented, in spelling, by the digraph "th." This is the only spelling representation of these two phonemes. Therefore, it is confusing at first for students learning how to transcribe words with /θ/ and /ð/. You may need to practice listening for the difference in voicing between the two phonemes since the spelling is the same for both sounds. Take a look at the *sample words* on page 143. Practice saying them aloud while listening to the voicing differences of the two phonemes.

Lower-Case s
Lower-Case z

Description

| /s/ | voiceless, alveolar fricative |
| /z/ | voiced, alveolar fricative |

Sample Words

/s/	/z/	/s/	/z/
sew	zenith	lesson	xylophone
centaur	azalea	cease	pays
assert	fuzzy	awesome	Aztec

Minimal Pairs

/s/	/z/		/s/	/z/
seal	zeal		brace	braise
lacy	lazy		spice	spies
sip	zip		seek	Zeke
close	close		sue	zoo
loose	lose		noose	news
race	raise		purse	purrs

Allographs

/s/		/z/	
Grapheme	*Example*	*Grapheme*	*Example*
s	sink	z	zone
ss	press	zz	fizz
sc	science	s	was
c	ice	ss	scissors
		x	Xanadu

Discussion   The constriction for the alveolar fricatives is formed in one of two ways, depending on the individual speaker. The first involves the articulation of either the tongue apex or blade and the alveolar ridge. The tongue is raised so that it only approximates the ridge; the tongue does not make direct contact. At the same time, the tongue forms a tapering groove along its central or midline portion as the back of the tongue contacts the upper molars.

The second method for producing the alveolar fricatives is by placing the tip of the tongue behind the lower central incisors while the front of the tongue is raised to approximate the alveolar ridge. The tongue is still grooved along its central portion, and the sides of the tongue make contact with the upper molars. For both articulations, the channel formed by the tongue and teeth helps to direct the airstream anteriorly through the closely held upper and lower teeth.

In terms of transcription, the biggest problem for students is learning the correct use of /s/ and /z/ to represent the plural "s" morpheme in words. Examine the word pairs below. Is the final phoneme transcribed as /s/ or /z/?

taps	seats	walks	chicks
tabs	seeds	runs	hogs

Whenever the final consonant of a word is voiceless, its plural marker will be transcribed as the voiceless phoneme /s/. The words "taps," "seats," "walks," and "chicks" all have a voiceless phoneme immediately preceding the plural morpheme /s/. The remaining words, which all have a voiced phoneme prior to the plural marker, are transcribed with /z/. Whenever the plural form of a word is "es" as in "babies" or "ladies," the plural phoneme is also represented by /z/, because it follows a (voiced) vowel. (The singular form of these words "baby" and "lady" ends with the vowel /ɪ/.) This rule should seem familiar to you because similar practice is involved in using the phonemes /t/ and /d/ to indicate the "-ed" morpheme.

The phoneme /z/ is used by some speakers in pronunciation of words that are normally transcribed with an /s/. Examples include:

resource → /rizɔrs/   greasy → /grizɪ/   absurd → /æbzɝd/

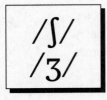

Esh
Yogh

Description

| /ʃ/ | voiceless, palatal (post alveolar) fricative |
| /ʒ/ | voiced, palatal (post alveolar) fricative |

Sample Words

/ʃ/	/ʒ/
shook	fusion
sure	casual
mansion	profusion
machine	measure
cashier	regime
pressure	television
national	seizure
omniscient	erosion

Allographs

	/ʃ/		/ʒ/
Grapheme	*Example*	*Grapheme*	*Example*
sh	shape	z	azure
ss	pressure	g	garage
sci	conscience	s	measure
ce	ocean	si	vision
ch	machine	zi	brazier
ci	social		
s	sugar		
si	pension		

Discussion   These two fricatives are created when the breath stream is forced through a constriction formed in a manner quite similar to the alveolar fricatives. The tongue has a groove along its central portion (although it is broader), and the sides of the tongue contact the upper molars. The airstream is directed anteriorly toward the front teeth. The more open constriction for /ʒ/ and /ʃ/ is formed by the closely held tongue blade and the hard palate. This articulation is posterior to the constriction formed for the alveolar fricatives /s/ and /z/. Therefore, /ʃ/ and /ʒ/ are considered by many phoneticians and linguists to have a **post alveolar** or **palatoalveolar** articulation (see Figure 5.11). (The IPA chart lists these phonemes as *post alveolar*.) Unlike /s/ and /z/, the lips are rounded in production of /ʃ/ and /ʒ/.

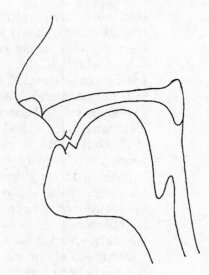

FIGURE 5.11 Palatal articulation.

The transcription of the phonemes /ʃ/ and /ʒ/ is a bit tricky at first. Students will often confuse them with the two affricates /tʃ/ as in "cheap" and /dʒ/ as in "jam." Compare the following words:

sheep	/ʃip/	—	cheap	/tʃip/
shoe	/ʃu/	—	chew	/tʃu/
leisure	/lɛʒɚ/	—	ledger	/lɛdʒɚ/

Hopefully, you hear the difference in the pronunciation of these words. An explanation of the affricate manner of production will follow this section.

Lower-Case h

Description

/h/ voiceless, glottal fricative

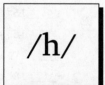

Sample Words

/h/

hook	whose
helium	behave
hairy	ahead
Harold	unhook

Allographs

/h/

Grapheme	**Example**
h	hit
wh	who

Discussion The fricative /h/ is created when the breath stream is forced through a constriction formed by the abducted vocal folds (the glottis). Because the vocal folds are not vibrating during production of this phoneme, it is considered to be voiceless. /h/ is the only fricative without a voiced cognate. In some phonetic contexts, however, it may take on a voiced quality. For instance, in the word "ahead" /əhɛd/, a vowel precedes and follows the /h/, causing it to become voiced because the vowels are both voiced. When /h/ precedes the high vowels /i, ɪ, u, and ʊ/, the friction noise is created entirely, or nearly so, at the constriction formed by the tongue and palate, not at the glottis. Say the words "he" /hɪ/ and "who" /hu/ and you will see that this is so.

During the production of /h/, the articulators will take on the shape of whichever vowel follows. For example, compare the shape and position of your lips for the words "hoop" and "heap." You will immediately notice that your lips are rounded—even before you produce the /h/ phoneme—in the word "hoop." Similarly, your lips are unrounded before the production of /h/ in "heap." The transcription of /h/ should pose few problems for students, because the only allographs of /h/ are "h" and "wh."

EXERCISE 5.3–THE FRICATIVE CONSONANTS

A. Place an "X" by the words with a fricative phoneme in their transcription.

_____ 1. push	_____ 6. brazen	_____ 11. Montana	_____ 16. hombre
_____ 2. thesis	_____ 7. cares	_____ 12. pleasure	_____ 17. leaks
_____ 3. loom	_____ 8. burlap	_____ 13. leather	_____ 18. worthy
_____ 4. happy	_____ 9. croissant	_____ 14. marrow	_____ 19. crouton
_____ 5. caution	_____ 10. vender	_____ 15. other	_____ 20. rajah

B. Indicate which of the following words have /ʃ/ or /ʒ/ in their transcription. Write the correct phoneme next to the word. (Hint: Watch out for /tʃ/ and /dʒ/!)

_____ 1. mishap	_____ 8. badge	_____ 15. Sean
_____ 2. usually	_____ 9. lesion	_____ 16. passion
_____ 3. decision	_____ 10. lotion	_____ 17. ricochet
_____ 4. cheese	_____ 11. corsage	_____ 18. college
_____ 5. largest	_____ 12. changed	_____ 19. allusion
_____ 6. reason	_____ 13. friction	_____ 20. inject
_____ 7. election	_____ 14. juice	_____ 21. Persia

C. For the following words, indicate whether the "th" sound is voiced (/ð/) or voiceless (/θ/) by placing the correct IPA symbol in the blank.

_____ 1. smoothly	_____ 7. wrath	_____ 13. thimble
_____ 2. method	_____ 8. writhe	_____ 14. booth
_____ 3. other	_____ 9. lathe	_____ 15. oath
_____ 4. those	_____ 10. thought	_____ 16. scathing
_____ 5. moth	_____ 11. clothes	_____ 17. another
_____ 6. gather	_____ 12. weather	_____ 18. anything

Continues

EXERCISE 5.3 (*cont.*)

____ 19. withstand   ____ 21. author   ____ 23. bothers

____ 20. wither   ____ 22. smother   ____ 24. atheist

D. For each item, create real words (or proper names) by placing one of the nine fricatives in the blank. Write your answers in the blank at the right of each item. More than one answer is possible for each item.

/f, v, θ, ð, s, z, ʃ, ʒ, h/

Example:

/__u/   /s/, /z/, /ʃ/, /h/ _____

(The words created are "sue," "zoo," "shoe," and "who.")

1. /mu__/   _____
2. /wɪ__/   _____
3. /ʌ__ɚ/   _____
4. /lɛ__ɚ/   _____
5. /__ɛrɪ/   _____
6. /ru__/   _____
7. /__aɪ/   _____
8. /__ɪr/   _____

E. For each item, select the word(s) that have the specified criterion in their transcriptions.

them   beige   hug   wreath   tape   cash   soon   vend

1. Begins with a voiceless fricative _____
2. Begins with a voiced obstruent _____
3. Ends with a voiceless obstruent _____
4. Contains a front vowel and a
   voiceless fricative   _____
5. Contains an alveolar sound   _____
6. Contains all voiced phonemes _____
7. Contains a stop and a fricative _____
8. Contains a nasal and a fricative _____
9. Contains a fricative and a
   central vowel   _____
10. Contains no fricatives   _____

F. Indicate whether the following words should be transcribed with a final /s/ or a final /z/.

_____ 1. babes   _____ 7. bananas   _____ 13. dramas

_____ 2. chafes   _____ 8. drinks   _____ 14. croaks

_____ 3. cars   _____ 9. passes   _____ 15. meats

_____ 4. books   _____ 10. throws   _____ 16. affairs

_____ 5. carpets   _____ 11. loaves   _____ 17. loafs

_____ 6. pushes   _____ 12. roasts   _____ 18. birds

Continues

EXERCISE 5.3 (*cont.*)

G. Circle the words that represent real English words.

1. /ʃʊk/   5. /vɛrɪ/   9. /pɝs/   13. /feɪvɚ/
2. /ʒɪŋ/   6. /ðaɪ/   10. /ʃɑrk/   14. /kreɪzd/
3. /zɔrt/   7. /θrʊ/   11. /ɪrðu/   15. /bɪʒɚ/
4. /θɝd/   8. /vɔɪnz/   12. /ʃæku/   16. /hoʊðɚ/

H. In the blanks, write each of the words using English orthography.

1. /eɪʒən/   _____   9. /sɝvəst/   _____
2. /vɔrtɛks/ _____   10. /ʌðɚz/   _____
3. /vɑrnɪʃ/   _____   11. /froʊzn̩/   _____
4. /bɑðɚ/   _____   12. /ʃɪvɚd/   _____
5. /spɛrd/   _____   13. /fæʔn̩/   _____
6. /θæŋks/   _____   14. /hɔrɚ/   _____
7. /hɪrseɪ/   _____   15. /gəziboʊ/   _____
8. /ɝbən/   _____   16. /bɝθdeɪz/   _____

I. For each item below, correct any vowel or consonant transcription errors by marking out the incorrect IPA symbol and placing the correct symbol above it. If no error is present, so indicate by circling "no error."

1.	bijou	/biʃu/	no error
2.	neither	/niθɚ/	no error
3.	verify	/vɛrifaɪ/	no error
4.	hosed	/hosd/	no error
5.	Hoosier	/huʒɚ/	no error
6.	panther	/pænðɚ/	no error
7.	assure	/əʃur/	no error
8.	favored	/fevɚd/	no error
9.	shining	/shaɪnɪŋ/	no error
10.	earthy	/ɛrθɪ/	no error
11.	amnesia	/æmniʒə/	no error
12.	unthinking	/ʌnθɪnkɪŋ/	no error

J. Transcription Practice
Transcribe the following words using the IPA.

1. Garth   _____   10. haste   _____
2. fence   _____   11. perhaps   _____
3. sure   _____   12. shorter   _____
4. dozed   _____   13. perused   _____
5. soared   _____   14. unversed _____
6. hives   _____   15. mother   _____
7. shout   _____   16. consumed _____
8. thorns   _____   17. mirage   _____
9. those   _____   18. potions   _____

Continues

EXERCISE 5.3 (*cont.*)

19.	overt	_____	30. third base	_____
20.	Tarzan	_____	31. goiter	_____
21.	thunder	_____	32. terror	_____
22.	heather	_____	33. thousand	_____
23.	satin	_____	34. contour	_____
24.	sheepish	_____	35. shortcake	_____
25.	surrounds	_____	36. varied	_____
26.	Horton	_____	37. defies	_____
27.	thirty	_____	38. discussed	_____
28.	vision	_____	39. shorthand	_____
29.	pharynx	_____	40. muttered	_____

Complete Assignment 5-3.

The Affricate Consonants

Pronunciation Guide

/tʃ/   as in "chair"   /tʃɛr/
/dʒ/   as in "jar"   /dʒɑr/

The **affricate** manner of production involves a combination of the stop and fricative manners. For this reason, affricates are obstruents. Both English affricates are considered to have a palatal place of articulation. During production of the two affricates, the articulation begins as an alveolar stop. The tongue tip contacts the posterior alveolar ridge; there is a corresponding increase in intraoral pressure in the oral cavity. However, when the breath stream is released (voiced or voiceless), the air is forced through the constriction formed by the tongue and palate, creating a turbulent noise. (The constriction is similar to that formed during production of the palatal fricatives /ʃ/ and /ʒ/, that is, palatal, or post alveolar.)

Acoustic Information   Figure 5.12 shows spectrograms of the two English affricates in the words "batch" /bætʃ/ and "badge" /bædʒ/. Note the expected presence of the stop gaps prior to the release of /t/ and /d/ in both words. Also, because the place of articulation is the same for the two affricates, their frequency spectra are similar. A major difference in the two spectrograms is the greater intensity of the fricative component associated with the voiceless affricate when compared to the voiced affricate. This is due to greater airflow through the constriction in the oral cavity during production of /ʃ/. Also, as expected, the spectrogram of the voiced affricate shows a voice bar prior to release of the stop component /d/.

Description

/tʃ/   voiceless, palatal affricate
/dʒ/   voiced, palatal affricate

/tʃ/
/dʒ/

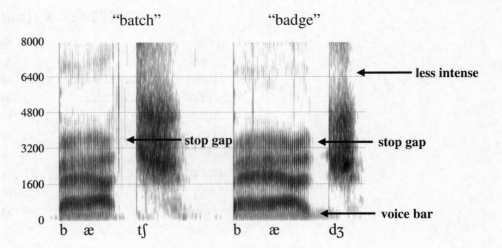

FIGURE 5.12 Spectrograms of the words "batch" and "badge."

Sample Words

/tʃ/	/dʒ/
chick	jelly
righteous	adjoin
nature	injure
crutch	badger
chimney	Jake
hatchet	refrigerate
wretched	generous

Minimal Pairs

/tʃ/	/dʒ/	/tʃ/	/dʒ/
etch	edge	chin	gin
batch	badge	cherry	Jerri
match	Madge	cheap	jeep
rich	ridge	chalk	jock
"H"	age	choke	joke

Allographs

	/tʃ/		/dʒ/
Grapheme	**Example**	**Grapheme**	**Example**
ch	check	j	joke
tch	witch	g	gem
t	nature	gg	exaggerate
te	righteous	d	educate
ti	question	dg	lodge
		di	soldier

Discussion   Although English has only two phonemic affricates, different languages possess others, such as /ts/. This affricate combines the voiceless alveolar stop /t/ and the voiceless alveolar fricative /s/. The phonemes /t/ and /s/ do appear together in some English words and phrases such as "cats" /kæts/ and "let's go" /lɛtsgoʊ/. In these contexts, /ts/ is not a distinct phoneme. It is actually the result of the phoneme /t/ plus the morpheme /s/. (In these contexts, /s/ is used as a plural morpheme in "cats" and as a contraction in "let's.") Be careful not to confuse the affricates /tʃ/ and /dʒ/ with the fricatives /ʃ/ and /ʒ/!

EXERCISE 5.4—THE AFFRICATE CONSONANTS

A. Indicate the words below that have /tʃ/ or /dʒ/ in their transcription. Write the correct phoneme next to the word.

_____ bon voyage	_____ fantasia	_____ cabbage
_____ barrage	_____ touches	_____ exertion
_____ arrange	_____ pasture	_____ sabotage
_____ charming	_____ nitrogen	_____ gender
_____ vulture	_____ riches	_____ glacier
_____ mushroom	_____ charade	_____ eject
_____ gerbil	_____ rigid	_____ unchained

B. For each item, create as many real words (or proper names) as possible by placing one of the following fricatives or affricates in the blank. Write your answers to the right of each item. More than one answer is possible for each item.

/f, v, θ, ð, s, z, ʃ, ʒ, h, tʃ, dʒ/

1. /__ɛr/ _____
2. /__æt/ _____
3. /__oʊ/ _____
4. /__ɑrm/ _____
5. /__ɪn/ _____
6. /ri__/ _____
7. /bæ__/ _____
8. /bi__/ _____

C. For each item, select the word(s) that have the specified criterion in their transcriptions.

other   shrunk   none   jeans   hedge   churned   measure

1. Contains an initial voiced phoneme _____
2. Contains a fricative _____
3. Contains an affricate and a front vowel _____
4. Contains an affricate and a nasal _____
5. Contains a palatal obstruent _____
6. Contains an obstruent and a central vowel _____
7. Contains a stop, nasal, and affricate _____
8. Contains all voiced sounds _____

Continues

EXERCISE 5.4 (*cont.*)

D. Circle the words that represent real English words.

1. /skrʌntʃ/	5. /muʒd/	9. /ouðən/	13. /fæʃtɚ/
2. /pʊdʒɪ/	6. /kɪtʃən/	10. /dʒeɪd/	14. /gautʃt/
3. /tʃɔrz/	7. /moutʃ/	11. /hʌdʒ/	15. /dʒʌmpɪ/
4. /harʃɚ/	8. /ʃarm/	12. /tʃɜn/	16. /partʃt/

E. In the blanks, write each of the words using English orthography.

1. /tʃɝpt/	_____	9. /ʃʊrlɪ/	_____
2. /dʒʌŋk/	_____	10. /dʒɝzɪ/	_____
3. /tʃɪt tʃæt/	_____	11. /pɝtʃəs/	_____
4. /wɪʃboʊn/	_____	12. /tʃaklət/	_____
5. /ədʒɔɪnd/	_____	13. /mətʃʊr/	_____
6. /matʃoʊ/	_____	14. /tʃʌmɪ/	_____
7. /gəraʒ/	_____	15. /ædʒəteɪt/	_____
8. /pæstʃɚ/	_____	16. /dʒɛzəbɛl/	_____

F. For each item below, correct any vowel or consonant transcription errors by marking out the incorrect IPA symbol and placing the correct symbol above it. If no error is present, indicate by circling "no error."

1. major	/meɪʒɚ/		no error
2. March	/martʃ/		no error
3. jumped	/dʒʌmpt/		no error
4. Wichita	/wɪtʃɪtɑ/		no error
5. wedged	/wɛdʒt/		no error
6. usher	/ʌʃɚ/		no error
7. sergeant	/sɝdʒənt/		no error
8. massage	/məsɑʒ/		no error
9. gorge	/dʒɔrʒ/		no error
10. manger	/mændʒɚ/		no error

G. Transcription Practice
Transcribe the following words using the IPA.

1. shocked	_____	11. vivid	_____
2. station	_____	12. shutter	_____
3. butcher	_____	13. excite	_____
4. knickers	_____	14. axon	_____
5. extra	_____	15. scoured	_____
6. tangent	_____	16. carved	_____
7. southern	_____	17. outshine	_____
8. necktie	_____	18. gender	_____
9. corsage	_____	19. careless	_____
10. spirits	_____	20. nurture	_____

Continues

EXERCISE 5.4 (*cont.*)

21. cashmere	_____	31. exists	_____
22. chopping	_____	32. ginger	_____
23. cashbox	_____	33. thorny	_____
24. genders	_____	34. Egypt	_____
25. charming	_____	35. chow mein	_____
26. sharpened	_____	36. perverse	_____
27. cashier	_____	37. duchess	_____
28. garbage	_____	38. anxious	_____
29. orchids	_____	39. mischief	_____
30. strengthen	_____	40. capture	_____

Complete Assignment 5-4.

The Approximant Consonants: Glides and Liquids

Pronunciation Guide

Glides

/j/   as in "yet"   /jɛt/   /w/   as in "wet"   /wɛt/

Liquids

/r/   as in "rip"   /rɪp/   /l/   as in "lip"   /lɪp/

The **approximants,** the last group of consonants to be discussed, fall into a manner of production quite different from the others already discussed. In some respects, these four phonemes behave both like vowels, and in other respects like consonants. Even though these consonants are produced with an obstruction in the vocal tract, the articulators are only approximated during their production; the constriction in the vocal tract is less than that associated with the English obstruent consonants.

Because the approximants do not usually form the nucleus of a syllable, they cannot be categorized as vowels. (The phoneme /l/ may become syllabic in some contexts, however.) In a manner similar to vowels, all of the approximants are voiced, so their sound source originates in the larynx. Also, all approximants are produced with a closed velopharyngeal port.

Phoneticians have given various names to this group of consonants. The approximants have been termed *semivowels, frictionless continuants,* and *oral resonants.* The approximants are generally subdivided into two groups: *glides* and *liquids.*

Glides, as their name suggests, involve a gliding motion of the articulators, in a manner similar to the production of a diphthong. For this reason, glides are often referred to as semivowels (although some individuals use this term to refer to *all* approximants). The duration of an approximant glide is shorter (faster) than the duration of a diphthongal glide. Glides are always prevocalic. The glides /j/ and /w/ are characterized by continued movement of the articulators throughout their production into the following vowel.

The term **liquid** is used to categorize the oral resonant consonants /r/ and /l/. Some phoneticians have categorized the liquids as semivowels and also as glides. The term liquid is in no way a reference to the way in which these phonemes are produced. Liquid is simply a general term that has been adopted by phoneticians to categorize these two phonemes.

Acoustic Information   Figure 5.13 is a spectrogram of the glides /w/ and /j/ in the words "away" and "a yay." Note the similarities in the two spectrograms. Because of their formant structure, the glides look very much like vowels. However, glides are shorter in duration and less intense than vowels. The F_1 of both glides appear very similar on the spectrograms in terms of their low frequency specifications. However, the frequency specification of F_2 for the two glides is quite different, reflecting the place of articulation associated with each. /w/ has a low F_2. This is not surprising since /w/ has a similar place of articulation to the vowel /u/. Recall that because /u/ is a back vowel it has a low F_2. On the other hand, the F_2 for /j/ is high because its place of articulation is similar to the front vowel /i/, which also has a high F_2. There is also a difference in the higher formants as seen on the spectrograms. Whereas F_3 and F_4 are visible on the spectrogram during production of /j/, they are not during production of /w/ because of their lack of intensity.

Figure 5.14 depicts spectrograms of the liquids /l/ and /r/ in the words "allay" and "array," respectively. Similar to the glides, the liquids appear similar to the vowels in terms of formant structure. However, liquids are shorter in duration and have lesser intensity than vowels. The frequency range of F_1 is low in frequency for both liquids. F_2 for the liquids /r/ and /l/ also share similar F_2 patterns. However, there is a major difference when comparing the resonance patterns associated with F_3 for /r/ and /l/. F_3 for /l/ remains at a high frequency, whereas F_3 for /r/ decreases to around 1500 Hz. This is due to the constriction in the vocal tract associated with production of the liquid /r/.

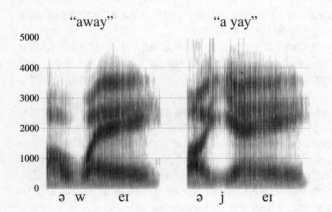

FIGURE 5.13 Spectrograms of the words "away" and "a yay."

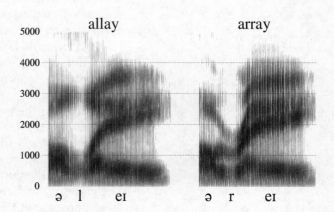

FIGURE 5.14 Spectrograms of the words "allay" and "array."

/j/

Lower-Case j

Description

/j/   voiced, palatal glide

Sample Words

/j/

your	feud
young	cured
yellow	mutate
Yale	onion
yes	fewer

Allographs

/j/

Grapheme	Example
y	yell
u	fuse
eu	feud
i	union

Discussion   /j/ is produced by raising the tongue blade toward the palate (see Figure 5.7). The tongue and lips are in a position similar to that for production of the vowel /i/. The articulators then glide away from the articulation for /j/ to the lip and tongue position necessary for production of the following vowel. The continual motion of the articulators is what characterizes this consonant as a glide. Because the articulators change while gliding from /j/ to the following vowel, a corresponding change occurs in relation to the resonance of the vocal tract.

To demonstrate the similarity in articulation for the glide /j/ and the vowel /i/, say the word "yam" /jæm/. Prolong the initial /j/ phoneme as you say the word. You should hear the phoneme /j/ being produced as you glide from /i/ to /æ/ (/iiiiæm/).

Lower-Case w

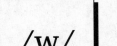

Description

/w/   voiced, labiovelar glide

Sample Words

/w/

when	swill
weed	Kuwait
quick	away
twins	penguin
square	quartz

Allographs

/w/

Grapheme	Example
w	we
wh	why
qu	quit
u	language

Discussion The phoneme /w/ is characterized by its two simultaneous places of articulation, bilabial and velar. During the production of this phoneme, the lips become rounded, and at the same time, the back of the tongue approximates the soft palate. (Say a word beginning with /w/ and see for yourself.) In the production of this phoneme, the lips and tongue begin in the aforementioned position and continue their gliding movement into the following vowel. The beginning articulatory position for /w/ is quite similar to the position for the vowel /u/. Try saying the word "week" /wik/ by prolonging production of /w/. You should hear the glide /w/ being produced as you glide from /u/ to /i/ (/uuuuik/).

Some individuals differentiate between the voiced phoneme /w/ and the voiceless phoneme /ʍ/. The phoneme /ʍ/ is used by some speakers who pronounce the first two letters in words such as "when," "where," and "which" as "hw." For example, /ʍɛn/ would indicate a pronunciation of /hwɛn/ for "when." Most speakers of American English do not distinguish between the voiced and voiceless /w/ in their speech habits. In this text, only the voiced /w/ will be adopted.

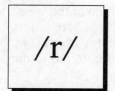

Lower-Case r

Description

/r/   voiced, palatal liquid

Sample Words

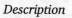

/r/

red	car	rhesus	more
stress	fear	carrot	pure
brown	there	revolt	stork

Allographs

/r/

Grapheme	Example
r	rose
rr	barren
rh	rhododendron

Discussion The official IPA symbol for this phoneme is actually /ɹ/ (known as "turned r"). As was mentioned earlier, /r/ is the symbol for a voiced alveolar trill, a sound found in Spanish and Finnish but not in English. As mentioned in Chapter 1, we will use the symbol /r/ to represent this particular phoneme. Since /r/ and /ɹ/ do not both exist in English, there will be no confusion as to its use. Also, /r/ is easier to write when doing transcription by hand. Of course, it is much easier to type /ɹ/ than it is to write it!

/r/ can be produced in one of two ways, depending on the speaker. Both methods employ a double constriction in the vocal tract. The **retroflexed** articulation of /r/ involves raising the tip of the tongue and curling it back toward the alveolar ridge (or the anterior portion of the palate) as the back of the tongue creates a second velar constriction. The second method of producing /r/, the **bunched** articulation, involves lowering the tip of the tongue and raising (or bunching) the blade of the tongue so that it closely approximates the hard palate, while the tongue root forms a second pharyngeal constriction. The voiced breath stream is forced through the constrictions formed by either method. In both cases, the tongue does not touch the other articulator involved. Both articulations are commonly used by English speakers.

When /r/ occurs at the beginning of a word or syllable (prevocalic), it is always considered to be a consonant. However, in words such as "her" /hɝ/ or "murder" /mɝdɚ/, postvocalic /r/ is actually a vowel. Nevertheless, it is possible to consider final /ɝ/ (or /ɚ/) as a syllabic consonant. That is, "her" and "murder" actually could be transcribed as /hr̩/ or /mr̩dr̩/. In this manner, /r/ becomes the nucleus of the syllable and therefore becomes a syllabic.

In the case of rhotic diphthongs (r-colored vowels), postvocalic /r/ is considered to be a consonant, as in "hair" /hɛr/ or "fear" /fɪr/. The final /r/ in a rhotic diphthong is not considered to be a syllabic; pronouncing "hair" or "fear" with a syllabic final consonant would change these one-syllable words into two-syllable words: /hɛr̩/ and /fɪr̩/.

In Eastern and Southern American dialects, some speakers delete postvocalic /r/, as in "star" /stɑ/. Some Eastern and Southern speakers also derhotacize the central vowels /ɚ/ and /ɝ/, as in "stir" /stɜ/ and "perhaps" /pəhæps/.

Lower-Case l

Description

/l/   voiced, alveolar liquid

Sample Words

/l/

lawn	jello
split	mulch
bowl	hollow
black	pistol
bottle	allure

Allographs

/l/

Grapheme	Example
l	lend
ll	ball

Discussion   Because the airstream for /l/ flows over the sides of the tongue, /l/ is classified as a **lateral** consonant. The phoneme /l/ has two separate articulations depending on whether the phoneme is pre- or postvocalic. Each of these results in a different allophone of /l/. For prevocalic /l/ (as in "lip" or "slip"), the tongue tip is raised in order to approximate the alveolar ridge. In this position, the back of the tongue remains low in the oral cavity, and the airstream is diverted over both sides of the tongue. This is the production for the so-called *light* /l/. Other examples of *light* /l/ include "clue," "police," and both /l/s in "Lulu."

When /l/ occurs in the postvocalic position of words, the tongue tip is lowered, and the back of the tongue is raised to approximate the palate as the airstream passes over both sides of the tongue. This is the production for the *velarized,* or *dark,* /l/. This allophone of /l/ is found in the words "tall," "chorale," "until," and "welcome." In *narrow* (allophonic) transcription, dark /l/ is transcribed as [ɫ], as in "tall" [tɑɫ] and "chorale" [kɔræɫ], and *light* /l/ is transcribed as [l], as in "let" [lɛt]. For now, however, we will not distinguish between the two allophones, and we will transcribe them both using the same IPA symbol, namely, /l/. The use of diacritics in narrow transcription will be addressed in much greater detail in Chapter 7.

In many words, postvocalic /l/ becomes a syllabic consonant. Recall that a syllabic consonant serves as the nucleus of a syllable as in the words "rotten" /rɑʔn̩/ and "happen" /hæpm̩/. Unlike syllabic nasals, syllabic /l/ does *not* have to follow a homorganic consonant in order for it to be syllabic.

Examine the examples of syllabic /l/ below. Listen to each of the words so that you are comfortable with its transcription.

legalize	[ligl̩aɪz]	bottled	[bɑɾl̩d]
hobble	[hɑbl̩]	hustle	[hʌsl̩]
cardinal	[kɑrdn̩l̩]	bundle	[bʌndl̩]

Note that all of the examples above have a velarized (dark) l in their transcriptions even though it is not indicated (e.g., [hʌsɫ̩] and [bʌndɫ̩]).

EXERCISE 5.5—THE APPROXIMANT CONSONANTS

A. Indicate which of the following words has an approximant in its transcription. Write the correct phoneme, that is, /w, j, r, or l/, next to the word.

_____ awkward	_____ reasoned	_____ suede	_____ jonquil
_____ bellow	_____ towered	_____ fewer	_____ screaming
_____ quick	_____ Jupiter	_____ peril	_____ barley
_____ today	_____ lazy	_____ swiped	_____ puny
_____ torpedo	_____ repaid	_____ yawned	_____ fired

B. Indicate with an "X" which of the following words have /j/ in their transcription.

_____ tune	_____ hood	_____ choosy
_____ jealous	_____ piano	_____ compute
_____ putrid	_____ maybe	_____ usual

Continues

EXERCISE 5.5 (*cont.*)

_____ loop _____ jar _____ yours

_____ fuel _____ adjourn _____ daisy

_____ keynote _____ Cupid _____ boysenberry

C. Indicate with an "X" which of the following words have /w/ in their transcription.

_____ awesome _____ why _____ warrior

_____ well _____ awry _____ swept

_____ stalwart _____ wrath _____ quirk

_____ how _____ rowboat _____ borrowed

_____ showed _____ reward _____ wrist

_____ lower _____ Howard _____ wayward

D. Indicate with an "X" the words that have /r/ in their transcriptions.

_____ lurk _____ surround _____ purchase

_____ barter _____ rewritten _____ perfected

_____ burgundy _____ tires _____ scorpion

_____ unreal _____ fourth _____ flirtatious

_____ guarded _____ spirited _____ grandiose

_____ grasp _____ curvature _____ divert

E. Circle the words that represent real English words.

1. /dʒɛloʊ/
2. /blaɪð/
3. /riljə/
4. /ɚoʊlɚ/
5. /dʒɑr/
6. /sɝkl̩z/
7. /fjɝt/
8. /kwɔrl̩d/
9. /wʊln̩/
10. /pjaɪd/
11. /spjud/
12. /wɑlʃat/
13. /swɪlz/
14. /riwɝd/
15. /poʊləs/
16. /fjunts/
17. /jɛlɪ/
18. /skjud/
19. /ɑkwəd/
20. /riɚən/

F. In the blanks, write each of the words using English orthography.

1. /jɛloʊ/ _____
2. /robʌst/ _____
3. /wɑrɪɚ/ _____
4. /jɝnd/ _____
5. /birl̩z/ _____
6. /graʊtʃt/ _____
7. /ripjut/ _____
8. /gwɑvə/ _____
9. /lɪkwəd/ _____
10. /taɪl̩d/ _____
11. /kəteɪl̩d/ _____
12. /kwɑrl̩/ _____
13. /lʌkl̩ɪ/ _____
14. /læʔn̩/ _____
15. /fjuʃə/ _____
16. /kwɛstʃən/ _____

G. For each item below, correct any vowel, diphthong, nasal, or stop consonant transcription errors by marking out the incorrect IPA symbol and placing the correct symbol above it. If no error is present, so indicate by circling "no error."

1. bowling /boʊwlɪŋ/ no error
2. wrongful /wrɑŋfʊl/ no error
3. warbled /wɑrbl̩d/ no error

Continues

EXERCISE 5.5 *(cont.)*

4. pewter	/piuɾɚ/	no error
5. quandary	/qwɑndrɪ/	no error
6. regional	/ridʒənl̩/	no error
7. lawyer	/l̩ɔjɚ/	no error
8. flurries	/flɝis/	no error
9. fuming	/fjumɪŋ/	no error
10. baloney	/bʌloʊnɪj/	no error
11. relish	/ɚɛlɪʃ/	no error
12. confusion	/kənfuʒən/	no error

H. Transcription Practice
Transcribe the following two-syllable words, using the IPA.

1. quicksand _____	21. bugle	_____
2. slouched _____	22. chisel	_____
3. jury _____	23. eunuch	_____
4. acquaint _____	24. Charles	_____
5. shoulder _____	25. belonging	_____
6. slither _____	26. rubric	_____
7. sergeant _____	27. unique	_____
8. skewer _____	28. bequeathed	_____
9. cordial _____	29. kayak	_____
10. useful _____	30. billiards	_____
11. withdrew _____	31. eyewash	_____
12. worship _____	32. lingual	_____
13. enshrined _____	33. quarreled	_____
14. fumed _____	34. anguished	_____
15. luncheon _____	35. outward	_____
16. junior _____	36. rupture	_____
17. unscathed _____	37. shoe wax	_____
18. shrivel _____	38. quotient	_____
19. Yankees _____	39. strangler	_____
20. quarter _____	40. allure	_____

Complete Assignment 5-5.

Review Exercises

A. For the following words, determine whether a *tap* (ɾ), a *glottal stop* (ʔ), or *nasal plosion* (np) is found in its transcription. Fill in the blank with the appropriate answer. If none of these are apparent in the transcription, leave the answer blank.

_____	1. writin'	_____	6. certain
_____	2. rudder	_____	7. crater
_____	3. about	_____	8. winter
_____	4. nutty	_____	9. Martin
_____	5. harden	_____	10. sudden

B. Indicate with an "X" which of the following words or phrases have a syllabic consonant in their transcription.

_____	1. wheel	_____	6. pull
_____	2. written	_____	7. contagious
_____	3. regal	_____	8. that'll
_____	4. Seton Hall	_____	9. grab 'em by the neck
_____	5. candles	_____	10. hold 'er by the tail

C. For all of the consonant phonemes below, indicate their manner, place, and voicing.

	Manner	*Place*	*Voicing*
Example:			
/d/	stop	alveolar	voiced
/k/	_____	_____	_____
/r/	_____	_____	_____
/θ/	_____	_____	_____
/ŋ/	_____	_____	_____
/dʒ/	_____	_____	_____
/b/	_____	_____	_____
/ʃ/	_____	_____	_____
/j/	_____	_____	_____
/f/	_____	_____	_____
/n/	_____	_____	_____

D. Create at least two minimal pairs for the underlined phoneme so that they match the differing features given.

Differing Features

Example:

p̲it	mit, wit	voice	manner	
1. s̲eed	_____	voice	manner	
2. cop̲e	_____	voice	manner	place
3. s̲ome	_____	place		
4. z̲ip	_____	voice	place	
5. b̲ag	_____	place	manner	

E. Each of the following pairs of words differ by one phoneme. Determine how the phonemes differ in terms of manner, place, and/or voicing. Then list the differing features for each pair given.

Differing Features

Example:

none-ton _____ voice, manner _____

1. sin-sing _____

2. jaw-raw _____

3. sue-shoe _____

4. tin-tip _____

5. clue-crew _____

6. cop-mop _____

7. choke-joke _____

8. pet-met _____

9. done-gun _____

10. even-Eden _____

11. Yale-rail _____

12. late-lake _____

13. fame-shame _____

14. cat-cad _____

15. pass-pad _____

F. Identify the words that contain an affricate. If the word has an affricate, indicate the position in the word (pre-, post-, or intervocalic), and whether the affricate is voiced or voiceless.

Word	Transcribed Affricate	Voicing	Position in Word
Example:			
<u>ch</u>arm	/tʃ/	voiceless	prevocalic
1. jester			
2. version			
3. itchy			
4. cash			
5. switched			
6. January			
7. regime			
8. mashing			
9. crush			
10. urgent			

G. Transcribe the underlined consonant allographs in the following words and indicate the appropriate voicing, place, and manner of articulation.

Word	Transcribed Phoneme	Voicing	Place	Manner
Example:				
cab	/k/	voiceless	velar	stop
1. celery				
2. breech				
3. phase				
4. wreck				
5. call				
6. method				
7. yes				
8. crude				
9. chasm				
10. edge				
11. walk				
12. cohesion				

H. Transcription Practice

Transcribe the following words, using the IPA.

CD #2
Track 1

1. birthmarks	_____	21. cosmos	_____
2. conjuring	_____	22. chimpanzees	_____
3. beachcomber	_____	23. discarded	_____
4. otherwise	_____	24. prestigious	_____
5. George Bush	_____	25. charming	_____
6. Vatican	_____	26. Turkish bath	_____
7. zinc oxide	_____	27. bothersome	_____
8. handkerchief	_____	28. jackknife	_____
9. expedite	_____	29. enzyme	_____
10. foundation	_____	30. tooth fairy	_____
11. admitted	_____	31. cherry pie	_____
12. thereafter	_____	32. coauthor	_____
13. injunction	_____	33. hyacinth	_____
14. convergence	_____	34. enjoyment	_____
15. sabotage	_____	35. pharmacist	_____
16. physician	_____	36. unworthy	_____
17. buttonhole	_____	37. 100th	_____
18. discouraged	_____	38. pasteurized	_____
19. evolved	_____	39. fidgety	_____
20. indigent	_____	40. Father's Day	_____

I. Transcription Practice

Transcribe the following words (containing three syllables) using the IPA.

CD #2
Track 2

1. aorta	_____	21. sequential	_____
2. airliner	_____	22. portrayal	_____
3. congealed	_____	23. Thanksgiving	_____
4. Caucasian	_____	24. xylophone	_____
5. vocation	_____	25. artichoke	_____
6. funeral	_____	26. pigeonhole	_____
7. registered	_____	27. Williamsburg	_____
8. yesterday	_____	28. undergrowth	_____
9. November	_____	29. humorous	_____
10. troublesome	_____	30. weariness	_____
11. upholstered	_____	31. universe	_____
12. impudent	_____	32. ungathered	_____
13. torrential	_____	33. manuscript	_____
14. distribute	_____	34. obscurely	_____
15. diaphragm	_____	35. nucleus	_____
16. appetite	_____	36. quadrangle	_____
17. persevere	_____	37. harmonize	_____
18. courageous	_____	38. registrar	_____
19. muscular	_____	39. parboiled	_____
20. papyrus	_____	40. structural	_____

J. Acoustics of Speech/Spectrogram Interpretation

1. Examine the spectrogram of the three words below. The words are "pad," "mad," and "bad" (not in that order). Identify which word is which. Which acoustic characteristics helped you make your decisions?

_____

_____

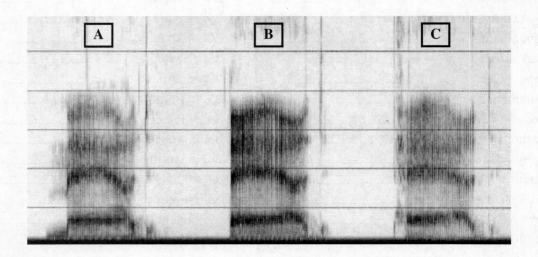

2. Examine the two spectrograms of the words "song" and "thong." Which is which? Which acoustic characteristics helped you make your decisions?

_____

_____

_____

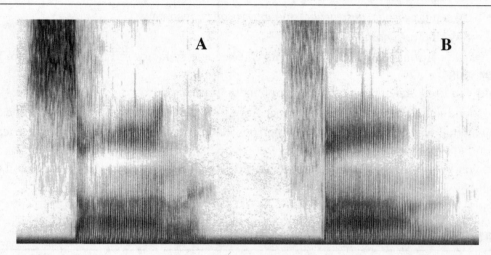

3. The following spectrogram is of the word "cod." Label each of the following directly on the spectrogram.

   a. a voice bar   d. a stop gap
   b. a formant transition e. aspiration
   c. F_2

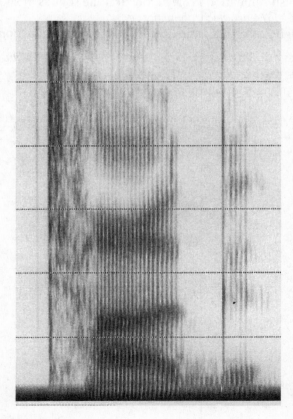

Complete Assignments 5-6 and 5-7.

Study Questions

1. What is a consonant? How do vowels and consonants differ?
2. Define the terms *sonorant* and *obstruent*.
3. Define the terms *manner, place,* and *voicing.*
4. Distinguish between *prevocalic, postvocalic,* and *intervocalic* consonants.
5. What is meant by the term *nasal plosion?*
6. What is a *syllabic* consonant? Which consonants can become syllabics in English? What are the rules that govern their usage?
7. When would you use a *tap* and a *glottal stop* in phonetic transcription?
8. Indicate the sound source for each of the following: vowels, stops, nasals, fricatives, affricates, and approximants.
9. Describe the actual ways in which the following consonant manners are produced: stops, fricatives, nasals, affricates, and approximants.
10. How would you be able to tell the difference between stops, fricatives, affricates, nasals, and approximants when looking at a spectrogram?

Online Resources

Hall, Daniel, University of Toronto, Interactive vocal tract (nd). Retrieved from:
   www.chass.utoronto.ca/~danhall/phonetics/sammy.html
   (interactive visual display of the vocal tract for all English phonemes)

University of Iowa Phonetics Flash Animation Project: fənɛtɪks: the sounds of spoken English (2001–2005).
   Retrieved from: *www.uiowa.edu/~acadtech/phonetics/#*
   (video and animation of English, German, and Spanish consonant production)

University of Victoria Department of Linguistics: Linguistics IPA Lab (nd). *Public IPA Chart.* Retrieved from:
   http://web.uvic.ca/ling/resources/ipa/charts/IPAlab/IPAlab.htm
   (interactive IPA chart with pronunciations of all IPA consonant symbols)

Assignment 5-1

Name _____

Stop consonant transcription.

Transcribe the following two- and three-syllable words.

CD #2
Track 3

1. deadbeat _____
2. darker _____
3. diode _____
4. packing _____
5. Vicky _____
6. backup _____
7. taboo _____
8. decoy _____
9. Cape Cod _____
10. tugboat _____
11. bedbug _____
12. bobcat _____
13. decode _____
14. doted _____
15. diaper _____
16. buckeye _____
17. dugout _____
18. tiptoe _____
19. beaded _____
20. khaki _____
21. co-op _____
22. edit _____
23. dittoed _____
24. tip top _____
25. guide dog _____
26. agape _____
27. go cart _____
28. goodbye _____
29. bagpiper _____
30. katydid _____
31. operate _____
32. terrier _____
33. peapod _____
34. boycotted _____
35. period _____
36. irrigate _____
37. gaiety _____
38. cataract _____
39. gadabout _____
40. carpeting _____
41. dedicate _____
42. barbaric _____
43. caterer _____
44. attitude _____
45. poetic _____
46. corrected _____
47. biotic _____
48. doorkeeper _____
49. bugaboo _____
50. corridor _____

Assignment 5-2

Name _____

Stop and nasal consonant transcription.

Transcribe the following two- and three-syllable words.

CD #2

Track 4

1. minute	_____	26. animate	_____
2. windbag	_____	27. enduring	_____
3. cranky	_____	28. Canada	_____
4. mustard	_____	29. incarnate	_____
5. coyness	_____	30. ionic	_____
6. downtime	_____	31. entire	_____
7. condone	_____	32. cantata	_____
8. bookmark	_____	33. torpedoed	_____
9. tune-up	_____	34. mitigate	_____
10. benign	_____	35. pinto bean	_____
11. magnet	_____	36. piranha	_____
12. bunker	_____	37. bandana	_____
13. curtain	_____	38. motorcade	_____
14. negate	_____	39. Montana	_____
15. omit	_____	40. dignity	_____
16. kidney	_____	41. myopic	_____
17. pontoon	_____	42. commando	_____
18. mundane	_____	43. accountant	_____
19. coward	_____	44. pyramid	_____
20. pointing	_____	45. binary	_____
21. inert	_____	46. nominate	_____
22. command	_____	47. mnemonic	_____
23. bumpkin	_____	48. dogmatic	_____
24. airman	_____	49. interrupt	_____
25. tenant	_____	50. gabardine	_____

Assignment 5-3

Name _____

Stop, nasal, and fricative consonant transcription.

Transcribe the following three- and four-syllable words.

CD #2
Track 5

1. succinctness _____
2. Alzheimer's _____
3. ambition _____
4. commercial _____
5. unsanctioned _____
6. decomposed _____
7. visionary _____
8. cathartic _____
9. admonish _____
10. systemic _____
11. ombudsman _____
12. redemption _____
13. Zambia _____
14. schematic _____
15. horrific _____
16. aversion _____
17. vehemence _____
18. Venetian _____
19. thoroughfare _____
20. orthodox _____
21. zucchini _____
22. xenophobe _____
23. fluorescent _____
24. excavate _____
25. symphonic _____
26. seventeenth _____
27. thereabouts _____
28. homeopath _____
29. understanding _____
30. uncertainty _____
31. vaporizer _____
32. thermometer _____
33. subconsciousness _____
34. sarcophagus _____
35. reservation _____
36. orthodontist _____
37. perversity _____
38. subdivision _____
39. weatherbeaten _____
40. unconvincing _____
41. chauvinism _____
42. innovative _____
43. impersonate _____
44. heterodyne _____
45. catechism _____
46. extortionist _____
47. disorganized _____
48. incandescence _____
49. criticism _____
50. conversation _____

Assignment 5-4

Name _____

Stop, nasal, fricative, and affricate consonant transcription.

Transcribe the following three- and four-syllable words.

CD #2

Track 6

1. repackaged _____
2. compassion _____
3. digestive _____
4. confiscate _____
5. injury _____
6. membranous _____
7. Egyptian _____
8. geosphere _____
9. foundation _____
10. intersperse _____
11. maturate _____
12. exertion _____
13. effervesce _____
14. matchmaker _____
15. chimpanzee _____
16. astonish _____
17. gestation _____
18. omniscient _____
19. amateur _____
20. chastisement _____
21. advantaged _____
22. pasteurized _____
23. x-axis _____
24. disparage _____
25. educate _____

26. affectionate _____
27. contortionist _____
28. menagerie _____
29. moisturizing _____
30. notorious _____
31. pessimistic _____
32. North Dakota _____
33. unimportant _____
34. terrifying _____
35. punctuation _____
36. potassium _____
37. jurisdiction _____
38. pedagogy _____
39. participant _____
40. overshadow _____
41. homogenized _____
42. indigestion _____
43. damaged goods _____
44. thundershower _____
45. graduation _____
46. juxtaposing _____
47. photogenic _____
48. designation _____
49. sandwiches _____
50. pathologies _____

Assignment 5-5

Name _____

Stop, nasal, fricative, affricate, glide, and liquid consonant transcription.

Transcribe the following three- and four-syllable words.

CD #2
Track 7

1. quietly	_____	26. glorified	_____
2. wondrous	_____	27. flamboyant	_____
3. Hercules	_____	28. chromium	_____
4. cultural	_____	29. extrapolate	_____
5. koala	_____	30. employee	_____
6. rebellious	_____	31. legalized	_____
7. quantify	_____	32. delinquency	_____
8. subsequent	_____	33. accumulate	_____
9. withering	_____	34. chlorinated	_____
10. aquarium	_____	35. Asiatic	_____
11. inquiry	_____	36. ballerina	_____
12. curious	_____	37. quagmire	_____
13. worldly	_____	38. inflammable	_____
14. strategy	_____	39. legislation	_____
15. pressurized	_____	40. futuristic	_____
16. puberty	_____	41. burglarize	_____
17. symbolic	_____	42. slovenly	_____
18. refusal	_____	43. nonchalant	_____
19. wonderfully	_____	44. liquidate	_____
20. journalism	_____	45. infuriate	_____
21. disgruntled	_____	46. bureaucracy	_____
22. visualize	_____	47. exquisitely	_____
23. Yosemite	_____	48. acquittal	_____
24. malicious	_____	49. bulimia	_____
25. illustrious	_____	50. ridicule	_____

Assignment 5-6　　Name _____

Transcribe the following geographic locations in IPA.

1. Bowling Green, Kentucky _____
2. Wheeling, West Virginia _____
3. Albuquerque, New Mexico _____
4. Tallahassee, Florida _____
5. Chattanooga, Tennessee _____
6. Joplin, Missouri _____
7. Honolulu, Hawaii _____
8. Anaheim, California _____
9. Thunder Bay, Ontario _____
10. Rochester, Minnesota _____
11. Prague, Czechoslovakia _____
12. Helsinki, Finland _____
13. Raleigh, North Carolina _____
14. Tijuana, Mexico _____
15. Omaha, Nebraska _____
16. Denton, Texas _____
17. Geneva, Switzerland _____
18. Istanbul, Turkey _____
19. Johannesburg, South Africa _____
20. Hiroshima, Japan _____
21. Antwerp, Belgium _____
22. Montreal, Quebec _____
23. Boise, Idaho _____
24. Boston, Massachusetts _____
25. Stockholm, Sweden _____

CD #2
Track 8

Assignment 5-7

Name _____

Transcribe the following.

CD #2
Track 9

1. curious savage _____
2. transmission fluid _____
3. terrible twos _____
4. lightning 'n' thunder _____
5. persuasive argument _____
6. apparent dilemma _____
7. algebra equation _____
8. legal document _____
9. implausible idea _____
10. perplexed child _____
11. veritable fortune _____
12. grapefruit juice _____
13. watermelon rind _____
14. Wuthering Heights _____
15. torrential downpour _____
16. Scranton, PA _____
17. very tranquil _____
18. butterscotch pudding _____
19. patchwork quilts _____
20. oxygen cycle _____
21. anxious parent _____
22. earthquake rumble _____
23. pasteurized milk _____
24. privileged character _____
25. punitive damages _____
26. pharyngeal inflammation _____

Connected Speech

Learning Objectives

After reading this chapter you will be able to:

1. Explain the effects of assimilation as they relate to speech production and phonetic transcription.
2. Contrast the effects of *elision, epenthesis, metathesis,* and *vowel reduction* as they relate to connected speech.
3. Explain how the suprasegmental aspects of speech impact speech production and phonetic transcription.

The exercises in the previous chapters were designed so that you would learn to recognize all of the individual English speech sound segments and how to determine which IPA symbols best represent them. By now, you should feel fairly comfortable transcribing individual words using the correct IPA symbols in broad transcription. In Chapters 4 and 5, the words given in all of the examples and in all of the exercises were transcribed as isolated items, as if they were excised from a sentence. When a word is pronounced carefully as a single item, it is said to be spoken in its **citation form.** The identity of a word spoken in citation form may differ markedly from its identity in **connected speech.** Connected speech results from joining two or more words together in the creation of an utterance. In Chapter 5, some of the exercises involved transcription of items consisting of two words. However, these two-word utterances were transcribed as if each word was produced in citation form. The production of a particular utterance may vary drastically when comparing its citation form with its form in connected speech. In citation form, the word "him" would be transcribed as /hɪm/. The same word in connected speech might be transcribed as /əm/ as in the phrase "I caught him" /aɪkɔtəm/. Also, in connected speech, the production of any particular utterance will most likely vary from speaker to speaker due to differences in dialect and speaking style.

In clinical practice, speech-language pathologists transcribe isolated words when administering phonological tests to their clients to determine which speech sounds are in need of remediation. More often than not, clinicians need to transcribe entire utterances as spoken by their clients. For example, after obtaining a language sample from a child, a clinician will need to analyze the utterances not only in terms of the specific syntactic (grammatical) structures being used, but also in terms of the particular phonemes the child is using correctly or incorrectly. To perform a thorough phonological analysis of a client's speech patterns, the speech-language pathologist may need to transcribe entire utterances of connected speech.

Several major issues make transcribing connected or continuous speech much different from transcribing isolated words. In connected speech, the phonetic identity of words often changes. As already mentioned, the way a word sounds in citation form varies greatly from the way it might sound in a sentence. In connected speech, phonemes are eliminated and/or completely altered once words are strung together in an utterance. In addition, connected discourse is characterized by continuous changes in the stress, intonation, and timing of phonemes, words, and complete sentences. Listening to, and transcribing, words in continuous discourse requires a lot of concentration. It takes a good ear to be able to hear the subtle nuances associated with connected speech. This chapter will focus on two major issues associated with the transcription of connected speech: (1) assimilation and (2) the suprasegmental aspects of speech.

Assimilation

In citation form, each word is spoken in a fairly deliberate manner. That is, the phonemes are pronounced quite carefully, keeping the inherent length of each phoneme fairly intact. Once words are produced in conversation, the deliberateness of speech disappears. Phonemes are not produced in a strictly serial order as we speak; the onset of one phoneme will occur before the previous one has been completely articulated. This often results in an overlapping of the individual phonemes of English. For instance, the utterance, "Where did you go?" might be produced as /wɛrdʒəgoʊ/. The question, "What in the world are you going to do?" might be spoken as /wəʔn̩ðəwɝldəjəgʊnədu/. The syllable boundaries often become obscured in conversational, or casual, speech, even though listeners have little difficulty understanding what is being said. Also, notice that the quality of the vowels changes quite markedly in connected speech.

While we talk, it is necessary to overlap the production of the various phonemes to maintain the rapidity of connected speech. The overlapping of the articulators during speech production is termed **coarticulation.** Coarticulation is a time-efficient process; there is simply not enough time for the articulators to produce each phoneme in its intended isolated form. In addition, coarticulation makes connected speech easier for the speaker to produce. Speech would become quite laborious and slow, indeed, if each individual phoneme was produced in its full, isolated form in every syllable of every word.

An example of coarticulation can be found in the production of the word "soon." In this word, the lips are already rounded at the beginning of the word in anticipation of the rounded vowel /u/. That is, the normally unrounded phoneme /s/ becomes rounded due to the phonetic environment provided by the vowel. Say the word "soon," paying particular attention to the position of your lips for the phoneme /s/. This rounded version of /s/ (written as [sʷ] in narrow transcription) is an allophone of the /s/ phoneme. Another example of coarticulation can be seen by examining the articulation of the phoneme /n/ in the word "tenth." In "tenth," the tongue is placed against or between the teeth in production of /n/ instead of at the alveolar ridge. That is to say, /n/ will become *dentalized* in this particular phonetic environment. Dentalized /n/ is an allophone of /n/ indicated by the dental diacritic [̪], as in "tenth" [tɛn̪θ].

It should be apparent (from the examples above) that a particular phoneme will be articulated differently if that phoneme is preceded or followed by a particular sequence of consonants and vowels. Also, the effects of rapid, continuous speech often will change the phonetic identity of phonemes. It is possible for a particular phonetic context to cause a phoneme to be replaced by a completely different phoneme. Sometimes it is even possible for the phonetic context to result in the complete deletion of a phoneme.

Examine the following utterance: /wʌz ʃi/ ("was she"). In conversation, this utterance is typically produced as /wʌʒ ʃi/. In this case, the /z/ phoneme is produced farther back in the mouth than normal due to the palatal fricative /ʃ/ found in the word "she." Notice that in this example, the change from /z/ to /ʒ/ (due to /ʃ/) occurs across the boundary between the two words. The process whereby phonemes take on the phonetic character of neighboring sounds is referred to as **assimilation.** Some phoneticians suggest that assimilation is brought about as a direct result of coarticulation during the production of connected speech (Calvert, 1986; Ohde & Sharf, 1992).

Some individuals support the notion that coarticulation and assimilation are two separate processes (MacKay, 1987), while others use the terms synonymously (Cruttenden, 2001). When viewed as separate processes, coarticulation would be defined as a change in the phonetic identity of a sound that results only in an allophonic variation of a phoneme, whereas assimilation would refer specifically to articulatory changes that result in the production of a completely different phoneme.

In this text, coarticulation will be viewed as the articulatory process whereby individual phonemes overlap one another due to timing constraints and simplicity of production. Assimilation will be viewed as the realized changes in the identity of phonemes brought about by coarticulation. The term assimilation will be used here to refer to *both* allophonic changes and phonemic changes brought about by phonetic environment.

There are two basic forms of assimilation, regressive and progressive. **Regressive assimilation** occurs when the identity of a phoneme is modified due to a phoneme following it. This is also referred to as *right-to-left* or *anticipatory assimilation.* That is, the articulators anticipate the production of a phoneme occurring later in time. On the other hand, **progressive assimilation** occurs when a phoneme's identity changes as the result of a phoneme preceding it in time. This type of assimilation is also called *left-to-right* or *perseverative assimilation.* That is, the articulators persevere in their production of a particular phoneme and maintain a particular posture for a later phoneme.

Consider the utterance "Would you like to go?" How might you say this utterance? One acceptable pronunciation of this utterance might be /wʊdʒəlaɪkrəgoʊ/. Notice that "would you" is transcribed as /wʊdʒə/. The environment provided by the palatal glide /j/ of "you" alters the pronunciation of /d/ in the word "would," resulting in a right-to-left assimilation of /d/ to /dʒ/. In this case, the alveolar plosive /d/ becomes palatal, inducing articulation of the affricate /dʒ/. A similar example involves production of the word "question." This word can be pronounced one of two ways: /kwɛstʃən/ or /kwɛʃtʃən/. Notice that in the second example, the /s/ has been assimilated to /ʃ/ due to the palatal affricate /tʃ/ in the second syllable of the word. This is a clear demonstration of right-to-left assimilation.

Many of the assimilations brought about by phonetic environment are seen as a change in the *place of articulation* of a particular phoneme. Most of these assimilations are regressive; the phonemes become similar in place of articulation to later-occurring phonemes. The following examples demonstrate regressive assimilation resulting in a change in alveolar place of articulation (from Cruttenden, 2001).

that guy → /ðæk˺ gaɪ/	phone booth → /foʊm buθ/
win more → /wɪm mɔr/	hat box → /hæp˺ bɑks/
tin cup → /tɪŋ kʌp/	Miss Universe → /mɪʃunɪvɚs/
bad boy → /bæb˺ bɔɪ/	cross check → /krɑʃ tʃɛk/
I'll bet you → /aɪlbɛtʃə/	

(Note: [˺] indicates an unreleased plosive.)

An example of progressive, or left-to-right, assimilation can be seen when the plural morpheme /s/ is pronounced as /z/ when it follows a voiced phoneme, for example, /dɑgz/ "dogs" or /ɑrmz/ "arms." In these examples, the voiced phoneme has a left-to-right (progressive) effect on the following /s/ phoneme, causing it to be produced as /z/. Similarly, production of the past tense morpheme "ed" is produced as /t/ when preceded by a voiceless phoneme, for example, /wɑkt/ "walked." Note the effect of progressive assimilation brought about by the /k/ phoneme.

Another example of progressive assimilation occurs when a nasal phoneme follows a plosive with the same place of articulation as in /hæpm̩/ "happen." In this case, the place of articulation of the plosive is preserved in production of the nasal, that is, left-to-right, assimilation (see Cruttenden, 2001).

Elision

In English, it is common for phonemes to be eliminated during production due to particular phonetic contexts. For example, the word "exactly" may be spoken as /əgzæklɪ/. Notice that the /t/ has been eliminated in this particular pronunciation. Omission of a phoneme during speech production is called **elision.** Another example of elision occurs in the word "camera." It is not uncommon for speakers to pronounce this word as /kæmrə/ as opposed to /kæmɚə/. Note that in /kæmrə/, an entire syllable has been deleted, or *elided.*

Elision often results as a historical process as a language develops over time. Elision also occurs as a result of coarticulation associated with connected speech. In addition, elision is found to occur across word boundaries due to certain phonetic environments. Examine the words and phrases (along with their transcriptions) in Table 6.1 to see the resultant elision brought about by effects of phonetic context.

TABLE 6.1   Examples of Elision

Utterance	Transcription	Elided Phoneme
aptly	/æplɪ/	/t/
asthma	/æzmə/	/ð/
fifths	/fɪfs/	/θ/
glands	/glænz/	/d/
used to	/juztu/	/d/
cup of tea	/kʌpəti/	/v/
What's his name?	/wətsəzneɪm/	/h/
Give me that.	/gɪmɪðæt/	/v/

EXERCISE 6.1

Examine each of the following utterances and their transcriptions. Indicate, in the blank, the phoneme that has been elided.

1. lengths   /lɛŋks/   _____

2. friendship   /frɛnʃɪp/   _____

3. countess   /kaʊnəs/   _____

4. bands   /bænz/   _____

5. kept quiet   /kɛpkwaɪət/   _____

6. I caught her.   /aɪkɔɾɚ/   _____

7. word of mouth   /wɝɾəmaʊθ/   _____

8. Where did he go?   /wɛrdɪɾigoʊ/   _____

Epenthesis

In connected speech, additional phonemes are sometimes inserted in words during their production. The addition of a phoneme to the production of a word is termed **epenthesis.** Epenthesis can be the result of factors related to (1) coarticulation, (2) variation in production, or (3) speech disorders.

In terms of coarticulation, the glides /j/ and /w/ may sometimes *seem* to appear between two adjacent vowels, either in the same word or in two different words. For example, it may seem that the glide /j/ is inserted after a front vowel (or diphthong) in words such as "Leo" /lijoʊ/, "Ohio" /ohaɪjoʊ/, or "we own" /wijoʊn/. Similarly, it may seem that the glide /w/ is inserted after a back vowel, as in the words "cooing" /kuwɪŋ/, "going" /goʊwɪŋ/, or "to each" /tuwitʃ/. In these examples, the tongue is gliding in transition from one vowel nucleus to another. The addition of these "transitional" phonemes often result as "native speakers correctly pronounce their own language" (MacKay, 1987, p. 147).

Epenthesis sometimes occurs in words in which a nasal consonant precedes a voiceless fricative. In the words "tense" /tɛnts/, "lengths" /lɛŋkθs/, and "Amsterdam" /æmpstɚdæm/, it may appear that a homorganic voiceless stop is added during production, even though the stop does not actually occur in the word. These added phonemes are the result of physiological constraints on the articulators (due to coarticulation) when producing the phoneme sequence of nasal + fricative, that is, /ns/ (tense), /ŋθ/ (lengths), and /ms/ (Amsterdam).

Due to individual speaking style or dialectal variation, some speakers do not make a true distinction in production of words such as "chance"/"chants" or "tense"/"tents." For these individuals, both productions would be identical and therefore would be transcribed the same, that is, /tʃænts/ or /tɛnts/. However, many speakers *do,* in fact, make a clear distinction between the two pronunciations of these words, that is, /tʃæns/ – /tʃænts/ or /tɛns/ – /tɛnts/. You will have to listen carefully during transcription to determine whether a speaker is actually inserting a stop following the nasal in these contexts.

Other examples of epenthesis occur in the idiosyncratic or dialectal production of certain words. For instance, the words "elm" and "film" are pronounced by some individuals (including my father) as /ɛləm/ and /fɪləm/. Also, some speakers in the southern United States insert the vowel /i/ before /u/ in words such as "Tuesday" /tiuzdeɪ/ or "due" /diu/. Speakers in the East also sometimes insert an /r/ at the end of some words that normally end with schwa, for example, "soda" /soʊdɚ/ or "Cuba" /kjubɚ/.

Finally, epenthesis is sometimes observed in individuals with speech sound disorders. For instance, some children will insert /ə/ in the middle of a consonant blend. Examples include "break" /bəreɪk/ and "glad" /gəlæd/. Schwa insertion is also prevalent in the speech of some deaf individuals.

EXERCISE 6.2

Examine each of the following words and their corresponding transcriptions. Indicate with an "X" the transcriptions that illustrate epenthesis.

1.	noon	/nuən/	_____
2.	pants	/pænts/	_____
3.	choose	/tʃiuz/	_____
4.	friends	/frɛndz/	_____
5.	lamb	/læm/	_____
6.	straw	/strɔr/	_____
7.	rinse	/rɪns/	_____
8.	milk	/mɛlk/	_____
9.	clam	/kəlæm/	_____
10.	Wednesday	/wænzdeɪ/	_____

Metathesis

The transposition of sounds in a word is known as **metathesis.** Metathesis can occur as a result of a "slip of the tongue," personal speaking style, dialectal variation, or a speech disorder. Some examples include:

elephant	→ /ɛfələnt/	spaghetti	→ /pəsgɛɾɪ/
ask	→ /æks/	cinnamon	→ /sɪmənən/
realtor	→ /rilətɚ/	animal	→ /æmɪnḷ/

Vowel Reduction

Another issue commonly encountered when transcribing connected speech involves the phenomenon called **vowel reduction.** Often, the full form (full weight) of a vowel (such as /æ/) becomes more like the mid-central vowel /ə/ when spoken in connected speech. Compare the following transcriptions of the utterance "I can go."

/aɪ kæn goʊ/	*citation form with full vowel /æ/*
/aɪkəngoʊ/	*casual form with reduced vowel /ə/*

The first transcription would be indicative of very careful pronunciation, as if all three words were spoken in isolation. Contrast the citation form with the second transcription, the more casual form. Notice that the vowel /æ/ has been reduced to /ə/. In other words, the articulation of the vowel shifted from low-front to mid-central. In this case, the tongue does not meet the true articulatory target for /æ/ in the low front portion of the mouth. Instead, the body of the tongue remains toward the center of the oral cavity. You have already experienced vowel reduction in certain isolated words such as "feasible." When transcribing this word, it would be possible to transcribe the second vowel with /ɪ/ as in /fizɪbl̩/ or with /ə/ as in /fizəbl̩/, depending on the pronunciation. In the second transcription, the /ɪ/ vowel reflects reduction to /ə/.

What causes vowel reduction? In connected speech, there is often not time for the articulators to achieve their target positions because speech occurs so rapidly. Therefore, the articulators adopt new positions that are still acceptable to the ear. These vowel reductions are not considered to be "bad," "lazy," or "sloppy" articulations. They are simply considered to be the product of connected speech. Below is a list of words demonstrating the process of vowel reduction. Each word is transcribed twice, first using a particular vowel in its full form, and second, using the reduced vowel form. Notice that the two pronunciations for each word are acceptable depending upon the way a person might say the words.

Examples of Vowel Reduction

	Full Vowel	**Reduced Vowel**
t**o**morrow	/tumɑroʊ/	/təmɑroʊ/
d**e**cide	/disaɪd/	/dəsaɪd/
tr**i**bunal	/traɪbjunl̩/	/trəbjunl̩/
obscene	/ɑbsin/	/əbsin/
excel	/ɛksɛl/	/əksɛl/
d**o**mestic	/domɛstɪk/	/dəmɛstɪk/

The following six word pairs are comprised of words sharing the same morpheme. Note the difference in pronunciation between the vowels (in bold) in each pair. The first word in each pair has a vowel with full weight, that is, not reduced. The second word of each pair has the reduced form of the vowel. In each pair, the change in vowel form from full to reduced is due to a change in primary word stress *away from the syllable* in question.

transf**o**rm	/trænsˈfɔrm/	c**o**ncept	/ˈkɑnsɛpt/
transf**o**rmation	/trænsfɚˈmeɪʃən/	c**o**nception	/kənˈsɛpʃən/

excrete	/ɛksˈkrit/	**i**mpose	/ɪmˈpoʊz/
excretory	/ˈɛkskrətɔrɪ/	**i**mposition	/ɪmpəˈzɪʃən/

s**e**quence	/ˈsikwəns/	cond**e**mn	/kənˈdɛm/
s**e**quential	/səˈkwɛnʃəl/	cond**e**mnation	/kɑndəmˈneɪʃən/

Each of the following word pairs demonstrates more than one vowel undergoing a change in vowel quality. Examine each pair in order to see the changes from the full to the reduced vowel form, or vice versa.

dem**o**n	/ˈdimən/	ge**o**metry	/dʒiˈɑmətri/
dem**o**nic	/dəˈmɑnək/	ge**o**metric	/dʒiəˈmɛtrɪk/

m**e**tab**o**lism	/məˈtæbəlɪzm̩/	par**a**meter	/pɚˈæmɚɚ/
m**e**tab**o**lic	/mɛtəˈbɑlɪk/	par**a**metric	/pɛrəˈmɛtrɪk/

EXERCISE 6.3

Transcribe each of the following word pairs, paying attention to the changes in vowel quality (for the bold letters) inherent in their pronunciations.

Example:

valid	/vælɪd/
validity	/vəlɪdɪɾɪ/

1. m**i**racle _____
   m**i**raculous _____
2. **a**ccuse _____
   accusation _____
3. auth**o**rize _____
   auth**o**rity _____
4. dem**o**lish _____
   dem**o**lition _____
5. mechan**i**cal _____
   mechan**i**stic _____

In connected speech, several English monosyllabic words undergo a change in pronunciation when compared to the way they might be spoken in isolation. The change in pronunciation of these words is brought about by vowel reduction associated with changes in word stress. An example can be demonstrated with the pronunciation of the word "as," as in the phrase *as soon as possible* (/əz sun əz pɑsəbl̩/). The reason for this change in the pronunciation of "as" (from /æz/ to /əz/) is due to the fact that, in isolation, the word "as" could be spoken as a stressed monosyllable. In connected, casual speech, it would rarely be stressed. The change in the pronunciation of "as" demonstrates a shift from what is called the *strong form* of the word (/æz/) to the *weak form* of the word (/əz/). Table 6.2

CD #2
Track 10

EXERCISE 6.4

Transcribe each phrase twice: first in citation form and then in casual form.

Example:

bigger than me	/bɪgɚ ðæn mi/	/bɪgɚ ðən mi/
1. your mother	_____	_____
2. right and left	_____	_____
3. food for thought	_____	_____
4. What will they do?	_____	_____
5. Thank him.	_____	_____
6. as big as	_____	_____
7. of mice and men	_____	_____
8. What is her name?	_____	_____

TABLE 6.2 Examples of Strong and Weak Forms of Some English Monosyllabic Words (adapted from Cruttenden, 2001)

Strong (Stressed) Form		Weak (Unstressed) Form(s)
a	/eɪ/	/ə/
an	/æn/	/ən/, /n̩/
and	/ænd/	/ən/, /ənd/, /n̩/
are	/ɑr/	/ɚ/
as	/æz/	/əz/
but	/bʌt/	/bət/
can	/kæn/	/kən/
does	/dʌz/	/dəz/, /əz/
for	/fɔr/	/fɚ/
had	/hæd/	/həd/, /əd/
has	/hæz/	/əz/
her	/hɚ/	/ɚ/
him	/hɪm/	/ɪm/, /əm/, /m̩/
his	/hɪz/	/ɪz/, /əz/
of	/ʌv/	/əv/, /ə/
than	/ðæn/	/ðən/
to	/tu/	/tə/
will	/wɪl/	/l̩/
you	/ju/	/jə/

provides a list of some of these monosyllabic English words, in both their strong and weak forms. The strong form would indicate the word has been stressed. In conversational speech, these words rarely receive stress. For example, the word "the" is rarely pronounced with full stress on the vowel, as in /ðʌ/. More commonly, the pronunciation would be unstressed, that is, /ðə/.

The following examples help to demonstrate pronunciation changes inherent in continuous speech. Compare the first transcription, the citation form of each utterance, with the second transcription, the more casual pronunciation. Keep in mind that the examples given are only *one* possible way of saying each utterance in connected speech. Pay particular attention to the inherent vowel reduction, as well as the assimilation, associated with the more casual form. Note the use of the double bar symbol in the transcriptions below. It is used to represent punctuation marks in transcription of connected speech. Specifically, the double bar /‖/ replaces semicolons, periods, and question marks.

Did you eat yet? I could eat a horse.

/dɪd ju it jɛt ‖ aɪ kʊd it eɪ hɔrs‖/
/dʒitjɛt ‖ aɪkədiɾəhɔrs‖/

What in the world are you going to do?

/wʌt ɪn ðə wɝld ɑr ju goʊɪŋ tu du‖/
/wəʔn̩ðəwɝldɚjəgʊnədu‖/

What has your brother done with my cat and dog?

/wʌt hæz jɔr brʌðɚ dʌn wɪθ maɪ kæt ænd dɑg‖/

/wətʃɚbrəðɚdʌnwɪθmaɪkæʔn̩dɔg‖/

When does the train arrive with her luggage?

/wɛn dʌz ðʌ treɪn əraɪv wɪθ hɚ lʌgədʒ‖/

/wɛnzðətrenəraɪvwɪðɚlʌgədʒ‖/

CD #2
Track 11

EXERCISE 6.5

Transcribe the following utterances, first in citation form, and then in casual form.

1. I bet you I can help them get out of that mess.

   _____

   _____

2. I caught you cheating on that test. I am going to tell the teacher.

   _____

   _____

3. What is his reason for not being able to come to the party?

   _____

   _____

4. What's the matter with Thelma? Let me see if I can cheer her up.

   _____

   _____

5. What did you do to your car? I should be able to get it going.

   _____

   _____

Complete Assignment 6-1.

Suprasegmental Aspects of Speech

In contrast with isolated words, connected speech is characterized by continual modifications or alterations in stress, in the timing of words, and in intonation. It is these alterations that give connected speech its natural characteristic rhythm. Stress, timing, and intonation variations do not affect solely the individual speech sound segments of words. These modifications span entire syllables, words, phrases, and sentences. For this reason, stress, timing, and intonation are generally referred to as the **suprasegmental** aspects of speech production. The prefix *supra-* means *above, beyond,* or *to transcend.* Therefore, the suprasegmental features of speech go beyond or transcend the boundaries of the individual speech sound segment or phoneme, affecting an entire utterance.

Stress Revisited

The preceding discussion should not imply that isolated words are immune from the effects of the suprasegmental features of speech. In Chapter 2, the importance of identifying word stress for purposes of phonetic transcription was discussed. As you recall, a stressed syllable in a word is generally spoken with more articulatory force, resulting in a syllable that is louder, longer in duration, and higher in pitch than an unstressed syllable. Word stress is a suprasegmental feature of speech because entire syllables are stressed, not just individual phonemes. Your transcription practice in the previous chapters has helped you to clearly understand the importance of being able to identify the syllables with primary stress in any word. During transcription, you know when to accurately use /ə/ versus /ʌ/ and /ɚ/ versus /ɝ/. Without this knowledge, it would not be possible to transcribe English accurately using the IPA.

In Chapter 2, we were concerned only with identifying primary stress in words. It is time to turn our attention to the other degrees of word stress. Multisyllabic words have syllables with more than one degree or level of stress. For instance, the word "pretense" has two levels of stress: primary and secondary. This word would be transcribed as /ˈpriˌtɛns/. Note that the IPA symbol for indicating secondary stress is a small mark below and to the left of the syllable receiving secondary stress. The following two-syllable words each have two levels of stress.

ˌmainˈtain	ˌtranˈscend	ˈvalˌue
ˌinˈclude	ˌalˈthough	ˈproˌnoun
ˌtranˈscribe	ˈeˌgo	ˈcouˌpon
ˌsarˈdine	ˈmoˌped	ˈpayˌroll

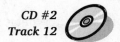

CD #2
Track 12

EXERCISE 6.6

The following words have two levels of stress, primary and secondary. Mark each syllable's stress pattern accordingly, using the appropriate IPA symbols for stress.

1. intense
2. falsehood
3. Lucite
4. rosette
5. teabag
6. frostbite
7. obese
8. entree
9. erode
10. handshake
11. react
12. household

Not all multisyllabic words have syllables with both primary and secondary stress. Some multisyllabic words have only one (primary) stressed syllable. When the nucleus of the other syllable(s) contains either /ə/, /ɚ/, /m̩/, /n̩/, or /l̩/ (or sometimes /ɪ/ and /ʊ/ when produced in a reduced form), the syllable is said to be unstressed. We already know that /ə/ and /ɚ/ are never found in a syllable receiving primary stress. According to Carrell and Tiffany (1960), the schwa vowel is considered an indefinite vowel because it is more of a "murmur" than a full vowel. Its indefinite status makes it a nonprominent nucleus, so much so that it receives no stress at all. The following bisyllabic words have only one stressed syllable (marked appropriately). The other syllable is unstressed.

'riddle	'person	sur'round
'button	'zebra	pre'tend
'melon	'happy	con'tain
'manage	se'date	re'mind

Note that when /ɪ/ is the nucleus of a final open syllable (as in "happy") or the nucleus of the syllable /ɪŋ/, it is unstressed (and lax) as well.

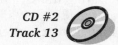

CD #2
Track 13

EXERCISE 6.7

The following bisyllabic words have only one syllable that receives stress; the other syllable is unstressed. Mark the stressed syllable using the correct IPA symbol for primary stress.

1. leopard	5. murky	9. scary
2. sweater	6. anoint	10. naked
3. rhythm	7. magnet	11. extreme
4. contend	8. belief	12. parade

The following three-syllable words have only one stressed syllable:

con'tagious	ba'loney	a'lerted
fer'ocious	'calendar	'constable
a'version	'terrible	'shivering
con'cession	be'havior	'interval

The following four-syllable words also have only one stressed syllable:

'literacy	'passionately	vol'uminous
'definitely	'knowledgeable	chro'nology
'speculative	chry'santhemum	cou'rageously
'personable	to'getherness	ex'perience

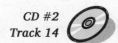

CD #2
Track 14

EXERCISE 6.8

The following three- and four-syllable words have only one stressed syllable. Mark each one correctly using the IPA symbol for primary stress.

1. measuring	5. courageous	9. sorority
2. statistics	6. Germany	10. fraternity
3. laryngeal	7. unbearable	11. Albuquerque
4. warranted	8. Canadian	12. dysphonia

Now contrast the following three- and four-syllable words that each have syllables with primary and secondary stress (in addition to unstressed syllables).

ˌplanˈtation	ˌreimˈburse	ˌmorˈphemic
ˈinterˌnet	ˌtranˈsistor	ˈtantaˌmount
ˌtranˈscription	ˌMonˈtana	ˈpeneˌtrate
ˈsaxoˌphone	ˈtermiˌnate	ˈzodiˌac
ˈmandaˌtory	ˌparaˈplegia	disˈcrimiˌnate
ˈrepliˌcate	ˌeduˈcation	ˈgeneralˌize

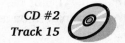

CD #2
Track 15

EXERCISE 6.9

The following three- and four-syllable words have two levels of stress (in addition to some unstressed syllables). Mark primary and secondary stress using the appropriate IPA symbols.

1. myopic
2. cyberspace
3. architect
4. idea
5. citation
6. circumstance
7. bacteria
8. effervescent
9. alimony
10. communicate
11. elevator
12. Indiana

Complete Assignment 6-2.

Sentence Stress

In addition to word stress, each sentence a speaker produces also has inherent **sentence stress.** Examine the following: "Cheryl drove to school." Say this sentence aloud in a natural manner, the way you might say it while conversing with a friend. In this manner, you may have noticed that the last word in the sentence tends to stand out or have more emphasis. Say the sentence again, and see if you notice the emphasis on the last word, "Cheryl drove to ˈschool." Many sentences and phrases are spoken with the primary emphasis or stress on the last word. Examine the following phrases and sentences. Listen for the emphasis on the final word. Notice the words that receive primary stress, especially in the last two examples.

I like his ˈstyle.
Bill and Jane went ˈhome.
If I get ˈcaught, I will get in ˈtrouble.
In order to get good ˈgrades, you will have to study ˈharder.

Phrases and sentences do not always end with a stressed word. Certain words in a sentence will usually receive emphasis or stress depending on (1) the level of importance of that word in the sentence and (2) the speaker's intent of the message being conveyed. Words that contain salient information in a sentence are called **content words.** Content words are generally nouns, verbs, adjectives, and adverbs. The less important words in a sentence, including pronouns, articles, prepositions, and conjunctions, are called **function words.** Content words tend to (but do not always) receive sentence stress; function words usually do not receive stress. In the sentence "Cheryl drove to school," the content words are "Cheryl," "drove," and "school." Although "school" tends to receive stress when this sentence is produced in a neutral manner, it would be possible to stress the other content words, depending on the speaker's intent. When the final word of the sentence, "school," is stressed, the speaker denotes the location to which Cheryl drove—she drove to school, not the library. Compare these variations of the sentence:

Cheryl 'drove to school.   'Cheryl drove to school.

What is the speaker's intent in each of these sentences? In the first sentence, the speaker stressed the word "drove" to indicate Cheryl's mode of transportation; Cheryl drove to school; she did not walk. In the second sentence, the speaker stressed the word "Cheryl" to indicate that Cheryl, not her brother Ethan, drove to school. Notice that in each case, stress was placed on a content word.

The use of sentence stress to indicate a speaker's particular intent is termed *contrastive stress*. Examine the stress shifts in the following statements. In each case, the speaker uses stress contrastively to indicate the particular intent desired.

Sentence:	*Intent:*
Sheila purchased a new red sedan.	*Kennedi* didn't buy the car.
Sheila *purchased* a new red sedan.	Sheila didn't *sell* the car.
Sheila purchased a *new* red sedan.	Sheila didn't buy a *used* car.
Sheila purchased a new *red* sedan.	Sheila didn't buy the *green* car.
Sheila purchased a new red *sedan*.	Sheila didn't buy the *SUV*.

EXERCISE 6.10

Underline the word in each of the following sentences that would receive primary sentence stress, based upon the given intent.

Example:

	Intent:	I didn't buy pants.
	Sentence:	I bought a <u>shirt</u> last week.
1.	Intent:	We did not go to a play last night.
	Sentence:	Carol and I went to a matinee.
2.	Intent:	David doesn't live on West Brooklyn.
	Sentence:	My neighbor David lives at 4555 East Brooklyn Avenue.
3.	Intent:	Sam doesn't care for taffy.
	Sentence:	Flo ate the taffy from the circus.
4.	Intent:	Jason and Andrea talked to their grandmother.
	Sentence:	Jason and Andrea did not get a chance to talk to their uncle.
5.	Intent:	They liked Mrs. Harlan's husband.
	Sentence:	The third graders really liked Mr. Harlan.

CD #2
Track 16

EXERCISE 6.11

Listen to each of the following sentences on the audio CD. <u>Underline</u> the word that is given primary sentence stress. Then, write the intent of the utterance on the blank line.

Example:

Mary had a little <u>lamb</u>.

<u>She didn't have a goat.</u>

1. The girl's name was Mary.

   _____

2. Jared only forgot to get the toothpaste at the store.

   _____

3. Why did they walk to the playground?

   _____

4. Why did they walk to the playground?

   _____

5. Mark got a new blue bike for his birthday.

   _____

6. Mark got a new blue bike for his birthday.

   _____

7. Mark got a new blue bike for his birthday.

   _____

Sentence stress also plays an important role in distinguishing the *type* of information being presented by a speaker. When conversing with someone, the conversation usually volleys back and forth between the two participants. Two types of information are provided during a conversation, **given information** and **new information.** When people converse, each person will typically provide new information to the conversation, adding to the given (old) information previously discussed. For instance, a friend might ask, "What did you have for lunch?" Your reply might be, "I had a hamburger and french fries for lunch." *Hamburger* and *french fries* would be considered new information, since this is your addition to the conversation. Since these words provide new information to the listener, these words would typically be stressed. The phrases "I had a . . ." and "for lunch" would be given information since the information refers back to the prior question; these phrases would not receive stress. Suppose your friend responds, "Oh, I only had a cheeseburger." In this case *cheeseburger* would be the new information in the dialog; it would correspondingly receive stress.

Examine the following conversation between Sally and Jane. They are discussing Sally's most recent purchase. As you read the dialogue, it is easy to see that each participant's response advances the conversation. New information is in italic.

Sally: You got a new *purse*.

Jane: Yeah, I got it at the *mall*.

Sally: *Which* mall?

Jane: The one *downtown*.

Sally: Which *store*?

Jane: Oh. I got it at *Green's*.

Sally: Was it *expensive*?

Jane: It was on *sale*.

Sally: Was it more than *fifty dollars*?

Jane: It was only *twenty*!

As the conversation ensues, each participant stresses or emphasizes the new information she wishes to convey. Of course, neither participant is consciously stressing these words; it happens as a result of knowing how sentence stress is utilized in conversation. The use of sentence stress (as well as other suprasegmental features) is behavior that is the direct consequence of learning language and being familiar with the way language operates in conversation.

CD #2
Track 17

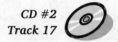

EXERCISE 6.12

The following dialogue is between a waitress and a customer in a restaurant. Circle the words in the dialogue that are stressed in order to convey new information.

Waitress: Would you like something to drink?

Customer: Lemonade, please. I would also like to order.

Waitress: Would you like an appetizer?

Customer: No, thank you.

Waitress: Would you like to hear about our specials?

Customer: Please.

Waitress: We have grilled salmon and fettuccine alfredo.

Customer: I'll have the fettuccine.

Waitress: Would you like our house dressing on your salad? It's Italian.

Customer: I would like to have blue cheese, please.

Waitress: I'll also bring out some fresh rolls.

Customer: Thank you.

Waitress: You're welcome.

When marking sentence stress in transcription, you will first need to identify the word(s) that receive sentence stress. Then, you will need to identify the other content words in the utterance. The word(s) receiving primary sentence stress will be marked with the traditional IPA symbol (') preceding the syllable that normally receives word stress. The stressed syllables of the other content words will be marked using the IPA symbol for secondary stress (₁). For example, the sentence "I want iced coffee" would be marked for sentence stress in the following manner (depending on the speaker's intent):

ˌI want ˈiced ˌcoffee. (I want cold coffee.)
ˌI want ˌiced ˈcoffee. (I do not want tea.)

Now contrast the following sentence pairs:

*The **boys** jumped into the pool.*   ***I'll** be married in September.*
The ˈboys ˌjumped into the ˌpool.   ˈI'll be ˌmarried in Sepˌtember.

*The boys **jumped** into the pool.*   *I'll be **married** in September.*
The ˌboys ˈjumped into the ˌpool.   ˌI'll be ˈmarried in Sepˌtember.

*The boys jumped into the **pool**.*   *I'll be married in **September**.*
The ˌboys ˌjumped into the ˈpool.   ˌI'll be ˌmarried in Sepˈtember.

Foreign speakers who are learning English as a second language may have trouble with English stress patterns, both in words and in sentences. Word stress is not predictable in English as it is in some other languages. Therefore, it is difficult for new users of English to learn to use stress patterns correctly. Improper use of word and sentence stress may add to the "accent" of an individual learning English as a second language.

Hearing-impaired individuals with a severe or profound hearing loss may experience difficulties producing stress patterns correctly because their auditory channel is diminished. One common characteristic of "deaf speech" is incorrect placement of stress on function words, because the rules of stress placement are not fully understood. A speaker who stresses function words has speech patterns that appear unintelligible to normal hearing listeners because normal listeners are not accustomed to hearing this type of spoken stress pattern.

CD #2
Track 18

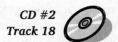

EXERCISE 6.13

Mark sentence stress for each of the following items using the appropriate IPA notation. Each sentence will be spoken by two different speakers. Pay attention to differences in stress between the two speakers. You will need the optional audio CD for this exercise.

Example:

    a. The ˌcow ˌjumped over the ˈmoon.

    b. The ˌcow ˈjumped over the ˌmoon.

  1. a. Steve's roommate is from Minneapolis.

    b. Steve's roommate is from Minneapolis.

  2. a. Tim went skydiving on Saturday.

    b. Tim went skydiving on Saturday.

  3. a. The answer on the exam was "false."

    b. The answer on the exam was "false."

  4. a. Susan's birthday is next Tuesday.

    b. Susan's birthday is next Tuesday.

Continues

EXERCISE 6.13 (*cont.*)

5. a. I'd like a steak for dinner.
    b. I'd like a steak for dinner.

6. a. I went to New York City to see some plays.
    b. I went to New York City to see some plays.

7. a. My professor shaved his mustache.
    b. My professor shaved his mustache.

8. a. I need potatoes from the store.
    b. I need potatoes from the store.

Intonation

It is often difficult to talk about sentence stress without addressing the topic of intonation, another suprasegmental feature of speech. Because stress involves changes in voice pitch, speakers continually modify the fundamental frequency of their voice while speaking in order to stress particular words in an utterance. The modification of voice pitch is known as **intonation.** A speaker's intonation pattern cues a listener as to the type of utterance being spoken, that is, a statement of fact, a question, an exclamation, and so forth. When someone asks a question requiring a yes/no answer, voice pitch generally rises at the end of the utterance. Intonation is also responsible, at least in part, for indicating a speaker's particular mood.

Consider the short sentence "I did." This statement can be spoken in several ways, depending upon the speaker's intent and the corresponding intonation pattern. For instance, "I did" could be spoken as a casual, matter-of-fact reply to the question "Did you read the paper today?" The statement could be spoken with emphasis on the word "did" in response to the never-ending parental question "Have you cleaned your room yet?" In response to "Who ate the pie?" a speaker would probably emphasize the word "I." With each change in speaker intent, there would be a corresponding change in the intonation applied to the utterance. Note that in each version of the utterance, there is both a change in sentence stress *and* a corresponding increase in the fundamental frequency of the voice.

An **intonational phrase** is made up of all changes in fundamental frequency spanning the length of a meaningful utterance. An intonational phrase may consist of an entire sentence, a phrase, or simply one word. Long sentences will usually have more than one intonational phrase. Intonational phrases in longer sentences are signaled by a slight pause in the utterance (indicated in writing with a comma, hyphen, or semicolon). Below are several utterances comprised of one, two, and three intonational phrases.

One intonational phrase:	*Two intonational phrases:*
Yes!	*You took my umbrella, didn't you?*
I want to go home.	*I got a blue scarf, not a red one.*

Three intonational phrases:

The boys, who ate the candy, got sick.
Pete, my best friend, took me to the ball game.

There are two intonational phrases in the accusation "You took my *umbrella, didn't* you?" The words in italic type would most likely have the highest voice pitch. Say the sentence out loud, paying particular attention to the changes in the pitch of the voice. You will notice that the highest voice pitch occurs on the words "umbrella" and "didn't." Similarly, in the sentence "The boys, who ate the candy, got sick," there are three distinct intonational phrases (separated by commas). You should notice that the highest voice pitch occurs on the words "boys," "candy," and "sick."

The syllable that receives the greatest pitch change in any particular intonational phrase is called the **tonic syllable** (Ladefoged, 2001) or **nuclear syllable** (Fudge, 1984). Likewise, the emphasis given to this syllable is referred to as the **tonic accent** or the **nuclear accent.** Each intonational phrase is characterized by only one tonic accent. In the question "Are you done?" the tonic accent would fall on the final word "done." The tonic accent would be located on the second syllable of the word "confused" in the statement "He was confused," because word stress is normally found on the second syllable of that word. In the sentence "You took my umbrella, didn't you?" the tonic accent is on the second syllable of umbrella (um'brella) in the first intonational phrase, and the first syllable of didn't ('didn't) in the second intonational phrase.

The tonic accent most often is located at the end of an intonational phrase (Ladefoged, 2001). However, when a speaker uses contrastive stress to draw attention to a particular word in an utterance, the tonic accent would be located on the stressed syllable. Compare the two pronunciations of the following sentence.

It won't rain *today*.
It *won't* rain today.

In the first example, the tonic accent would be located on the last syllable of the utterance ("It won't rain to'day"). In the second example, the tonic accent would be located on the second word ("It 'won't rain today").

Intonational phrases are characterized by the *direction* of their pitch change; they are generally classified as falling or rising. If a waiter asks you, "Would you like some soup?" you would hear a rise in intonation at the end of the question. If a waiter states, "We have two special soups tonight," you would probably not hear a rising intonation pattern. The voice pitch would most likely fall at the end of this statement.

Falling intonational phrases accompany complete statements and commands and are indicative of the finality of an utterance (Jones, 1963). In the sentence "The boys went home" (spoken as an unemotional statement), the voice pitch falls throughout the utterance. There is a general fall, or declination, in the pitch of the voice over the length of most neutrally spoken statements. Some other examples of falling intonational phrases would be evident in utterances such as the following:

I guess.   That should do it.   It's time to go.   I like riding roller coasters.

Falling intonational phrases also are typical in utterances comprised of Wh-questions. Wh-questions are those that begin an utterance with the words "where," "what," "why," "when," "which," and "how." Examples include:

Why did you go?   What's your favorite color?
Where is your friend?   When did you arrive?

Rising intonational phrases (typical of questions and incomplete thoughts) usually indicate some uncertainty on the speaker's part (Jones, 1963; Pike, 1945). As previously indicated, yes/no questions have a rising intonation pattern. Examples include:

Are you coming?   Is it time yet?

He did?   Can you?

Rising intonational phrases also occur with *tag questions*.

His name is Bill, isn't it?   They're watching reruns

I am gonna just hang out, okay?   again, aren't they?

                                       He likes Lady Gaga, doesn't he?

Rising intonational phrases also are common when reciting a list of items. For example:

My favorite colors are red, blue, and green.

Say the above sentence aloud. Listen to the rise in the pitch of your voice, following the words "red" and "blue." The voice pitch then falls toward the end of the sentence.

The examples given above represent only a few of the more common intonation patterns seen in American English. In addition, the various examples given are only suggestions of the way the utterances could be spoken. It would be possible to pronounce any of the examples in a variety of ways. For instance, the sentence "I can't" could be spoken as a statement (falling intonation) or as a yes/no question (rising intonation), depending on the speaker's intent.

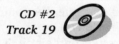

CD #2
Track 19

EXERCISE 6.14

Indicate whether the intonational phrases in the following utterances are generally rising or falling. Circle the appropriate response.

1.	When will you leave?	Rising	Falling
2.	Is your brother home?	Rising	Falling
3.	I need to go the library.	Rising	Falling
4.	What's your favorite season?	Rising	Falling
5.	Did you get paid yet?	Rising	Falling
6.	The dog ran away.	Rising	Falling
7.	Sophie is my oldest friend.	Rising	Falling
8.	How did you know about that?	Rising	Falling
9.	Honest?!?	Rising	Falling
10.	I'm sure!!!	Rising	Falling

Tempo

Tempo is the term used to describe the durational aspect of connected speech. Because timing, or duration of articulatory events, affects entire utterances, tempo also is considered to be a suprasegmental feature of speech. Obviously, the overall rate of speech plays a role in determining the tempo of speech. For adults, the average speech rate is on the order of approximately 5 to 5.5 syllables per second (Calvert, 1986). Tempo also is determined by the duration of individual phonemes and the duration of pauses located between syllables, words, phrases, and sentences.

Duration of Individual Phonemes

Each of the phonemes in English, when spoken in isolation, has an inherent duration. As a rule, diphthongs have a greater duration than vowels, and vowels have a greater duration than the consonants. Among the consonants, the glides and liquids have the greatest duration; the stop consonants have the shortest duration. The duration of any individual phoneme will change once placed in connected speech. For instance, you already know that the stressed syllable of a word is longer in duration than an unstressed syllable. Obviously, the syllable is lengthened due to the increased duration of its individual phonemes. Refer back to Figure 4.18 in Chapter 4. This figure shows spectrograms of the words ['probate] and [pro'test]. Inspection of the spectrograms reveals that although both syllables begin with the same phonemic sequence /pro(ʊ)/, the diphthong in the first (stressed) syllable of "probate" is longer in duration (129 msec.) than the vowel in the first (unstressed) syllable of "protest" (76 msec.). It follows then that the first syllable in "probate" would be longer in duration than the first syllable in the word "protest."

The inherent length of individual phonemes also varies depending upon phonetic context. For instance, vowels preceding voiceless consonants are shorter in duration than vowels preceding voiced consonants. That is, the vowel /æ/ in "batch" is shorter than /æ/ in the word "badge." Turn back to Chapter 5 and examine the spectrograms in Figures 5.1 (comparing "ape" and "Abe"), 5.8 (comparing "leash" and "liege"), and 5.12 (comparing "batch" and "badge"). You can readily see that the vowels preceding the voiceless consonant in each minimal pair is indeed shorter than the vowel preceding its voiced cognate.

Vowels in open syllables also are longer than vowels in closed syllables. Compare the length of the vowel /i/ in the words "beet" and "bee" by saying them aloud. It should be evident that /i/ in the open syllable "bee" is longer in duration. The IPA uses a colon to indicate that a phoneme has been lengthened. Therefore, in the preceding examples, the words "batch" and "badge" could be transcribed as [bætʃ] and [bæːdʒ], respectively. Similarly, the words "beet" and "bee" could be transcribed as [bit] and [biː].

In connected speech, the final phoneme of one word and the initial phoneme of the following word may often be the same, as in "Yes, Susie." Say this phrase aloud. You will notice that there is really no break in the production of the two /s/ phonemes. Instead, you most likely hear a prolonged /s/ phoneme. This phrase would be transcribed [jɛsːuzɪ] using the colon diacritic to indicate the lengthened /s/ phoneme. Note that the syllable boundary disappears due to the prolonged /s/. Some other examples of this phenomenon include:

but, Terry	[bʌtːɛrɪ]	with them	[wɪðːɛm]
men know	[menːoʊ]	call Linda	[kɑlːɪndə]

EXERCISE 6.15

Select the one word from each pair that would have the longer vowel. Transcribe that word using the diacritical marking [ː].

Example:

key   keep   _____[kiː]_____

1. peace   peas   _____   4. spa   spot   _____
2. leave   leaf   _____   5. lack   lag   _____
3. rude   root   _____   6. toot   too   _____

EXERCISE 6.16

Transcribe the following utterances, using the [ː] diacritic where appropriate.

Example:

kite tail   [kaɪtːeɪl]

1. rice soup   _____
2. cotton netting   _____
3. big guns   _____
4. tail light   _____
5. calm morning   _____
6. bar room   _____
7. leaf fire   _____
8. push Sherri   _____

Pauses and Juncture in Connected Speech

Pauses occur in connected speech for a number of reasons. First, a pause may simply indicate that the speaker is taking a breath. Second, pauses may indicate hesitations on the part of a speaker as in the following, "His name was . . . um . . . um . . . oh, I remember . . . Charlie." Third, pauses are used in conversation to indicate the presence of a new thought or to emphasize a particular point. Examine the utterance "I want to go to the movies, but I don't have any money." The comma, which separates the two clauses, marks a pause in the utterance when it is said aloud. The speaker pauses because two ideas are being presented. The speaker needs to emphasize the importance of each idea, especially the latter. Similarly, there would be a pause at each of the commas in the utterance "I need to buy shampoo, tissue, bath soap, and deodorant," signaling the identity of each of the items. Recall that each comma also indicates the beginning of a separate phrase, with an accompanying change in intonation.

Juncture is the term used to indicate the way in which syllables and words are linked together in connected speech. **External juncture** is the term given to a pause that connects two intonational phrases. (That is, the connecting pause is external to the phrase.) The IPA symbols /|/ and /||/ are used to mark external juncture in connected speech. These symbols replace the commas, semicolons, and periods that mark the juncture on the printed page. The single bar IPA symbol /|/ is used to indicate the presence of a short pause (represented in print as a comma). As you recall, longer pauses, represented in print by a period or semicolon, would be represented with a double bar /||/. The sentence "Yes, I would like to go, but I can't," would be transcribed as /jɛs|ɪaɪ wʊd laɪk tə goʊ|bət aɪ kænt||/.

When transcribing connected speech, it sometimes becomes necessary to indicate the presence of a pause between words in the same intonational phrase because the transition between syllables may become blurred. Consider the utterances "I scream" and "ice cream." They share an identical phoneme string, i.e., /aɪskrim/. To indicate the pause between "I" and "scream" in the first utterance, the /+/ diacritic is used, that is, /aɪ + skrim/. The syllables /aɪ + skrim/ are said to have **open internal juncture** because there is a pause between the syllables. The transcription of the second utterance, /aɪskrim/ has no pause between the two syllables. Therefore, /aɪskrim/ has **close internal juncture.** No special symbols are needed to indicate close internal juncture because there is no pause between the syllables. Another example of open and close internal juncture occurs with the utterances, *night rate* → /naɪt + reɪt/ and *nitrate* → /naɪtreɪt/.

EXERCISE 6.17

Use the single-bar [|] and double-bar diacritics [||] to indicate external juncture in the following utterances. All punctuation marks have been omitted.

Example:

   [When I'm sleepy | I go to bed ||]

1. I want hot dogs ice cream and cotton candy
2. They left didn't they
3. The family who lived next door moved away
4. What is her problem
5. My uncle the dentist is 34 years old

Complete Assignment 6-3.

Review Exercises

A. For each of the following pronunciations, indicate the phonemic change that occurred as a result of assimilation. Also indicate the change in place in articulation.

Example:	Pronunciation	Phoneme change	Change from alveolar to:
bad boy	[bæb:ɔɪ]	b/d	bilabial
1. can make	[kæm:eɪk]	_____	_____
2. How's your mother?	[haʊʒɚ mʌðɚ]	_____	_____
3. gin game	[dʒɪŋ geɪm]	_____	_____
4. lead pipe	[lɛb paɪp]	_____	_____
5. has shaken	[hæʒ ʃeɪkn̩]	_____	_____
6. red gown	[rɛg gaʊn]	_____	_____

B. Transcribe each of the following items after eliding the indicated phoneme.

Example:	Elided phoneme	Transcription
aptly	/t/	/æplɪ/
1. bends	/d/	_____
2. winter	/t/	_____
3. land mine	/d/	_____
4. can of worms	/f/	_____
5. counter	/t/	_____
6. twelfths	/θ/	_____
7. What's her problem?	/h/	_____
8. wept loudly	/t/	_____

C. Transcribe each of the following utterances, first in citation form, and then in casual form.

CD #3
Track 1

1. I want to go home.

   _____

   _____

2. Let me see your book.

   _____

   _____

3. Could you move a little to the right?

   _____

   _____

4. Did John ever get paid?

   _____

   _____

5. Why did she leave so early?

   _____

   _____

6. It is raining cats and dogs.

   _____

   _____

7. When are you going to leave?

   _____

   _____

8. You have got to be kidding!

   _____

   _____

9. Who is going to rake the leaves tonight?

   _____

   _____

10. I want to wax my truck tomorrow morning.

    _____

    _____

D. Rewrite each of the following in English orthography (citation form).

1. /dʒɛvəgorəðəsɝkəs‖/

   _____

2. /wɛndədʃilivdʒɔrdʒə‖/

   _____

3. /maɪsɪsɹɚgɑrənubɔɪfrɛnd‖/

   _____

4. /gɪmɪədeɪɚtutədəsaɪd‖/

   _____

5. /aɪmgʊnəhæftəseɪnofɚnaʊ‖/

   _____

6. /aɪθɪŋkɪtsgʊnəreɪmɪðɚtədeɪɚtəmɑroʊ‖/

   _____

7. /wʊdʒɚɛvɚθɪŋkəduənðætfɚmi‖/

   _____

8. /dujəθɪŋkðətsuzn̩tʊkənəfəvəm‖/

   _____

9. /əmʃɚðətðɝgʊnəteljəwətʃənidtəduət‖/

   _____

10. /traɪəzimaɪt│hidʒɝstkʊdəntduwətʃiwɑnəd‖/

    _____

E. Indicate primary and secondary stress, where appropriate, in each of the following three- and four-syllable words. Keep in mind that some syllables in the words are unstressed. Use a dictionary to help identify any syllable boundaries of which you are unsure.

CD #3 Track 2

1. courageous
2. terrified
3. majestic
4. asthmatic
5. Plexiglas
6. plurality
7. mandatory
8. clandestine
9. flamboyant
10. creation
11. computation
12. cranberry
13. bulletin
14. surrendered
15. semantics
16. colonial
17. mercenary
18. independent
19. October
20. ballerina

F. 1. Transcribe each of the following word pairs. Be sure to indicate primary and secondary stress.

2. Compare your vowel transcriptions in each pair (for the vowels represented by the bold letters). If vowel reduction results when going from the first to the second word, place an "X" in the "reduced" column. If your transcription indicates a change from a reduced vowel to the full form of the vowel, place an "X" in the "full" column.

		Reduced	Full
Example:			
valid	validity		
/ˈvælɪd/	/vəˈlɪdɪɾi/	X	
1. **o**rigin	**o**riginate		
2. micr**o**scope	micr**o**scopy		
3. arist**o**crat	arist**o**cracy		
4. strat**e**gy	strat**e**gic		
5. man**i**ac	man**i**acal		
6. homog**e**nous	homog**e**neous		
7. paral**y**ze	paral**y**sis		
8. fel**o**ny	fel**o**nious		

9. perspire   perspiration

_____

10. repeat   repetitious

_____

G. Indicate with an "X" whether the following utterances have an overall rising or falling intonation contour.

	Rising	Falling

CD #3
Track 3

1. I got a sweater for my birthday.   ____   ____
2. Are you happy?   ____   ____
3. The girls had spaghetti for supper.   ____   ____
4. Are you positive?   ____   ____
5. When you're finished, go to bed.   ____   ____
6. Were you late for work today?   ____   ____
7. Let me get back to you.   ____   ____
8. Did you buy a new CD?   ____   ____
9. What do you mean?   ____   ____
10. Is that your idea of a joke?   ____   ____

H. Use the diacritical markings [|] or [||] to indicate external juncture for each of the following utterances. All punctuation marks have been omitted.

CD #3
Track 4

1. If I want your help you'll be the first to know
2. Maybe I will maybe I won't
3. They bought a new house didn't they
4. The girls who went swimming all got a cold
5. I can't really make up my mind
6. I scream you scream we all scream for ice cream
7. When are you leaving on vacation
8. Are your cousins coming for a visit or not
9. Do you have ants in your pants
10. I quit my job but only when I was sure I could get another

I. Transcribe each of the following utterances in casual form, indicating a lengthened phoneme [:] where appropriate. Also use the diacritical markings [|] or [||] to indicate external juncture where appropriate.

CD #3
Track 5

Example:

Did you have a good day?

[dɪdʒəhævəgʊd:deɪ||]

1. I caught my cat Tom by the tail.

_____

2. Which shampoo did you buy at the store?

_____

3. Would you put the white tablecloth on the table, please?

_____

4. Mom might take me shopping, if I get good grades.

_____

5. Have you finished taping the TV special yet?

_____

6. With them, it's hard to tell what they are thinking.

_____

7. Please give me your phone number before you leave.

_____

8. Clem made a home run at the big game last Tuesday.

_____

9. Teddy and Farrell love to play outside with the water sprinkler.

_____

10. I won't take any more of the junk Ken hands out.

_____

J. Each of the following sentences will be spoken by two different speakers. Transcribe each of the utterances in casual form. Be sure to use single-bar or double-bar diacritics to indicate external juncture.

CD #3
Track 6

1. Why can't you ever act your age?

_____

_____

2. Why, oh why did I ever leave Iowa?

_____

_____

3. When did they say their flight was?

_____

_____

4. I will probably go home tomorrow, or the day after.

_____

_____

5. Where did she ever get an idea like that?

_____

_____

6. You have got to be pulling my leg.

_____

_____

7. My friends S.B. and Dale are going to pick me up at 3:00.

_____

_____

8. Why did you repaint the barn already?

_____

_____

9. They are going to tell you what you need.

_____

_____

10. Did she take two of them? Nah, she took four.

_____

_____

Study Questions

1. What is coarticulation, and what is assimilation? What is the difference between these two processes?

2. What is the difference between regressive and progressive assimilation? What are other terms that could be used to represent the same processes?

3. Define the following processes associated with connected speech:

   a. elision   b. epenthesis   c. metathesis

4. Describe the process of vowel reduction.

5. What is the cause of the change in the casual pronunciation of the following words?

   was shared → /wʌʒ ʃɛrd/   tan car   → /tæŋ kɑr/

   bat girl   → /bæk gɝl/   would you → /wʊd ʒu/

6. What is the difference between a syllable that receives secondary stress and a syllable that is unstressed? What is the difference in the way these levels of stress are marked?

7. How is sentence stress marked?

8. What is the difference between given and new information?

9. What is a content word? What is a function word?

10. Define the terms *intonation* and *intonational phrase.*

11. When would you observe (1) a rising intonational phrase and (2) a falling intonational phrase?

12. How does phonetic environment affect vowel duration?

13. What is the difference between internal and external juncture?

14. What is the difference between open and close internal juncture?

15. What role do pauses play in connected speech?

Online Resources

Intonation and stress: Key to understanding and being understood, by Kenneth Beare (2010). Retrieved from:
   http://esl.about.com/od/speakingadvanced/a/timestress.htm
   (basic introduction to stress and intonation in English)

Pronunciation strategies, by Carolyn Samuel (2003). Retrieved from:
   http://individual.utoronto.ca/English/SGSPronunciation.htm
   (information relating to word stress and sentence stress)

Teaching English intonation and stress patterns, by Ted Power (nd). Retrieved from:
   www.btinternet.com/~ted.power/esl0108.html
   (resource guide for teachers of English as a second language)

Assignment 6-1

Name _____

Transcribe each of the following utterances, first in citation form, and then in casual form. Only the casual form will be presented on the CD.

CD #3
Track 7

1. I bet you that you are going to win the race.

   _____

   _____

2. We really have to study tonight for the phonetics test.

   _____

   _____

3. Tell Sherry that she will have to go to the store to get some bacon and eggs.

   _____

   _____

4. My friend Caroline is having a party on the third of next month.

   _____

   _____

5. Bob can always finish his homework when he gets home.

   _____

   _____

6. Let me think about your answer for a minute.

   _____

   _____

7. We have just got to clean the house tomorrow.

   _____

   _____

8. Don't forget to pick up our cleaning on the way to work.

   _____

   _____

9. I am going to miss you when you move to the country.

   _____

   _____

10. Please share those ideas with the rest of the group.

    _____

    _____

Assignment 6-2

Name _____

Indicate primary and secondary stress (where appropriate) for the following words.

CD #3
Track 8

1. stethoscope
2. zoology
3. synchronized
4. latitude
5. execute
6. conversion
7. voyager
8. triangle
9. nomadic
10. infinite
11. fluoridate
12. December
13. detonate
14. vulcanize
15. bronchitis

16. automate
17. symmetrical
18. stupendous
19. flirtatious
20. distribute
21. chlorinate
22. magazine
23. openness
24. kitchenette
25. gullible
26. flamingo
27. evasive
28. caravan
29. modernize
30. comprehend

Assignment 6-3

Name _____

CD #3

Track 9

Each of the following items will be spoken by two different speakers. Transcribe the following utterances in casual form. Be sure to use single-bar and/or double-bar diacritics to indicate external juncture. Also use the lengthening diacritic [:] when appropriate.

1. You can lead a horse to water, but you can't make him drink.

   _____

   _____

2. I am not sure we have those shoes in your size; they only come in sizes seven, eight and one-half, or nine.

   _____

   _____

3. That man said he would drive around back to pick up his packages.

   _____

   _____

4. My professor remembered to bring in the model of the larynx; it was really helpful.

   _____

   _____

5. When you are finished typing the paper, remember to come over so we can celebrate.

   _____

   _____

6. Miss Smith thinks that her cousin Neil will be coming over for a visit today.

   _____

   _____

7. My niece Sarah's favorite colors have always been magenta, turquoise, and chartreuse.

   _____

   _____

8. Don't tell her I told you, but Jeannene said she has always been neutral when it comes to that topic.

   _____

   _____

9. If you stay a little while longer, I'll give you a piece of that terrific carrot cake.

   _____

   _____

10. Now, remember, the game begins sharply at 4:30. Don't forget to bring your bat and glove.

   _____

   _____

Clinical Phonetics: Transcription of Speech Sound Disorders

Learning Objectives

After reading this chapter you will be able to:

1. Describe the basic steps involved in the clinical process.
2. Describe normal developmental data relating to speech sound acquisition in children.
3. Explain how phonological process analysis and nonlinear phonology contrast in the assessment of a client's phonological system.
4. Perform allophonic transcription of disordered speech utilizing appropriate diacritics and non-English IPA symbols.
5. List and discuss factors you need to consider to assure accuracy in the practice of phonetic transcription.

The purpose of this chapter is to introduce you to the application of phonetics in a clinical setting. The focus of the book thus far has been to acquaint you with the process of transcribing typically developing speech patterns (at least what is considered to be typical in Standard American English). As future clinicians, you will be faced with the task of evaluating a client's speech behavior to determine whether that client is in need of intervention. Therefore, you should have an understanding of the process of typical speech-language development. In addition, you will need to know how to evaluate your client to determine whether there is a problem with speech-language production. Ultimately, if the client is in need of intervention, you will need to know how to generate a plan for treatment. These topics will be briefly introduced in this chapter. A thorough discussion of these topics is beyond the scope of this text. This material will be covered in other courses in your curriculum that focus on phonological development and disorders.

Overview of the Clinical Process

The terms **articulation disorder** and **phonological disorder** both have been used by hearing and speech professionals over the years to characterize a client who experiences difficulty with speech sound production. The term *articulation disorder* usually refers to a person who only has a problem producing a few phonemes, or whose speech errors are tied to the motoric aspects of speech production. *Phonological disorder,* on the other hand, generally refers to an individual who has difficulty with the sound system of a language and utilizing the rules that govern the combination and order of phonemes in words (Elbert & Gierut, 1986). More recently, professionals have adopted the use of the term **speech sound disorder** to include *all* disorders involving speech sound production. In this text, the term *speech sound disorder* will be used in this manner.

To evaluate the speech production capabilities of your clients in a clinical setting, you will need to administer a battery of tests to assess articulatory competency. The test battery usually includes the administration of articulation tests and elicitation of a spontaneous speech sample. Once testing is completed, you will be able to analyze your client's speech productions in utterances of varying length (i.e., syllables, words, phrases, and sentences). The results of testing will ultimately help determine the therapeutic approach you select for your clients.

Articulation tests attempt to systematically identify the correct/incorrect usage of phonemes in a child's repertoire by having the child name objects, or pictures of objects, with which they are familiar. Consonants and consonant clusters (and sometimes vowels) are evaluated in various positions of words to determine whether the individual phonemes of English can be produced correctly in differing phonetic contexts in an age-appropriate manner. Spontaneous, connected speech samples are elicited by engaging the client in conversation about hobbies, favorite activities, or a favorite TV show or movie. With very young children, spontaneous speech samples may be obtained while children describe pictures in a book or while they play with toys. The spontaneous, connected speech samples are transcribed and analyzed for age-appropriate behavior.

Articulation tests are usually scored on a phoneme-by-phoneme basis to determine whether the client displays any speech errors, or **misarticulations.** The errors are then categorized as errors of *substitution, omission, distortion,* and/or *addition.* An example of a **substitution** would be producing the word "hello" as /hɛwoʊ/, substituting /w/ for /l/; this would be written as a w/l substitution. An example of an **omission** would be producing the word "big" as /bɪ/, leaving off the final /g/. A **distortion** would involve the production of an allophone of the intended phoneme. If a client produced the word "sit" with a *dentalized* /s/, that is, [s̪ɪt] (which sounds somewhat like /θɪt/), it would be considered a distortion. An **addition** error involves the insertion of an extra phoneme in a word, as in /dɑgə/ for "dog." Analyzing speech sound errors on a phoneme-by-phoneme basis may be appropriate when a child displays only a few phonemic errors. Should a child have several speech sound errors, other methods of analysis may prove to be more favorable. One such method would involve analyzing speech sound errors in terms of the *phonological processes* the child is exhibiting. To understand the concept of phonological processes, we must first turn our attention to the process of typical phonological development in children.

Typical Phonological Development

Over the past 70 years, many studies have attempted to delineate the order of phoneme acquisition in typically developing children (Poole, 1934; Prather, Hedrick, & Kern, 1975; Sander, 1972; Smit, Hand, Freilinger, Bernthal, & Bird,

1990; Templin, 1957; Wellman, Case, Mengert, & Bradbury, 1931). These developmental studies all examined a large number of children in order to answer a basic question: "What is the age at which children typically develop and master English speech sounds?" Without this knowledge, it would be difficult to know whether a child is developing speech in a typical manner.

Smit and colleagues (1990) examined phoneme development in 997 children between the ages of 3 and 9 by using a picture naming task. They presented developmental data for 75 and 90 percent correct phoneme production (mastery) in the initial and final positions of words. Interestingly, Smit and her colleagues found some differences between girls and boys in terms of their phonological development; girls less than 6 years of age tended to develop some phonemes earlier than boys in the same age group. Therefore, the data from their study is presented separately for boys and girls in Table 7.1, both for 75 percent and 90 percent mastery.

TABLE 7.1 Developmental Phonological Data from Smit, Hand, Freilinger, Bernthal, and Bird (1990). Data are presented as years and months. For example, 6;0 means 6 years and 0 months.

	75% Mastery		90% Mastery	
Phoneme	**Girls**	**Boys**	**Girls**	**Boys**
m	≤3;0	≤3;0	3;0	3;0
p	≤3;0	≤3;0	3;0	3;0
h	≤3;0	≤3;0	3;0	3;0
w	≤3;0	≤3;0	3;0	3;0
b	≤3;0	≤3;0	3;0	3;0
n	≤3;0	≤3;0	3;6	3;0
k	≤3;0	≤3;0	3;6	3;6
d	≤3;0	≤3;0	3;0	3;6
g	≤3;0	≤3;0	3;6	4;0
t	≤3;0	≤3;0	4;0	3;6
f	≤3;0	3;6	3;6–5;6	3;6–5;6
j	3;6	3;6	4;0	5;0
ŋ	5;6	6;0	7;0–9;0	7;0–9;0
r	6;0	5;6	8;0	8;0
l	4;6	6;0	5;0–6;0	6;0–7;0
s	3;0	5;0	7;0–9;0	7;0–9;0
tʃ	4;0	5;0	6;0	7;0
ʃ	4;0	5;0	6;0	7;0
z	5;0	6;0	7;0–9;0	7;0–9;0
dʒ	4;6	4;0	6;0	7;0
v	4;0	4;6	5;6	5;6
θ	5;6	6;0	6;0	8;0
ð	4;0	5;6	4;6	7;0

EXERCISE 7.1

Examine the findings from the data presented in Table 7.1. Answer the following questions:

1. Which manners of articulation do children appear to develop first?

2. Which places of articulation do children appear to develop first?

3. Which manners of articulation still appear to be problematic for typical 5-year-old children?

4. For which manner of articulation do children first use voiceless/voiced pairs?

The data from Smit and her colleagues reveal certain important findings relative to children's phoneme mastery. These findings include:

1. Ninety-percent mastery of several phonemes occurs by the age of 3 years. The mastery of all English phonemes may not be complete until a child is at least 7 to 9 years of age.

2. In relation to manner of articulation, the nasal and stop consonants are acquired first, followed, in order, by the glides, fricatives, liquids, and affricates.

3. In relation to place of production, sounds produced in the front of the mouth (e.g., labial and alveolar) are usually developed first, followed by velar and palatal articulations.

Developmental speech sound studies all focused on segmental (phoneme-by-phoneme) acquisition. Another method used in the analysis of the phonological development of children is to examine production in terms of underlying patterns or processes children may use in the production of speech sounds. Stampe (1969) proposed a theory of **natural phonology** that supports the idea that young children are born with innate processes necessary for the production of speech. Because young children are not capable of producing adult speech patterns, they often simplify the adult form. These simplifications are termed **phonological processes.** As children mature, they learn to suppress these processes. When this happens, children then are able to produce the more appropriate adult form of the articulation. If only segmental development is considered, a child who is not capable of producing a certain phoneme may be viewed as not having that sound in her phonetic inventory. When viewed in terms of phonological processes, the child may be using a phonological process that results in the deletion or modification of that sound. Adults may have difficulty understanding the speech patterns of a young child with whom they are not familiar. This is often due not to missing sounds in the child's phonetic repertoire, but is most likely due to the fact that adults are not accustomed to the simplifications, or processes, being produced by the child (Hodson & Paden, 1991).

Phonological Processes

Many phonological processes are found to occur in the speech patterns of typically developing children. These processes can be divided into three general categories: **syllable structure processes, substitution processes,** and assimilatory processes (Ingram, 1976). Some of the more common processes associated with these subdivisions are presented below and are summarized in Table 7.2. Developmental data (the age when specific processes are suppressed) in the following sections are from Grunwell (1987). Make sure to pay particular attention to the examples given *in terms of their phonetic transcription.*

Syllable Structure Processes

These processes, as a group, affect the production of syllables so that they are simplified, usually into a consonant-vowel (CV) pattern (Ingram, 1976). CV patterns are among the first syllable types to be used in the speech patterns of developing infants.

Weak Syllable Deletion

Weak syllable deletion, or simply *syllable deletion,* is a phonological process that involves the omission of an unstressed (weak) syllable either preceding or following a stressed syllable. This process may persist until a child is nearly 4;0. It is also common in some adult productions (Hodson & Paden, 1991). Examples include:

telephone → /tɛfon/	probably → /prɑblɪ/ or /prɑlɪ/
tomato → /meɪɾo/	above → /bʌv/

TABLE 7.2 Examples of Some Common Phonological Processes of Children

Syllable Structure Processes	Example Word	Production
Weak syllable deletion	surprise	/praɪz/
Final consonant deletion	look	/lʊ/
Reduplication	baby	/bibi/
Cluster reduction	clean	/kin/
Substitution Processes		
Stopping	sand	/tænd/
Fronting	kite	/taɪt/
Deaffrication	jump	/ʒʌmp/
Gliding	lake	/weɪk/
Vocalization	help	/hɛʊp/
Assimilatory Processes		
Labial assimilation	put	/pʊp/
Alveolar assimilation	mine	/naɪn/
Velar assimilation	garden	/gɑrgən/
Prevocalic voicing	cop	/gɑp/
Devoicing	ride	/raɪt/

EXERCISE 7.2

Indicate with an "X" the transcriptions that are examples of weak syllable deletion.

Examples:

	Intended Word	Transcription
_____	please	/piz/
X	elephant	/ɛfənt/

_____	1.	yes	/ɛs/
_____	2.	baby	/beɪ/
_____	3.	banana	/nænə/
_____	4.	mama	/mə/
_____	5.	today	/deɪ/
_____	6.	milk	/mɪk/
_____	7.	mitten	/mɪt/
_____	8.	lady	/di/
_____	9.	scissors	/sɪ/
_____	10.	juice	/dʒu/

Final Consonant Deletion

Final consonant deletion effectively reduces a syllable to a CV pattern, that is, to an open syllable. Typically developing children begin to use most consonants in the coda (final) position of words by the time they reach the age of 3 years, 0 months (3;0). This process is generally suppressed completely by age 3;6. Examples include:

$$\text{bake} \rightarrow \text{/beɪ/} \qquad \text{mouse} \rightarrow \text{/maʊ/} \qquad \text{cat} \rightarrow \text{/kæ/}$$

EXERCISE 7.3

Which of the following words could be affected by final consonant deletion? Indicate those words with an "X" and then transcribe the word in IPA, applying the process of final consonant deletion.

Examples:

shoe		_____	_____
foot		X	/fʊ/

away	1.	_____	_____
cup	2.	_____	_____
through	3.	_____	_____
clown	4.	_____	_____
bread	5.	_____	_____

Continues

EXERCISE 7.3 (*cont.*)

say	6. _____	_____
phone	7. _____	_____
black	8. _____	_____
stop	9. _____	_____
go	10. _____	_____

Reduplication

Reduplication involves the repetition of a syllable of a word. Total reduplication involves a repetition of an entire syllable, as in "mommy" → /mɑmɑ/. Partial reduplication involves repetition of just a consonant or vowel, as in "bottle" → /bɑdɑ/ (Lowe, 1996). Reduplication is common in the early speech development of some children. It is generally suppressed before 2;6. Other examples include:

daddy → /dædæ/ or /dɑdɑ/   doggy → /dɑdɑ/
movie → /mumu/   baby → /beɪbeɪ/

EXERCISE 7.4

For the words given, indicate with an "X" the transcriptions that indicate the process of reduplication.

_____ 1. wagon   /wægə/   _____ 4. pencil   /pɛpɛ/

_____ 2. children /dɪdɪ/   _____ 5. water   /wɑwɑ/

_____ 3. jacket   /dækɪ/   _____ 6. yellow   /jɛdo/

Cluster Reduction

Cluster reduction results in the deletion of a consonant from a consonant cluster (adjacent consonants in the same syllable). If the cluster contains three consonants, one or two of the consonants may be deleted, as in "spray" → /preɪ/ or /reɪ/. Cluster reduction may persist until approximately 4;0. Other examples include:

snow → /noʊ/   play → /peɪ/   stripe → /traɪp/, /taɪp/, or /raɪp/

EXERCISE 7.5

For the words given, indicate with an "X" the transcriptions that indicate the process of cluster reduction.

_____ 1. blue   /bu/   _____ 6. stop   /tɑp/

_____ 2. spot   /spɑ/   _____ 7. crayon   /keɪɑn/

_____ 3. stripe /raɪp/   _____ 8. milk   /mɪk/

_____ 4. path   /pæt/   _____ 9. wish   /wɪs/

_____ 5. spring /rɪŋ/   _____ 10. grape   /geɪp/

Substitution Processes

Substitution processes involve the replacement of one class of phonemes for another. For instance, the phonological process known as **stopping** involves the substitution of a stop for a fricative or affricate. Similarly, the process known as **fronting** involves the substitution of an alveolar phoneme for a velar or palatal articulation.

Stopping

As just mentioned, stopping involves the substitution of a stop for a fricative or an affricate. This is a commonly occurring process because stops are acquired before most fricatives in typically developing speech (see Table 7.1). The substitution is usually for a stop produced with the same, or similar, place of articulation:

Fricative/affricate		Substituted stop	Fricative		Substituted stop
/s, ʃ, tʃ, θ/	→	/t/	/f/	→	/p/
/z, ʒ, dʒ, ð/	→	/d/	/v/	→	/b/

Sometimes children produce a stop for a fricative or affricate along with a change in voicing, for example, /sɪp/ → /dɪp/. The change in voicing is a phonological process called *prevocalic voicing* and will be discussed in more detail below. Stopping of fricatives and affricates may continue for some phonemes until 4;0 or 5;0. Examples include:

sake → /teɪk/   (voiceless alveolar fricative → voiceless alveolar stop)

zoo → /du/   (voiced alveolar fricative → voiced alveolar stop)

fat → /pæt/   (voiceless labiodental fricative → voiceless bilabial stop)

ship → /tɪp/   (voiceless palatal fricative → voiceless alveolar stop)

The last example ("ship") demonstrates not only stopping, but also a more forward place of production of the affected consonant phoneme. That is, place of production shifted from palatal to alveolar. This process is called fronting and is discussed in the next section.

EXERCISE 7.6

Place an "X" in front of the following transcriptions that represent an example of the process of stopping.

_____ 1. shoe → /zu/	_____ 6. comb → /goʊm/
_____ 2. thank → /tæŋk/	_____ 7. summer → /tʌmɚ/
_____ 3. raisin → /weɪzn̩/	_____ 8. yellow → /wɛloʊ/
_____ 4. march → /mɑrt/	_____ 9. bath → /bæt/
_____ 5. shave → /seɪv/	_____ 10. shop → /tɑp/

Fronting

It is common for young children to substitute velar and palatal consonants with an alveolar place of articulation. This substitution process is commonly referred to as *fronting*. The alveolar substitutions typical of fronting are given below:

Velar		Alveolar	Palatal		Alveolar
/k/	→	/t/	/ʃ/	→	/s/
/g/	→	/d/	/tʃ/	→	/ts/
/ŋ/	→	/n/	/ʒ/	→	/z/
			/dʒ/	→	/dz/

Fronting usually disappears in typically developing children's speech by the age of 2;6 to 3;0. Examples include:

cat → /tæt/ (voiceless velar stop → voiceless alveolar stop)
wash → /wɑs/ (voiceless palatal fricative → voiceless alveolar fricative)
juice → /dzus/ (voiced palatal affricate → voiced alveolar affricate)
mash → /mæt/ (voiceless palatal fricative → voiceless alveolar stop)

The affricate /dz/ (in /dzus/) is not a phoneme of English, but may occur in disordered speech patterns. Also note that the pronunciation of /mæt/ for "mash" displays both fronting and stopping of the final phoneme:

mash /mæʃ/ → /mæs/ (fronting, i.e., palatal /ʃ/ → alveolar /s/)

and

/mæs/ → /mæt/ (stopping, i.e., fricative /s/ → stop /t/)

EXERCISE 7.7

Place an "X" in front of the following transcriptions that are indicative of fronting.

_____ 1. candy → /gændɪ/ _____ 6. ridge → /rɪd/

_____ 2. rake → /reɪt/ _____ 7. fishing → /ʃɪʃɪŋ/

_____ 3. bring → /brɪn/ _____ 8. paper → /teɪpɚ/

_____ 4. clown → /kraʊn/ _____ 9. goose → /dus/

_____ 5. brush → /brʌs/ _____ 10. sing → /tɪŋ/

Deaffrication

Deaffrication occurs when a child substitutes a fricative for an affricate. Examples include:

chip → /ʃɪp/ (voiceless, palatal affricate → voiceless, palatal fricative)
juice → /ʒus/ (voiced, palatal affricate → voiced, palatal fricative)
ledge → /lɛz/ (voiced, palatal affricate → voiced, alveolar fricative)

The last example, ledge → /lɛz/, demonstrates two substitution processes: (1) deaffrication and (2) fronting. In addition to the substitution of the fricative for an affricate, that is, /dʒ/ → /ʒ/ (deaffrication), the palatal /ʒ/ is produced as the alveolar /z/ (fronting).

Suppose a child produced the word "June" as /dun/. How many substitution processes are occurring in this production? If you answered "three," you are correct. A change from /dʒ → d/ involves deaffrication, fronting, and stopping. Study this example to make sure you understand the three processes that are occurring:

June /dʒun/ → /ʒun/ (deaffrication)
/ʒun/ → /zun/ (fronting)
/zun/ → /dun/ (stopping)

EXERCISE 7.8

Place an "X" in front of the following transcriptions that are indicative of deaffrication.

_____ 1. shake → /seɪk/   _____ 6. gem → /tʃɛm/

_____ 2. choose → /tsuz/   _____ 7. witch → /wɪʃ/

_____ 3. brush → /brʌt/   _____ 8. chalk → /sɔk/

_____ 4. Jack → /ʒæk/   _____ 9. chase → /ʃeɪs/

_____ 5. mesh → /mɛs/   _____ 10. bridge → /brɪdz/

Gliding

Gliding is a substitution process that involves the substitution of the glides /w/ or /j/ for the liquids /l/ and /r/. Gliding is common in children displaying typical developmental patterns as well as in those with phonological disorders. This process is overused in some cartoons to depict characters with disordered speech, for example, /wæbɪt/ for "rabbit." This phonological process is seen in children as young as 2;0, and may persist until a child is 5;0 or older. Examples include:

red → /wɛd/   blue → /bwu/
like → /jaɪk/   grow → /gwoʊ/

EXERCISE 7.9

Place an "X" in front of the following transcriptions that are indicative of gliding.

_____ 1. soap → /woʊp/   _____ 6. yes → /wɛs/

_____ 2. leaf → /wif/   _____ 7. loop → /wup/

_____ 3. ring → /jɪŋ/   _____ 8. grow → /gwoʊ/

_____ 4. lazy → /jeɪzɪ/   _____ 9. laugh → /jæf/

_____ 5. rice → /laɪs/   _____ 10. free → /fli/

Vocalization

Vocalization (vowelization) involves the substitution of a vowel for postvocalic or syllabic /l/ or /r/ (including the vowels /ɚ/ and /ɝ/). The vowels commonly substituted include /ʊ/, /ɔ/, and /o/ (or /oʊ/). Examples of vocalization include:

		Substitution
tiger	→ /tigʊ/	/ɚ/ → /ʊ/
turn	→ /tɔn/	/ɝ/ → /ɔ/
third	→ /θʊd/	/ɝ/ → /ʊ/
bear	→ /bɛʊ/	/r/ → /ʊ/
help	→ /hɛʊp/	/l/ → /ʊ/
fell	→ /fɛo/	/l/ → /o/
little	→ /wɪɾo/ or /wɪɾol/	/l̩/ → /o/ or /ol/

Note that the last example (little → /wɪɾo/) demonstrates both vocalization and gliding of /l/.

Some children may still produce the final /l/ following the vowel as in /wɪɾol/. You will have to listen carefully to determine if the /l/ was maintained in the child's articulation. This is a production especially prone to transcription error (see Louko & Edwards, 2001).

EXERCISE 7.10

Place an "X" in front of the transcriptions that are indicative of *vocalization.*

_____	1. middle → /mɪdo/		_____	6. belt → /bɛʊt/
_____	2. lamp → /wæmp/		_____	7. telephone → /tɛfon/
_____	3. answer → /ænsʊ/		_____	8. curtain → /kʊʔn̩/
_____	4. Kirk → /kɔk/		_____	9. bark → /bɑk/
_____	5. could → /kɔd/		_____	10. fire → /faɪ/

Complete Assignment 7-1.

Assimilatory Processes

Assimilatory processes involve an alteration in phoneme production due to phonetic environment (see Chapter 6 for a review of assimilation). Assimilatory processes involve labial, velar, nasal, and/or voicing assimilation. The assimilation in any of these instances may be either progressive or regressive. These processes are not present in all typically developing children. When they occur, they usually disappear before the age of 3. The assimilation processes associated with consonant production are also referred to as *consonant harmony.*

Labial Assimilation
Labial assimilation occurs when a non-labial phoneme is produced with a labial place of articulation. This is due to the presence of a labial phoneme elsewhere in the word. For example:

book → /bʊp/   (progressive assimilation)

(In this case, the non-labial /k/ is produced with a labial articulation due to the presence of the /b/ phoneme at the beginning of the word.)

mad	→ /mæb/	(progressive assimilation)
cap	→ /pæp/	(regressive assimilation)
swing	→ /ɸwɪŋ/	(regressive assimilation)

/ɸ/ is a voiceless bilabial fricative, a phoneme found on the IPA chart, but not common to English. It is found in African languages such as Hausa and Ewe. To produce /ɸ/, place your lips together and blow out so air escapes (but don't whistle). Pretend you are softly blowing out a candle. (Don't push air from the glottis, otherwise you will produce /h/.) Another way to produce /ɸ/ is to say the word "whew." When producing the word "swing" as /ɸwɪŋ/, the alveolar fricative /s/ undergoes labial assimilation due to the presence of /w/.

EXERCISE 7.11

Place an "X" in front of the words that correctly indicate the process of labial assimilation.

_____ 1. pie → /baɪ/		_____ 6. boat → /boʊp/
_____ 2. tap → /pæp/		_____ 7. train → /preɪn/
_____ 3. frog → /frɑk/		_____ 8. peg → /pɛb/
_____ 4. lip → /lɪb/		_____ 9. cause → /pɔz/
_____ 5. numb → /mʌm/		_____ 10. big → /bɪb/

Alveolar Assimilation

Alveolar assimilation occurs when a non-alveolar phoneme is produced with an alveolar place of articulation due to the presence of an alveolar phoneme elsewhere in the word. Examples include:

time	→ /taɪn/	(progressive assimilation)
shut	→ /sʌt/	(regressive assimilation)
bat	→ /dæt/	(regressive assimilation)

EXERCISE 7.12

Place an "X" in front of the words that correctly indicate the process of alveolar assimilation.

_____ 1. pig → /tɪg/		_____ 6. knife → /naɪs/
_____ 2. pat → /tæt/		_____ 7. that → /zæt/
_____ 3. short → /sɔrt/		_____ 8. phone → /soʊn/
_____ 4. Tom → /mɔm/		_____ 9. vat → /væp/
_____ 5. tune → /dun/		_____ 10. hard → /kɑrd/

It is not always easy to determine whether a child's speech productions are a result of assimilation or of a substitution process. For instance, a child who produces the word "cat" as /tæt/ might be demonstrating alveolar assimilation or may be fronting the /k/ phoneme. To determine whether a child is using assimilatory processes, it is necessary to evaluate several productions from the child's speech sample. In this manner, a particular phonological pattern may emerge. Examine two different children's productions of the following six words. What phonological pattern do you see?

Child #1		Child #2	
kite	/taɪt/	kite	/taɪt/
dog	/dɑd/	dog	/dɑd/
should	/sʊd/	should	/sʊd/
push	/pʊs/	push	/pʊʃ/
go	/doʊ/	go	/goʊ/
bike	/baɪt/	bike	/baɪk/

Child #1's productions of "kite," "dog," and "should" could be suggestive of either alveolar assimilation or fronting. However, productions of the words "push," "go," and "bike" reflect only fronting, because no alveolar phonemes exist in these words. Therefore, this child appears to be demonstrating the process of fronting. Contrast this pattern with child #2, who only mispronounces the first three words, words with alveolar phonemes. Child #2 appears to be demonstrating alveolar assimilation.

Velar Assimilation

Velar assimilation occurs when a non-velar phoneme is produced with a velar place of articulation due to the presence of a velar phoneme elsewhere in the word. Examples:

cup → /kʌk/ (progressive assimilation)
gone → /gɔŋ/ (progressive assimilation)
take → /keɪk/ (regressive assimilation)

EXERCISE 7.13

Place an "X" in front of the words that correctly indicate the process of velar assimilation.

_____ 1. turkey → /kɝkɪ/	_____ 6. ring → /wɪŋ/
_____ 2. kill → /gɪl/	_____ 7. bang → /gæŋ/
_____ 3. mouse → /maʊp/	_____ 8. shook → /ʃʊg/
_____ 4. grass → /kræs/	_____ 9. cap → /kæk/
_____ 5. fake → /keɪk/	_____ 10. brag → /græg/

Voicing Assimilation

There are two types of voicing assimilation. The first type, **prevocalic voicing**, involves voicing of a normally unvoiced consonant. This occurs when the consonant precedes the nucleus of a syllable. That is, the unvoiced consonant assimilates to the (voiced) nucleus. Examples include:

pig → /bɪg/ (regressive assimilation)
cup → /gʌp/ (regressive assimilation)

Another type of voicing assimilation involves the **devoicing** of syllable-final voiced phonemes that either precede a pause or silence between words, or occur at the end of an utterance. That is, the final phoneme "assimilates to the silence" following the word (Ingram, 1976, p. 35). Examples include:

bad → /bæt/   (regressive assimilation)

hose → /hos/   (regressive assimilation)

EXERCISE 7.14

Indicate whether the transcriptions of the following words indicate prevocalic voicing (P) or devoicing (D). Write P or D in the blanks. If neither process is demonstrated, leave the item blank.

_____ 1. pear → /bɛr/   _____ 6. gone → /kɔn/

_____ 2. led → /lɛt/   _____ 7. train → /dreɪn/

_____ 3. fair → /vɛr/   _____ 8. flag → /flæk/

_____ 4. card → /kɑrt/   _____ 9. shoe → /ʒu/

_____ 5. high → /haɪt/   _____ 10. chair → /ʃɛr/

Complete Assignments 7-2 and 7-3.

Not all of the processes outlined above necessarily occur in the speech patterns of all typically developing children. The processes that are most common in typical children's speech patterns include weak syllable deletion, final consonant deletion, gliding, and cluster reduction (Stoel-Gammon & Dunn, 1985). Also, suppression of a particular process does not happen all at once. Suppression may initially occur for only certain phonemes in a class. For instance, children who demonstrate stopping may suppress the process for /f/ and /s/ before they suppress it for the fricatives /v, z, ʃ, ð, and θ/ and also for the affricates /tʃ/ and /dʒ/ (Grunwell, 1987). Although most phonological processes disappear in the speech patterns of typically developing children by the age of 4 (Hodson & Paden, 1991), some processes disappear earlier.

Suppose you just evaluated a 7-year-old child using a picture-naming task, and you transcribed the following responses for seven of the words presented:

Picture	Child's Production	Picture	Child's Production
stove	/toʊb/	zipper	/dɪpʊ/
bird	/bʊd/	blue	/bu/
bath	/bæt/	drum	/dʌm/
sun	/tʌn/		

A phoneme-by-phoneme analysis would reveal several errors, including the following:

omission	/s/	(stove)
	/l/	(blue)
	/r/	(drum)

substitution	d/z	(zipper)	ʊ/ɚ	(zipper)
	t/θ	(bath)	ʊ/ɝ	(bird)
	t/s	(sun)	b/v	(stove)
distortions	none			
additions	none			

Because there are several speech sound errors present, a clearer picture of this child's phonological system may emerge if the speech productions are scrutinized in terms of phonological processes the child has not yet suppressed:

Picture	Child's production	Phonemic change	Phonemic process(es)
stove	/toʊb/	st → t; v → b	cluster reduction; stopping
bird	/bʊd/	ɝ → ʊ	vocalization
bath	/bæt/	θ → t	stopping
sun	/tʌn/	s → t	stopping
zipper	/dɪpʊ/	z → d; ɚ → ʊ	stopping; vocalization
blue	/bu/	bl → b	cluster reduction
drum	/dʌm/	dr → d	cluster reduction

Upon analysis of the child's responses, it now becomes evident that the child still has not suppressed the processes of *stopping, cluster reduction*, and *vocalization*. Because these phonological processes typically disappear by the age of 6, treatment would be indicated for this child, focusing on the reduction of these processes.

Children with Phonological Disorders

Children with speech sound disorders often display some of the same types of phonological processes as typically developing children. However, the processes would be suppressed *later* than typically observed, as in the example given above. The phonological processes used most consistently by children with speech sound disorders include cluster reduction, stopping, and liquid simplification (a combination of gliding and vocalization) (Stoel-Gammon & Dunn, 1985). These specific processes are among those consistently seen in typically developing children as well.

Children with disordered phonology also display several processes not usually found in the speech of typically developing children. These processes are called **idiosyncratic processes.** Several idiosyncratic processes include (from Stoel-Gammon & Dunn, 1985):

1. *Glottal replacement*—the substitution of a glottal stop for another consonant.

   pick → /pɪʔ/   butter → /bʌʔʊ/ (with vocalization)   lip → /ʔɪp/

   When the initial sound of a word is replaced with a glottal stop, it may sound as if the intial sound is simply deleted. You will need to listen carefully to make sure.

2. *Initial consonant deletion*—the omission of a single consonant at the beginning of a word.

   cut → /ʌt/   game → /eɪm/

   In the case of initial consonant deletion, you will need to determine whether the initial consonant truly is being deleted or is being replaced with a glottal stop.

3. *Backing*—the substitution of a velar stop consonant for consonants usually produced more anterior in the oral cavity. Backing usually involves alveolars and palatals; however, labial sounds may be affected.

   time → /kaɪm/   zoom → /gum/   push → /pʊk/

4. *Stops replacing a glide*—the substitution of a stop for a glide.

   yes → /dɛs/   wait → /beɪt/

5. *Fricatives replacing a stop*—the substitution of a fricative for a stop (frication).

   sit → /sɪs/   doll → /zɔl/

EXERCISE 7.15

For each of the given transcriptions, fill in the blank with the name of the appropriate idiosyncratic process just described. There may be more than one answer for each item.

Example:

| cat | → | /kæʔ/ | glottal replacement |

1. chairs → /ɛrz/   _____
2. letter → /lɛsɚ/   _____
3. witch → /dɪtʃ/   _____
4. tape → /keɪp/   _____
5. bunny → /ʌʔɪ/   _____
6. bad → /gæʔ/   _____

Another method of phonological assessment, quite different from phonological process analysis, involves performing an inventory of a child's speech sound system on multiple levels including words, syllables, segments, and features. In this type of analysis, the child's speech sample can come from both administration of phonological tests (naming pictures) and/or from elicitation of spontaneous speech (e.g., telling a story). The clinician then takes the recorded sample and transcribes each word the child produces. Some of the information the clinician can gather from such an analysis includes:

1. A complete inventory of the individual consonants and vowels the child produces.
2. An inventory of syllable shapes used by the child; in other words, whether a child produces open and/or closed syllables and consonant clusters at the beginning and/or end of syllables.
3. The combination of consonants (C) and vowels (V) the child uses to produce various syllable types: CV, VC, CVC, CCVC, CVCC, and so on.
4. The word shapes the child produces—the number and types of syllables in a word. (That is, can a child produce only one-syllable words, or can he also produce two-, three-, and four-syllable words?)
5. The stress patterns the child produces in bisyllabic and multisyllabic words with varying stress patterns, such as, lion, giraffe, elephant, orangutan.

This type of analysis is important because the child's sound system is evaluated not just in terms of the phonemes that are produced correctly/incorrectly relative to the adult model, but it is also analyzed independently, as a functional system in its own right in terms of phoneme production in words varying in phonetic composition, stress, and number of syllables. In other words, phonemes are identified without consideration of what is phonemic or contrastive in the target language (adult system), but rather which consonants and vowels are used contrastively in particular contexts in the child's system.

Analysis of a child's phonological system at more than one level is termed **nonlinear phonology.** That is, the child's phonological system is evaluated by looking at sound patterns at various levels including words, syllables, segments, and features. In this approach, phonological structure can be viewed in a hierarchical manner (i.e., nonlinearly) by utilizing tree diagrams to show the relationships between the differing levels. These tree diagrams are similar to those introduced in Chapter 2 to illustrate syllable structure in words. Only now, there are more branches in the trees.

Utilizing this nonlinear approach, the phonological structure of the word "window" is presented in Figure 7.1. Note the hierarchical arrangement of the various levels, or tiers, labeled "word tier," "syllable tier," "onset-rhyme tier," "CV tier," "segmental tier," and "feature tier." In nonlinear phonology, segments are further divided into a set of hierarchically arranged features known as *feature geometry.* For our purposes, the feature tier will be described in terms of manner, place, and voicing (after Stoel-Gammon, 1996).

How does nonlinear phonology help in remediation of a child with a phonological disorder? A simple example may help answer this question. Your client may produce the word "cat" as /kae/. At first glance, it appears that she may have problems producing the final /t/ phoneme. However, does she really have problems with final /t/, or does she generally have problems producing final consonants in all CVC words? Since nonlinear phonology looks at phoneme production at several levels, the answer may become more evident by analyzing the client's speech sample and looking for patterns of production across a number of words. If it is determined that the child cannot produce final consonants in

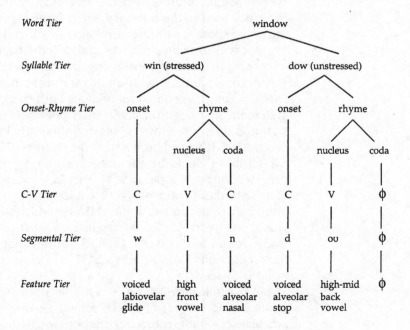

FIGURE 7.1 Hierarchical structure of the word "window."

words, it could be considered a "constraint" on a particular tier of her phonological system, whereas the absence of /t/ in "cat" but the presence of other consonants in coda position would be a constraint on a different tier.

Nonlinear phonology emphasizes the fact that all levels or tiers are connected hierarchically to each other and the interactions between segments and syllables can be observed by diagramming the client's phonological system. In order for your client's phonology to improve, therapy will need to consider what constraints exist and how remediation aimed at different tiers would improve her ability to produce the adult pattern.

EXERCISE 7.16

Draw the hierarchical structure of the word "platoon," making sure to indicate all of the following tiers: *word, syllable, onset-rhyme, C-V, segmental, and feature (place, manner, and voicing).*

Complete Assignments 7-4 and 7-5.

Transcription of Speech Sound Disorders: Diacritics

So far in this text we have been using *systematic phonemic transcription* as a method of recording on paper phonemes in words and sentences. We have paid little attention to allophonic variation in phoneme production. In this chapter, we will turn our attention to the use of *systematic narrow transcription* in order to more accurately describe the utterances of individuals who exhibit speech sound disorders. In the last chapter, you were introduced to some diacritics used in the transcription of some suprasegmental aspects of speech, including those for timing of phonemes [:], and for juncture [|] and [||]. This chapter will introduce diacritics used in the transcription of *segmental* aspects of speech, that is, for transcribing vowels and consonants. It is important that you become familiar with allophonic transcription of individual phonemes. Often, when transcribing individuals with speech sound disorders, the use of systematic phonemic (broad) transcription will not suffice because broad transcription does not allow for transcription of allophonic variation in phoneme production. If a child pronounces the word "red" as /wɛd/ (gliding), phonemic transcription would be adequate in capturing the production on paper. Now consider the speech patterns of a child who has a cleft palate and has problems with nasal emission (air escaping through the nasal cavity). Systematic phonemic transcription of the child's production of the word "smile," /smaɪl/, would not indicate the occurrence of nasal emission. A systematic narrow transcription of this word, [s̃maɪl], reveals that nasal emission occurred during production of /s/. (The symbol [˜] represents an allophone of [s], [s] with nasal emission.)

In the following section, several diacritics will be introduced as they relate to allophonic variants of speech sounds associated with (1) changes in place of articulation, (2) stop consonant production, (3) nasality, and (4) voicing. Only some of the more commonly used diacritics will be discussed on the following pages. The diacritic markings adopted in this text are from the 2005 revision of the IPA. Refer to Figure 2.1 for the complete list of the IPA diacritics.

Some of the diacritics can be used in transcribing typical pronunciation patterns. For instance, all voiceless stop consonants are aspirated when they occur in the initial position of a word. Narrow transcription of the word "teen" [tʰin] shows a raised "h" indicating that it has been produced with aspiration. In transcribing individuals with speech sound disorders, it might not be necessary to show the occurrence of aspiration in contexts where aspiration is expected to occur, as in the word "teen." Instead, you would need to indicate aspiration in transcription of phonetic contexts where it is not expected to occur. Also, you would need to indicate missing aspiration when it is expected to occur.

Place of Articulation

There are several IPA diacritics that are used to indicate allophonic variants related to changes in place of articulation of consonants and vowels. Some of these changes occur as a result of assimilation processes. Others occur as a result of dialect or phonological disorder.

Advanced/Retracted [k̟]/[t̠]

These two symbols are used to indicate a variation in tongue position associated with phoneme production. For example, when a consonant is produced with the tongue more forward in the oral cavity than normal (advanced), the symbol [₊] is used. For instance, the narrow transcription of the word "key" would be [k̟i] because the /k/ (normally produced with the body of the tongue in the velar region) is produced closer to the palate due to the environment provided by the front vowel /i/ (regressive assimilation).

When a consonant is produced with the tongue farther back than normal (retracted), the symbol [_] is used. When the alveolar stops /t/ or /d/ precede /r/, their place of articulation becomes postalveolar (closer to the palate) because /r/ is a palatal phoneme. Some examples include "true" [t̠ru] and "dry" [d̠raɪ] (regressive assimilation). Because of the backed articulation of these consonants, the words "true" and "dry" may appear to sound like /tʃru/ and /dʒraɪ/, respectively.

These two symbols may also be used to indicate a variation in tongue advancement associated with vowel production. The change in articulation may be due to dialectal variation (see Chapter 8) or a speech sound disorder. The change would involve the front/back dimension. For example, a retracted production of /æ/ would be transcribed as [æ̠], indicating that the vowel is farther back than would be expected, but not so far back as to result in the production of the vowel /ɑ/. Similarly, an advanced production of /ɑ/, that is, [ɑ̟], would be farther forward than normal, but not enough to result in production of /æ/.

EXERCISE 7.17

Place an "X" by the words that have a correct transcription using the diacritics [₊] and [_].

_____	1. could	[k̟ʊd]	_____	3. drop	[d̠rɑp]	_____	5. keep	[k̟ip]
_____	2. kiss	[k̟ɪs]	_____	4. clam	[kl̠æm]	_____	6. comb	[koʊm̟]

Raised, Lowered [ˌ , ˍ]

These diacritics can be placed beneath a vowel when there is a change in the height dimension associated with that vowel. The change in tongue height may be the result of a particular dialectal pronunciation of a vowel or as a result of a speech disorder. The symbol [ˌ] indicates that a vowel is produced with the body of the tongue raised more than expected for that particular vowel. For instance, if an adult attempts to produce the vowel /ɛ/, but raises the tongue higher than expected (but not so high as to produce /ɪ/), the transcription would be [ɛ̝]. Likewise, production of /ʊ/ with a lowered tongue position would be transcribed as [ʊ̞], as long as the production does not result in articulation of the vowel /o/.

EXERCISE 7.18

Examine each of the following vowels and their transcriptions. Then indicate which vowel would result if the articulation was raised, lowered, advanced, or retracted (depending on the diacritic used).

Examples:

vowel produced: resultant vowel is closer to:

    [i̞]   /ɪ/

    [ɑ̟]   /æ/

1. [ɛ̝] ___	5. [u̞] ___
2. [æ̝] ___	6. [ɛ̞] ___
3. [o̝] ___	7. [ɪ̞] ___
4. [o̞] ___	8. [u̟] ___

Labialized [ʷ]

A consonant that is not normally produced with lip rounding may become rounded in the presence of certain phonemes, for example, /u/, /ʊ/, or /w/. This phenomenon can be seen in the initial consonantal phoneme of "quick," "good," "zoo," and "rude." The additional articulation of lip rounding, associated with consonant production, is called **labialization.** The diacritic commonly used for a labialized phoneme is a "w" placed to the right of the normally unrounded phoneme as in [kʷwɪk], [gʷʊd], [zʷu], and [rʷud]. The transcriptions [kʷwɪk], [gʷʊd], [zʷu], and [rʷud] represent regressive, or right-to-left, assimilation, because the normally rounded phoneme follows the phoneme undergoing assimilation. Labialization may also occur in some cases of speech sound disorder when it is not expected to occur (not due to phonetic context).

EXERCISE 7.19

Transcribe these words, using the [ʷ] diacritic if the initial phoneme is labialized due to the phonetic environment. If the word does not have a labialized initial phoneme, leave the item blank.

Continues

EXERCISE 7.19 (cont.)

Examples:

swim	[sʷwɪm]
wood	_____ *

1. hood _____
2. shock _____
3. roof _____
4. thin _____
5. wool _____
6. plus _____
7. sweet _____
8. dune _____

*(/w/ is already a labialized consonant)

More Rounded/Less Rounded [i̹] / [u̜]

One variation in vowel production, sometimes seen in disordered speech, is the production of unrounded vowels as "more rounded" and the production of rounded vowels as "less rounded." The IPA symbol for an unrounded vowel produced with "more rounding" would be [i̹]. In the case where a normally rounded vowel becomes "less rounded," the appropriate IPA symbol (i.e., [u̜]) would be used.

Ball and Müller (2005) recommend the use of existing IPA vowel symbols when transcribing vowel rounding errors. For instance, if a child produces a rounded version of /i/, it would be appropriate to use the IPA symbol /y/, which is the symbol for a rounded, high front vowel (see Figure 2.1). This phoneme is not found in English, but can be found in other languages, such as German and French. Similarly, the IPA symbol for an unrounded version of the high back vowel /u/ would be /ɯ/, a vowel common in Korean. Since these IPA symbols are not common in English, you will need to refer to the IPA vowel chart in order to determine the rounded/unrounded counterparts of the English vowels.

EXERCISE 7.20

Use the appropriate IPA symbol for more or less liprounding for each of the following vowels.

Example:

/ɪ/   [ɪ̹]

1. /e/ _____		4. /ɛ/ _____
2. /o/ _____		5. /ɔ/ _____
3. /ʊ/ _____		6. /æ/ _____

EXERCISE 7.21

Using the IPA chart (Figure 2.1) as your guide, select the appropriate IPA vowel symbol for transcription of each of the following vowel conditions.

Example:

unrounded /i/ ___/y/___

1. unrounded /o/ _____   4. unrounded /u/ _____
2. rounded /ɛ/ _____   5. rounded /e/ _____
3. rounded /ɑ/ _____   6. unrounded /ɔ/ _____

Dentalization [t̪]

Alveolar consonants sometimes may be produced with a dental, instead of an alveolar, articulation. That is, the tongue tip makes contact with the upper front teeth (central incisors) during production. This process is termed **dentalization.** In the word "ninth," /n/ becomes dentalized in typical speech production. That is, the alveolar /n/ has a dental articulation brought about by the final phoneme /θ/ in "ninth." It would be possible to transcribe this word as [naɪn̪θ], given that the articulation is more forward than usual. However, when an alveolar phoneme is produced with a dental articulation, the dentalization symbol [̪] is preferred. Other words with dentalized alveolars include "filth" [fɪl̪θ] and "month" [mʌn̪θ]. These examples show regressive or right-to-left assimilation. The effect of dentalization crosses word boundaries as well. For instance, in the phrase "with Terry," the /t/ becomes dentalized, that is, [wɪθt̪ɛrɪ]. Notice that the plosive /t/ is released between the teeth. This is an example of progressive or left-to-right assimilation.

Dentalization occurs in some instances of disordered speech. Some young children produce dentalized /s/ and /z/ in words, such as "shoe" [s̪u] and "zoo" [z̪u] with the tongue tip touching the upper incisors during production of /s/. This is sometimes referred to as a *frontal lisp.* Some individuals transcribe this particular speech production as a /θ/ for /s/, or a /ð/ for /z/ substitution, as in "suit" /θut/ or "zebra" /ðibrə/. It is suggested that the correct transcription for this particular production should be [s̪] or [z̪], not /θ/ or /ð/, as long as the articulation retains a sibilant quality (Hodson & Paden, 1991).

Some children with phonological disorders also produce the affricates /tʃ/ and /dʒ/ as [t̪θ] and [d̪ð], respectively, as in "rich" [rɪt̪θ] and "jam" [d̪ðæm] (Powell, 2001). In this case, the articulation for the plosive portion of the affricate is no longer alveolar, it is dental, with the tongue tip between the front teeth. Also, note the substitution of the dental fricatives /θ/ and /ð/ for the palatal fricatives /ʃ/ and /ʒ/.

Some hearing-impaired children with cochlear implants may produce interdental fricatives as dentalized alveolar stops, as in "thumb" [t̪ʰʌm] and "mother" [mʌd̪ɚ], and labiodental stops may be produced in place of labiodental fricatives, as in "fish" [p̪ʰɪʃ] and "vase" [b̪eɪs] (Teoh & Chin, 2009). (Try producing /p/ with a labiodental articulation (instead of bilabial) by bringing your lower lip and upper incisors together.)

EXERCISE 7.22

Transcribe the following utterances, using the diacritic [̪] when necessary. Leave the item blank if it is not necessary to use the diacritic.

1. anthem   _____
2. moth   _____
3. either   _____
4. bathroom   _____
5. math time   _____
6. wealth   _____
7. rhythm   _____
8. panther   _____

Labiodental [ɱ]

In words in which the nasal consonants /m/ or /n/ are followed by /f/, the place of articulation is altered, due to the influence of the labiodental place of articulation for /f/ (regressive assimilation). Although English does not have a labiodental nasal phoneme, other languages do. The IPA symbol for this phoneme is /ɱ/. Because English does not make use of /ɱ/ phonemically, this assimilation may be considered an allophonic variant, not a phonemic change. Words in which this labiodental nasal occurs (depending on an individual speaker's pronunciation) include "comfort" /kʌɱfɚt/, "conference" /kɑɱfrəns/, "unfair" /əɱfɛr/, "emphasis" /ɛɱfəsəs/, and "symphony" /sɪɱfəni/. The diacritic for dentalization also may be used to transcribe labiodental assimilation, e.g., "comfort" /kʌm̪fɚt/.

EXERCISE 7.23

Transcribe the following words using /ɱ/ where appropriate. If not appropriate, leave the item blank.

1. inferential   _____
2. sphinx   _____
3. Memphis   _____
4. perform   _____
5. unfriendly   _____
6. camphor   _____
7. sunflower   _____
8. pharynx   _____
9. identify   _____
10. kinfolk   _____

Velarized [ɫ]

Velarization occurs when the alveolar consonant /l/ is produced in the velar region of the vocal tract. This production of /l/ is said to be *velarized* or "dark." /l/ becomes velarized in the postvocalic position of most words, as in "ball" and "eagle." The diacritic commonly used for velarization is a tilde through the middle of the phoneme, as in [bɑɫ] and [igɫ]. The velarized [ɫ] is found in all occurrences of syllabic [l̩], as in "little" [lɪɾɫ̩] and "bagel" [beɪgɫ̩]. Keep in mind that [ɫ] and [l̩] are separate allophones of /l/.

Velarized [ɫ] is sometimes found to occur at the beginning of words. This may occur as a matter of speaking style, or it may be associated with a speech sound disorder. Some hearing-impaired children produce [ɫ] at word onset as in "leave" [ɫiv] or "leg" [ɫɛg]. Word-initial [ɫ] may sound as if it is preceded by /g/ due to the velarized /l/, as in "love" [gɫʌv] (Teoh & Chin, 2009).

EXERCISE 7.24

Place an "X" next to the words that normally would *not* have a velarized /ɫ/ in their transcriptions.

1. _____ lake
2. _____ mingle
3. _____ loop
4. _____ beagle
5. _____ balding

6. _____ liked
7. _____ hilly
8. _____ Elton
9. _____ lady
10. _____ alone

Stop Consonant Production

In Chapter 5 you learned that stop consonants are comprised of an articulatory closure, an increase in intraoral pressure, and a release burst at one of three points of articulation: bilabial, alveolar, or velar. The manner in which stop consonants are produced (released, unreleased, aspirated, unaspirated) varies as a function of phonetic environment, dialect, and whether a person has a speech sound disorder.

Unreleased Stops [p̚]

An **unreleased** stop consonant is one that has no audible release burst associated with it. Unreleased stops occur quite often in English at the ends of words as in "leak," "put," "map," "hog," and "red." Contrast the production of the word "stop" first by releasing the final /p/ and then by not releasing it. The transcription of the unreleased production would be [stɑp̚]. Likewise, contrast the two productions of the word "bid," that is, [bɪd̚] and [bɪd]. When two voiceless stop consonants occur one after the other in the same syllable, the first one is not released, as in the words "stacked" [stæk̚t] and "reaped" [rip̚t].

Aspiration of Stops [pʰ]

Aspiration is often defined as a burst of air associated with the production of voiceless stop consonants (Calvert, 1986; MacKay, 1987). This definition may be somewhat misleading, because all stop consonants have a noise burst associated with their production. Aspiration involves the production of a frictional noise (similar to the glottal phoneme /h/) following the release of a voiceless stop and preceding the following vowel. There is, in a sense, a second burst of noise associated with voiceless stops. Keep in mind that aspiration occurs only in the presence of the voiceless stop consonants /p/, /t/, and /k/. Although there is an audible release burst associated with voiced stops, aspiration (the second frictional noise) is absent.

Aspiration occurs most often in released voiceless stops in the initial position of *stressed* syllables. Examples of aspiration occur in the words: "pass" [pʰæs], "torn" [tʰɔrn], "kiss" [kʰɪs], "atone" [ətʰoʊn], and "repay" [rəpʰeɪ]. Released voiceless stops at the ends of words may be aspirated as well, as in "leap" [lipʰ], "snake" [sneɪkʰ], and "right" [raɪtʰ]. Aspiration does *not* normally occur when a voiceless stop follows the fricative /s/, as in "spoon," "scat," or "stood." If an aspirated stop does occur in this phonetic environment due to a speech sound disorder, it should be marked appropriately, e.g., "spoon" [spʰun].

Unaspirated Stops [p⁼]

The symbol [⁼] is placed above and to the right of unaspirated voiceless stops. Unaspirated stops are most common when they occur immediately following the fricative /s/ as in the words "spin" [sp⁼ɪn] or "escape" [əsk⁼eɪp̚]. Although stops may be unaspirated, they may still be released. Both of the unaspirated stops in "spin" and "escape" are released.

Young children and children with phonological disorders may not aspirate initial stop consonants at the beginning of words as expected. When an aspirated stop is produced without aspiration, it may sound to a listener as a voiced stop. For instance "pan" [p⁼æn] might sound like "ban" /bæn/. Therefore, it is important to listen carefully to make sure your transcription is adequate. This is a misperception quite prone to transcription error (Louko & Edwards, 2001).

EXERCISE 7.25

Place an "X" next to each of the following words that normally contain an unaspirated phoneme.

1. ____ slack
2. ____ praised
3. ____ scorn
4. ____ despite

5. ____ excuse
6. ____ surprise
7. ____ stripe
8. ____ smooth

EXERCISE 7.26

Place an "X" next to the words that are typical transcriptions for the words given, using the diacritics for unreleased, unaspirated, and aspirated productions. If a transcription is given that is not typical in a particular phonetic context, correct it.

Examples:

| X | licked | [lɪk̚tʰ] | |
| ____ | cap | [kæp̚] | [kʰæp̚] |

Continues

EXERCISE 7.26 (cont.)

1. _____ skunk   [sk⁼ʌŋkʰ]   _____
2. _____ snacked   [snæk˺tʰ]   _____
3. _____ target   [tɑrgət˺]   _____
4. _____ brave   [bʰreɪv]   _____
5. _____ toga   [tʰoʊgʰə]   _____
6. _____ guarded   [gɑrdəd˺]   _____
7. _____ person   [pɝsʰən]   _____
8. _____ carefully   [kʰɛrfʊlɪ]   _____
9. _____ slope   [sl⁼oʊp˺]   _____
10. _____ great   [gʰreɪtʰ]   _____

Nasality

Several diacritics are used in narrow transcription to indicate changes in nasality associated with speech production. These include nasalization, nasal emission, and denasality.

Nasalization [æ̃]

Recall from Chapter 4 that vowels may become nasalized in the presence of nasal consonants. For example, in the word "mean," the vowel /i/ is surrounded by two nasal phonemes. The velum lowers during the production of the initial consonant /m/ and remains lowered throughout the word (for articulatory efficiency), because the final phoneme /n/ also is a nasal. The result is a nasalized vowel, as in [mĩn]. The following words also have nasalized vowels due to the nasal environment provided by /m/, /n/, or /ŋ/: "hang" [hæ̃ŋ], "in" [ĩn], "mom" [mãm], and both vowels in "roomy" [rũmĩ] and "any" [ɛ̃nĩ]. The effects of nasalization can also be seen across word boundaries as in "I can eat" [aɪ kæn ĩt]. Note that nasalization can be regressive, progressive, or a combination of both (as in the word "mom"). Some children with cochlear implants will show vowel nasalization preceding a nasal consonant, as predicted, but delete the consonant, as in "comb" [kʰõʊ̃] (Teoh & Chin, 2009).

In the transcription of disordered speech, this diacritic is also used to indicate the presence of excessive nasality associated with the production of non-nasal phonemes. This condition is known as hypernasal resonance or **hypernasality.** Hypernasality is usually due to improper velopharyngeal closure, as in cleft palate speech. Hypernasality may extend throughout an entire production of a word or an utterance.

Some hearing-impaired individuals with severe or profound loss may display hypernasality in their speech. In fact, deaf speech is often described as sounding "nasal." The problem in this case is not a physical one, since there is no structural deviation in the speech organs associated with velopharyngeal closure. Improper use of nasality is more likely due to faulty learning associated with the hearing loss. The auditory cues associated with nasality are difficult for deaf individuals to hear (Erber, 1983). Without having an appropriate auditory model of how oral versus nasal consonants should sound, it is difficult for deaf individuals to produce nasality correctly.

EXERCISE 7.27

Place an "X" next to the words where you might expect nasalization based upon the given phonetic context.

1. _____ mean   [m̃in]   4. _____ string   [strĩŋ]
2. _____ boon   [bũn]   5. _____ slam   [s̃læm]
3. _____ buddy   [bʌdĩ]   6. _____ thong   [θãŋ]

Nasal Emission [˜]

Nasal emission is the audible escape of air through the nares due to improper velopharyngeal closure. Airflow may escape through the velopharyngeal port itself or may escape through a cleft in the palate or velum. Individuals with cleft palate may exhibit nasal emission especially during the production of stops and fricatives (which require greater intraoral pressure) even if the cleft has been repaired. This is usually due to speaking habits learned prior to the surgery (Trost-Cardemone, 2009). The diacritic [˜] is used when nasal emission accompanies a phoneme that is *not* normally nasalized. Examples include "snail" [s̃neɪl], "nice" [naɪs̃], "zoo" [z̃u], and "pie" [p̃aɪ]. Keep in mind that nasal emission is not the same as nasalization. Nasalization of speech results when the velum is lowered in production of oral sounds, resulting in nasal resonance. Nasal emission is a process in which air escapes through the nares.

Denasality [˜]

Another condition related to nasality is **denasality,** also known as **hyponasality.** Denasality results when the nasal phonemes /m, n, and ŋ/ are produced *without* nasalization. Denasality is most often associated with the speech patterns of a person with a cold or upper respiratory tract infection. The utterance "My name is Matt" would sound like "By dabe is Batt," when spoken denasalized. Using the diacritic [˜] to indicate denasality, the above utterance would be transcribed as [m̃aɪ ñeɪm̃ ɪz m̃æt]. Children who do not have a cold but consistently sound like they do should probably be evaluated by a physician to determine whether a structural abnormality exists that may interfere with the production of nasal phonemes.

Voicing

These diacritics indicate a change in the manner of vocal fold vibration during the production of consonants and vowels. These changes include voicing and devoicing.

Voicing [t̬]

This diacritic is used when a voiceless phoneme is produced with partial voicing. A good example of voicing occurs when using the tap [ɾ] in the transcription of words such as "better" [bɛɾɚ] and "kitty" [kɪɾɪ]. In these words, the voiceless /t/ becomes partially voiced due to the voiced environment provided by the surrounding phonemes. However, the assimilation does not result in production of the voiced phoneme /d/. Some people use the diacritic for voicing instead of a tap when transcribing words such as "better" [bɛt̬ɚ] or "kitty" [kɪt̬ɪ]. Another example of partial voicing may occur in some pronunciations of the words "pester" [pɛs̬tɚ], "mister" [mɪs̬tɚ], and "Leslie" [lɛs̬lɪ].

EXERCISE 7.28

Transcribe the following words, using the diacritic for voicing instead of a tap (when necessary).

1. kettle _____   4. attempt _____
2. written _____   5. baton _____
3. water _____   6. battled _____

Devoicing [r̥]/[ʒ̥]

In certain phonetic environments, phonemes that are normally voiced become less voiced. This phenomenon is known as *devoicing*. Phonemes that become devoiced still have some voicing associated with them; they are not completely voiceless. The concept of devoicing is not really new to you. Recall that a word such as "ladder" is transcribed with the tap /ɾ/, indicating devoicing of the /d/ phoneme. You may recall that this assimilation results when /t/ or /d/ is intervocalic.

Devoicing also occurs when one of the approximants /w, l, r, or j/ follows a voiceless consonant. Examples include "pray" [p̥reɪ], "few" [fju̥], "clip" [kl̥ɪp], and "queen" [kw̥in]. Devoicing also may occur across word boundaries as in "thank you" [θæŋkju̥]. (Note the use of the diacritic *above* descending symbols such as /ʒ/.)

Words ending with a voiced fricative or affricate may become devoiced if silence follows the word, that is, if they are at the end of an utterance (Cruttenden, 2001). Examples include [bædʒ̥], [wʌz̥], and [lʌv̥]. In connected speech, when a word that ends with a voiced fricative is followed by a word that begins with a voiceless consonant, the fricative also may become devoiced (Cruttenden, 2001). For instance, the phrase "has seen" may be pronounced as [həz̥sin]. Other examples include "of course" [əv̥kɔrs], "she's sorry" [ʃiz̥sɑrɪ], and "I've passed" [aɪv̥pæst].

If a client is devoicing phonemes in contexts that are not expected, make sure to indicate that in your transcription using the [̥] diacritic. In cleft palate speech, voiceless plosives and fricatives may be produced as *voiceless* nasals (Grunwell & Harding, 1996). For example, "sun" [n̥ə̃n] or "pan" [m̥æ̃n].

EXERCISE 7.29

Using the diacritic for devoicing [̥], transcribe the following utterances.

1. pewter _____   5. he does _____
2. clearly _____   6. Ridge Street _____
3. he's stubborn _____   7. I lose _____
4. bathe Pam _____   8. they've played _____

Complete Assignments 7-6 and 7-7.

The extIPA and the VoQS

In 1994, an extension to the IPA was adopted by the International Clinical Phonetics and Linguistics Association (ICPLA) as the official set of diacritics to be used in the transcription of disordered speech. This extended version of the IPA is entitled the **extIPA** (Duckworth et al., 1990). The complete set of extIPA diacritics (revised to 2008) is located in Figure 7.2. You will notice that you are

extIPA SYMBOLS FOR DISORDERED SPEECH
(Revised to 2008)

CONSONANTS (other than on the IPA Chart)

	bilabial	labiodental	dentolabial	labioalv.	linguolabial	interdental	bidental	alveolar	velar	velophar.
Plosive	p̪ b̪		p̪̅ b̪̅	p̪ b̪	t̼ d̼	t̪̅ d̪̅				
Nasal			m̪̅	m̪	n̼	n̪̅				
Trill					r̼	r̪̅				
Fricative median			f̪̅ v̪̅	f̪ v̪	θ̼ ð̼	θ̪̅ ð̪̅	ħ̪̅ ɦ̪̅			f̦ŋ
Fricative lateral+median								ɬ̪ ɮ̪		
Fricative nareal	m̃							ñ	ŋ̃	
Percussive	w̬						ʭ			
Approximant lateral					l̼	l̪̅				

Where symbols appear in pairs, the one to the right represents a voiced consonant. Shaded areas denote articulations judged impossible.

DIACRITICS

labial spreading	s̒	„	strong articulation	f̬	͌	denasal	m̃
dentolabial	v̪̅	ˏ	weak articulation	v̞	˭	nasal escape	v̂
interdental/bidental	n̪̅	\	reiterated articulation	p\p\p	͌	velopharyngeal friction	s̆
alveolar	t̪	.	whistled articulation	s̩	↓	ingressive airflow	p↓
linguolabial	d̼	→	sliding articulation	θs̩	↑	egressive airflow	!↑

CONNECTED SPEECH

(.)	short pause
(..)	medium pause
(...)	long pause
f	loud speech [{f laʊd f}]
ff	louder speech [{ff laʊdɚ ff}]
p	quiet speech [{p kwaɪət p}]
pp	quieter speech [{pp kwaɪətɚ pp}]
allegro	fast speech [{allegro fɑst allegro}]
lento	slow speech [{lento sloʊ lento}]
crescendo, ralentando, etc. may also be used	

VOICING

̦	pre-voicing	̦z
̧	post-voicing	z̧
̨	partial devoicing	ꭧ
̧	initial partial devoicing	ꭧ
̧	final partial devoicing	z̧
̨	partial voicing	s̨
̧	initial partial voicing	ş
̧	final partial voicing	ş
˭	unaspirated	p˭
ʰ	pre-aspiration	ʰp

OTHERS

(◌), (C̈), (V̈)	indeterminate sound, consonant, vowel	ʞ	velodorsal articulation
(P̅l.v̅l̅s̅), (N̈)	indeterminate voiceless plosive, nasal, etc	꜊	sublaminal lower alveolar percussive click
( )	silent articulation (ʃ), (m)	!¡	alveolar and sublaminal clicks (cluck-click)
(( ))	extraneous noise, e.g. ((2 sylls))	*	sound with no available symbol

FIGURE 7.2 The extended IPA. © ICPLA 2008. Reproduced with permission.

already familiar with several of these symbols. The extIPA introduces several other symbols and terms for transcription of disordered speech. Several of the terms are described in Table 7.3.

The extIPA has several diacritics for indicating variations in intensity and tempo of connected speech as well as a notation system for indicating duration of pauses. As an example, normal intensity speech followed by very loud speech would be transcribed in the following manner:

[ðɪs ɪz nɔrməl ɪntɛnsɪtɪ spitʃ {*ff*falod baɪ spitʃ ðæt iz vɛrɪ laʊd*ff*}]

Note that *braces* are used to indicate the stretch of speech that is louder. The symbol *ff* stands for *fortissimo,* an Italian term used in music to denote a passage of music that is to be played very loud. Similarly, very soft speech would be indicated with the notation *pp,* from the Italian *pianissimo* for "very soft."

Diacritics are also provided in the extIPA to indicate variations in voicing patterns. The voicing diacritics allow for transcription of phonemes that are produced with pre-aspiration, as well as pre-, post-, or partial voicing.

Another extension to the IPA is the *Voice Quality Symbols,* or **VoQS** (Ball, Esling, & Dickson, 1995), see Figure 7.3. This extension was developed in order to provide speech pathologists with a more in-depth system of transcribing disorders associated with voice production, such as breathiness. Breathiness occurs when the vocal folds do not make sufficient contact during voicing, allowing

TABLE 7.3   Explanation of extIPA Terminology (from Duckworth et al., 1990)

ExtIPA Term	Description
Interdental	A phoneme produced with the tongue tip or blade between the teeth
Bidental	A voiceless or voiced glottal fricative produced with a constriction formed by the upper and lower teeth
Dentolabial	A plosive, fricative, or nasal phoneme produced when the lower lip contacts the upper teeth
Linguolabial	A plosive, fricative, nasal, or liquid (/l/) phoneme produced when the tongue contacts the upper lip
Labioalveolar	A plosive, fricative, or nasal phoneme produced when the alveolar ridge makes contact with the lower lip
Labial spreading	An abnormal degree of lip spreading associated with the production of a phoneme
Lateral + median fricative	The alveolar fricatives /s/ and /z/ produced with both a lateral and a medial airstream as in the production of some lateral lisps
Nareal fricative	Production of a nasal phoneme, /m, n, ŋ/, with accompanying nasal emission due to velopharyngeal incompetency
Velopharyngeal friction	The production of a frictional noise, or "snort," at the velopharyngeal port, due to velopharyngeal incompetency
Percussive	A stop produced by striking together two articulators, such as the cutting edges of the teeth or lips
Whistled articulation	Production of /s/ or /z/ with a very narrow tongue groove that creates a whistling sound
Reiterated articulation	An articulation that is repeated, as in stuttering
Silent articulation	A "mouthed" production of speech with no breath stream present
Extraneous noise	Speech or non-speech noise that obliterates the intended phonetic transcription
Indeterminate sound	An unrecognizable phoneme (circled); the extIPA has a notation system for indicating whether the indeterminate sound is a vowel, consonant, a voiceless plosive, etc. (see Figure 7.2)

VoQS: Voice Quality Symbols

Airstream Types

Œ	œsophageal speech	И	electrolarynx speech
Ю	tracheo-œsophageal speech	↓	pulmonic ingressive speech

Phonation types

V	modal voice	F	falsetto
W	whisper	C	creak
V̪	whispery voice (murmur)	V̬	creaky voice
Vʰ	breathy voice	Ç	whispery creak
V!	harsh voice	V!!	ventricular phonation
V̬!!	diplophonia	V̤!!	whispery ventricular phonation
V̟	anterior or pressed phonation	W̱	posterior whisper

Supralaryngeal Settings

L̝	raised larynx	L̞	lowered larynx
Vœ	labialized voice (open round)	Vʷ	labialized voice (close round)
V̪	spread-lip voice	Vᶹ	labio-dentalized voice
V̺	linguo-apicalized voice	V̻	linguo-laminalized voice
V˕	retroflex voice	V̪	dentalized voice
V̠	alveolarized voice	V̠ʲ	palatoalveolarized voice
Vʲ	palatalized voice	Vˠ	velarized voice
Vʁ	uvularized voice	Vˤ	pharyngealized voice
V̙ˤ	laryngo-pharyngealized voice	Vꞯ	faucalized voice
Ṽ	nasalized voice	Ṽ	denasalized voice
J̞	open jaw voice	J̝	close jaw voice
J̡	right offset jaw voice	J̢	left offset jaw voice
J̟	protruded jaw voice	Θ	protruded tongue voice

USE OF LABELED BRACES & NUMERALS TO MARK STRETCHES OF SPEECH
AND DEGREES AND COMBINATIONS OF VOICE QUALITY:

[ˈðɪs ɪz ˈnɔɹməl ˈvɔɪs {3V! ˈðɪs ɪz ˈvɛɹi ˈhaɹʃ ˈvɔɪs 3V} ˈðɪs ɪz ˈnɔɹməl ˈvɔɪs wʌns
ˈmɔɹ {L̝ 1V! ˈðɪs ɪz ˈlɛs ˈhaɹʃ ˈvɔɪs wɪð ˈlouəd ˈlæɹɪŋks 1V!L̝}]

FIGURE 7.3 The VoQS. © 1994 Martin J. Ball, John Esling, Craig Dickson. Reproduced with permission.

audible air to escape through the glottis. Causes of breathiness include growths, such as polyps or nodules, on the vocal folds. Some deaf speakers also display breathiness due to improper valving of air by the vocal folds, as air flows through the glottis from the lungs. The IPA diacritic [V̰] is used beneath specific phonemes that are produced with a breathy voice quality. If an entire utterance is breathy, it may be transcribed by using the symbol [V̰] preceding and following the breathy utterance. For example:

$$[\{V̰ \ aɪ \ hæv \ nɑdʒl̩z \ ɑn \ maɪ \ voʊkl̩ \ foldz \ V̰\}]$$

It is beyond the scope of this text to describe other conditions of the larynx that result in an alteration of voice quality. That material will be covered in coursework examining voice production (most likely at the graduate level).

Transcription of Speech Sound Disorders: Non-English Phonemes

Inspection of the IPA chart (Figure 2.1) indicates there are many consonant phonemes that do not appear in spoken English. Of the 58 pulmonic consonants listed (those produced with an egressive airstream from the lungs), only 22 occur in English. These do not include /w/ or the affricates /tʃ/ and /dʒ/. A couple of the IPA pulmonic consonants are produced only as allophones in English, namely, the glottal stop /ʔ/ and the alveolar tap /ɾ/. The lateral alveolar fricatives /ɬ/ (voiceless) and /ɮ/ (voiced) usually occur in English only in reference to disordered speech (see below). Although English has only two affricates, others such as /ts/, /dz/, and /pf/ do occur in other languages. The IPA chart also lists several non-pulmonic consonants (those not requiring an airstream from the lungs in their production), none of which are found in English. Finally, of the 28 vowels listed in the IPA chart, only 12 are produced in English (not counting /ɚ/, /ɝ/, or the diphthongs). Recall that some non-English IPA vowel symbols can be used when transcribing changes in liprounding associated with vowel production.

When transcribing disordered speech, it often becomes necessary to use some of the non-English phonemes represented in the IPA chart. This is because in some speech sound disorders, phonemes are produced with a place of articulation different from the intended target phoneme, such as substituting the voiceless velar fricative /x/ for the voiceless palatal fricative /ʃ/. Speech sound errors that require the use of non-English IPA characters in transcription generally involve changes in place of articulation of stops and fricatives. Also, some hearing-impaired speakers produce non-pulmonic implosive and ejective phonemes. Table 7.4 lists all of the non-English IPA symbols discussed in the following sections.

Glottal Stop [ʔ]

By now, you should be familiar with the use of the glottal stop in English, as in production of the word "button" /bʌʔn̩/. The glottal stop also appears in the speech of some children with phonological disorders, including those with hearing impairment (Levitt & Stromberg, 1983; Stoel-Gammon, 1983; Teoh & Chin, 2009). For instance, glottal stops may replace other stops or fricatives as in "puppy" /ʔʌʔi/, "sister" [ʔiʔʊ], or "maybe" [meʔi]. The glottal stop also may occur at the ends of words, as in "cat" /kʰæʔ/ or "caught" [kʰɔʔ]. You must

TABLE 7.4 Common Non-English IPA Symbols Used in Transcription of Speech Sound Disorders

Manner of Articulation	IPA Symbol Voiceless	Voiced	Example	
Glottal Stop	[ʔ]		puppy	[ʔʌʔɪ]
Fricatives				
Bilabial	[ɸ]	[β]	fat	[ɸæʔ]
Velar	[x]	[ɣ]	game	[ɣem]
Pharyngeal	[ʕ]	[ʕ]	sheep	[ʕip]
Lateral	[ɬ]	[ɮ]	zoo	[ɮu]
Affricates				
Bilabial	[pf]	[bv]	face	[pfes]
Alveolar	[ts]	[dz]	juice	[dzus]
Velar	[kx]	[gɣ]	ghost	[gɣos]
Approximant		[ʋ]	run	[ʋʌn]
Ejectives (voiceless)	[p', t', and k']		keep	[kip']
Implosives (voiced)	[ɓ, ɗ, and ɠ]		big	[ɓɪʔ]

learn to listen carefully to determine whether a glottal stop is being produced. For instance, in the word "cat," you would need to determine whether the final sound is /ʔ/, an omitted /t/ as in [kæ] or is being produced as an unreleased consonant, as in [kæt˺]. It should be noted that the presence of a glottal stop at the end of a word does not always signal the presence of a speech sound disorder. Glottal stops do occur naturally at the ends of words in some dialects of spoken English.

Cleft palate speakers also may produce glottal stops as substitutes for obstruents. In addition to possible problems with nasal emission and hypernasal resonance, cleft palate speakers may have difficulty producing stops due to decreased intraoral pressure in the oral cavity caused by the cleft. Substitution of a glottal stop assists in proper plosion with a place of articulation posterior to the cleft (so that no air escapes). Some examples include "top" [ʔɑ̃ʔʰ], "guess" [ʔɛ̃ʔ], and "comb" [ʔõm] (Trost-Cardemone, 2009). Glottal stop substitution may occur, even following surgery for the cleft, due to learned speaking habits.

Fricatives [ɸ, β, x, ɣ, ħ, ʕ, ʕ]
There are several IPA symbols for non-English fricatives that may be used in transcription of speech sound disorders. For example, *bilabial* and *velar* fricatives may be produced by some children with phonological disorders, including children with hearing loss (Louko & Edwards, 2001; Stoel-Gammon, 1983; Teoh & Chin, 2009). The bilabial fricatives [ɸ] (voiceless) and [β] (voiced) may be substituted for the labiodental fricatives /f/ and /v/, respectively. Similar to the labiodental fricatives, /f/ and /v/, the bilabial fricatives are non-strident (low intensity) and have a similar acoustic structure. Examples of bilabial fricative substitutions include "giraffe" [dəwæɸ] and "shovel" [dʌβoʊ] (Louko & Edwards, 2001).

Similarly, the velar fricatives /x/ (voiceless) and /ɣ/ (voiced) may be produced as a substitute for the velar stops /k/ and /g/. This is a substitution also seen in cleft palate speech. The velar fricatives are produced when full closure for the stops does not occur (Louko & Edwards, 2001). Some examples of velar fricative substitutions include "cat" /xæt/ or /ɣæt/, "game" /ɣem/, and "lecture" [lɛɣʒu].

In some cleft palate speakers, the fricatives /s, z, ʃ, or ʒ/ are backed and produced as pharyngeal fricatives (Trost-Cardemone & Bernthal, 1993). The IPA symbols for the pharyngeal fricatives are [ħ] (voiceless) and [ʕ] (voiced). Trust-Cardemone (2009) recommends the use of the symbol [ʕ] instead of [ħ] for the voiceless pharyngeal fricative. Some examples include "sheep" [ʕĩp] (or [ħip]) and "measure" [mɛ̃ʕɚ].

Lateral Fricatives [ɬ, ɮ]

Lateralization of the fricatives /s/ or /z/ occurs when the constricted airflow is diverted over the sides of the tongue, instead of being able to flow centrally. To produce a lateralized /s/, place your tongue in position for the initial phoneme in the word "let." Now, holding your tongue in place, try to produce an /s/ phoneme. Notice how the air flows over the sides of the tongue because it cannot escape anteriorly. This lateral production of /s/ or /z/ is sometimes referred to as a *lateral lisp* and is seen in some children with phonological disorders.

The IPA diacritic for a lateralized phoneme is a raised /l/, placed to the right of the indicated phoneme, as in [jɛsˡ]. There are other IPA symbols specifically used for transcription of a *lateral fricative*. The symbol [ɬ] represents a lateralized /s/, and [ɮ] represents a lateralized /z/. Examples include "yes" [jɛɬ] and "zoo" [ɮu]. Sometimes lateral fricatives are substituted for an affricate (deaffrication), as in "witch" [wɪɬ] and "jelly" [ɮɛlɪ].

The extIPA also lists two symbols for lateralized fricatives, [ʪ] (voiceless) and [ʫ] (voiced). These symbols are to be used when a fricative is produced with both a lateral *and* a central airstream.

Affricates [pf, bv, ts, dz, kx, gɣ]

Some individuals with phonological disorders may produce non-English affricates such as /pf/, /bv/ (bilabial), /ts/, /dz/ (alveolar), and /kx/, /gɣ/ (velar) (Louko & Edwards, 2001; Powell, 2001). The affricates /ts/ and /dz/ often replace /tʃ/ and /dʒ/ as in "watch" [wɑts] and "Jim" /dzɪm/. Other examples of non-English affricates include "fun" [pfʌn], "van" [bvæn], "ski" [kxi], and "go" [gɣo].

Approximant [ʋ]

Earlier in this chapter we discussed the fact that some children substitute /w/ for /r/ in a process commonly known as *gliding*. In some instances, however, the production is not truly a /w/, but somewhere between an /r/ and a /w/. What may occur in this case is the substitution of the voiced labiodental approximant [ʋ] for /r/ (Ball, 2008; Bauman-Waengler, 2008). This approximant is similar to /w/, however, it is labiodental, not labiovelar; there is no constriction of the tongue in the velar region. Instead, the lower lip and teeth are used in production of this sound. Because this phoneme is an approximant, the lower lip and teeth do not touch as would be the case for the labiodental fricative /v/.

Implosives [ɓ, ɗ, ɠ] and Ejectives [p', t', k']

An interesting phenomenon observed in the speech of some hearing-impaired speakers is the use of non-pulmonic **ejective** and **implosive** stop consonants. Both ejectives and implosive consonants rely on a *glottalic* airstream, as opposed to a pulmonic airstream. Both implosive and ejective consonants occur in some African and Native American languages. An ejective is produced in a manner similar to a pulmonic stop consonant. However, during its production, the vocal folds close and then are *raised,* causing a decrease in the area between the closed vocal folds and the constriction in the oral cavity formed by the tongue. This results in a greater amount of intraoral pressure than would be typical of a pulmonic stop. Then, when the stop is released, there is a large burst of air due to the increased intraoral pressure. Conversely, implosives are produced by *lowering* the vocal folds, thereby increasing the area of the vocal tract and decreasing the intraoral pressure between the vocal folds and the constriction in the oral cavity. When the stop is released, air flows *into* the vocal tract (an *ingressive* airstream).

It is not completely clear why hearing-impaired individuals produce ejectives and implosives. It is believed that these behaviors develop either due to the provision of increased tactile/kinesthetic feedback (Higgins et al., 1996), or as a result of faulty learning while developing the ability to produce voiced and voiceless stops (Monsen, 1983). The IPA symbols for the implosive and ejective stops (at the bilabial, alveolar, and velar places of articulation) are given below. The remaining implosive and ejective IPA symbols can be found in Figure 2.1.

	Implosive	Ejective
bilabial	/ɓ/	/p'/
dental/alveolar	/ɗ/	/t'/
velar	/ɠ/	/k'/

Implosives and ejectives have also been known to occur in individuals who stutter, and in people with phonological disorders not related to hearing impairment (Ball & Müller, 2007).

EXERCISE 7.30

Write the intended IPA symbol for each description given.

1. voiceless velar fricative   _____
2. voiceless bilabial affricate _____
3. voiced pharyngeal fricative   _____
4. voiced bilabial fricative   _____
5. voiceless lateral fricative   _____
6. velar ejective   _____
7. labiodental approximant   _____
8. alveolar implosive   _____
9. voiced velar fricative   _____
10. labiodental nasal   _____

Suggestions for Transcription

The complete set of combined diacritics from the revised 1996 IPA symbols, the extIPA, and from the VoQS seems extraordinarily overwhelming at first. The combined diacritic sets allow for the transcription of virtually all possible allophonic variants of English as well as most typical speech sound errors.

Obviously, not all of these symbols would be used routinely in the transcription of disordered speech. This raises an interesting question. Which symbols should be used routinely when transcribing disordered speech? This is not an easy question to answer. Undoubtedly, every speech-language pathologist would have a different answer to this question. The most important consideration is the accuracy of the transcription being performed. It is not necessarily important to indicate normal allophonic variations of phonemes if they do not disrupt the production of speech. For instance, there would be no need to indicate nasalized vowels, as long as the nasalization was appropriate. If, however, a client had inappropriate nasalization of speech, the appropriate diacritic [~] would then need to be indicated in the transcription.

When you begin transcribing both live and recorded samples of your clients, there are several factors you will need to consider so that your transcriptions will be as accurate as possible. Keep in mind that your clients' speech patterns often will be difficult to understand. This means that a good recording is necessary so that you will be able to replay the speech sample at a later time. Modern digital recorders are quite good at capturing your clients' speech. However, no matter how good the recording, certain phonemes may not always be audible during playback. This is due to the fact that some English phonemes are naturally low in intensity. This is especially true of the voiceless fricatives /f/, /θ/, and /ɸ/. This is one reason why it is extremely important for you to transcribe face to face during testing. Of course, wearing headphones (attached to your recorder) will aid in your transcription accuracy by reducing any background noise that might be present. Also, when you are performing a live transcription, you will be able to visually focus on the clients' articulators, especially in reference to lip rounding and tongue placement for certain phonemes. Although it is possible to make a video recording of your clients' diagnostic session, facial features may not always be clearly represented because video images only provide a two-dimensional view of the client.

Stoel-Gammon (2001, p. 15) suggests the following before beginning a transcription session:

1. Work in a quiet area.
2. Spend no more than 2–3 hours transcribing at any one time; take a 5–10 minute break every 45 minutes.
3. Before beginning, listen to an extended sample to become used to the speech patterns you will be transcribing.
4. Avoid being influenced by knowledge of the target words you are transcribing.
5. Listen to the vocalizations as many times as needed.

When listening to a recorded sample of a client's speech, it will become immediately apparent that certain speech segments will be easier to transcribe than others. Begin with the speech segments of which you are sure. You also may want to transcribe phonemes first, adding the diacritics later. Ohde and Sharf (1992, pp. 351–352) offer several beneficial suggestions to help the clinician focus on speech patterns that are particularly difficult to transcribe. Their transcription techniques include the following:

1. Count the number of syllables in each produced utterance and determine if it agrees with the number in the target utterance.
2. Identify the vowels, diphthongs, or syllabic consonants that constitute the nucleus of each syllable, using the minimal contrasts of front-back, high-low, tense-lax, and rounded-unrounded to zero in on the vowel.

3. Transcribe the syllable nuclei you are certain of, leaving space for preceding and following consonants.
4. Determine whether each vowel nucleus is initiated and terminated by a consonant or consonant cluster and if a target consonant is deleted.
5. Identify the consonants, using manner, voicing, and place feature analysis to zero in on them, and transcribe those you are certain of.
6. Decide which features of the remaining consonants you are uncertain about and how they differ from the target consonants.
7. Transcribe the consonants, using appropriate diacritics to indicate deviations from targets, if necessary.

Of course, it may not be possible for you to identify *every* phoneme that your client produces. When this happens, it may be necessary to use the appropriate symbols from the extIPA to indicate indeterminate sounds, that is sounds of which you are unsure. For instance, if you know a particular phoneme is a vowel, but you are not sure of the exact vowel, you would write V with a circle around it (i.e., Ⓥ to represent the phoneme in question). Or if you knew the phoneme was a voiceless plosive, but were not sure if it was /p, t, or k/, you would transcribe the phoneme as Pl, vls with a circle around it (i.e., ⟨Pl, vls⟩)

During transcription, you should be careful about "second guessing" or having expectations about what your client is attempting to say. In some instances, knowing what your client is saying may help you get a more accurate transcription. However, it is possible your expectations may be wrong and cause you to transcribe your client incorrectly. For example, Louko and Edwards (2001) report a case where a child was shown a picture of "twins" and the child responded ['tʰoːˌwĩn]. In reality, the child was attempting to say "children," *not* "twins." Upon additional exploration, the clinician did get the child to say [tʰɪnz], proving the child's first response was not at all a production of the word "twins." Had the clinician not investigated further, her transcription of "twins" as ['tʰoːˌwĩn] and not [tʰɪnz] could have turned out to be problematic when determining the specific phonological errors the child was exhibiting.

Review Exercises

A. Each of the following speech productions represent one type of *syllable structure process*. Match one of the processes given at the right to each transcription given.

Examples:

b	coat	/koʊ/	a. weak syllable deletion
c	kitty	/kɪkɪ/	b. final consonant deletion
			c. reduplication
			d. cluster reduction

____	1.	school	/kul/	____	6.	swing	/sɪŋ/
____	2.	candy	/kækæ/	____	7.	soap	/soʊ/
____	3.	lion	/laɪ/	____	8.	cookie	/kiki/
____	4.	mom	/mɑ/	____	9.	missed	/mɪt/
____	5.	running	/rʌn/	____	10.	water	/wɑ/

B. For each item, indicate whether the transcription indicates regressive (R) or progressive (P) assimilation.

Example:

   P   cup   /kʌk/

_____ 1. finger   /gɪŋgɚ/   _____ 6. feather   /fɛvɚ/
_____ 2. table   /peɪbl̩/   _____ 7. pillow   /pɪboʊ/
_____ 3. rabbit   /bæbɪt/   _____ 8. mat   /mæp/
_____ 4. map   /mæm/   _____ 9. sip   /zɪp/
_____ 5. park   /kɑrk/   _____ 10. grab   /græg/

C. Each of the following transcriptions reflects some form of assimilation. Match the type of assimilation to each transcription given.

Example:

   b   cup   /kʌk/   a. labial   d. prevocalic voicing
                                  b. velar   e. devoicing
                                  c. alveolar

_____ 1. pan   /tæn/   _____ 6. sunny   /zʌnɪ/
_____ 2. face   /veɪs/   _____ 7. green   /grɪŋ/
_____ 3. swim   /ɸwɪm/   _____ 8. sack   /sæt/
_____ 4. bad   /bæt/   _____ 9. park   /kɑrk/
_____ 5. numb   /mʌm/   _____ 10. nag   /næk/

D. For each of the following, match the transcription to the appropriate substitution process being demonstrated. There may be more than one correct answer per item.

_____ 1. mister   /mɪstʊ/   a. gliding
_____ 2. yellow   /jɛwoʊ/   b. deaffrication
_____ 3. matches   /mæʃəz/   c. vocalization
_____ 4. cage   /keɪʒ/
_____ 5. reel   /wiʊ/
_____ 6. little   /jɪroʊ/
_____ 7. choose   /ʃuz/
_____ 8. press   /pwɛs/

E. Match the transcriptions with the process being demonstrated. Each item has more than one correct answer.

_____ 1. jumped   /dʌmpt/   a. fronting
_____ 2. shampoo   /tæmpu/   b. stopping
_____ 3. watch   /wɑs/   c. deaffrication
_____ 4. feet   /bit/   d. prevocalic voicing
_____ 5. said   /dɛd/
_____ 6. thicker   /dɪkɚ/
_____ 7. shared   /zɛrd/
_____ 8. chops   /tɑps/

F. For each of the following words, apply the phonological process given and transcribe the resulting production.

    Example:

lean	final consonant deletion	/li/

   1. sleep   cluster reduction   _____

   2. brag   velar assimilation   _____

   3. jar   stopping   _____

   4. lemon   gliding   _____

   5. bake   labial assimilation   _____

   6. jelly   deaffrication   _____

   7. above   weak syllable deletion   _____

   8. pine   alveolar assimilation   _____

   9. came   fronting   _____

  10. crow   prevocalic voicing   _____

G. Indicate whether the given phonological process is possible for each of the words given. Circle "Yes" or "No."

   1. clown   weak syllable deletion   Yes   No

   2. pup   labial assimilation   Yes   No

   3. Jenny   reduplication   Yes   No

   4. cry   gliding   Yes   No

   5. shot   fronting   Yes   No

   6. play   devoicing   Yes   No

   7. stove   velar assimilation   Yes   No

   8. ship   stopping   Yes   No

   9. chew   deaffrication   Yes   No

  10. chair   cluster reduction   Yes   No

  11. penny   prevocalic voicing   Yes   No

  12. clay   final consonant deletion   Yes   No

H. Write the description for each of the following diacritics taken from the extIPA.

   1. m\m\m _____   5. θ̞ _____

   2. h̪ _____   6. s̰ _____

   3. ŋ̃ _____   7. r̰ _____

   4. ḇ _____   8. ƶ _____

I. Transcribe the following words as spoken by a 5-year-old male child who demonstrates *gliding*.

   1. lobster   _____   7. dentist   _____

   2. nurse   _____   8. refrigerator   _____

CD #3   3. soldier   _____   9. telephone   _____

Track 10   4. astronaut   _____   10. lamp   _____

   5. teacher   _____   11. toothbrush   _____

   6. truck driver   _____   12. bathtub   _____

13. toilet _____

14. hammer _____

15. alarm clock _____

16. vacuum cleaner _____

17. elephant _____

18. tiger _____

19. squirrel _____

20. spider _____

21. lion _____

22. dolphin _____

23. kangaroo _____

24. octopus _____

25. lawyer _____

J. Transcribe the following words and sentences as spoken by a 7-year-old female child who demonstrates *dentalization* of alveolar fricatives.

CD #3 Track 11

1. cherries _____

2. celery _____

3. cheese _____

4. cereal _____

5. grapes _____

6. ice cream _____

7. peas _____

8. pancakes _____

9. eggs _____

10. spider _____

11. octopus _____

12. squirrel _____

13. snake _____

14. skunk _____

15. jeans _____

16. sweater _____

17. pajamas _____

18. sandals _____

19. mittens _____

20. slippers _____

21. We went to Ben Franklin's and looked at the toys.

_____

22. I saw some dolls that I liked.

_____

23. They traveled to Maine from Nebraska.

_____

24. We do spelling and math.

_____

25. Sometimes we play mystery games.

_____

K. Transcribe the following words as spoken by a 7-year-old female child who demonstrates both *vocalization* and *dentalization* of alveolar fricatives.

CD #3 Track 12

1. frog _____

2. zebra _____

3. cookies _____

4. hamburger _____

5. skunk _____

6. strawberries _____

7. parakeet _____

8. carrots _____

9. cereal _____

10. hotdog _____

11. pancakes _____

12. celery _____

13. giraffe _____

14. lobster _____

15. rabbit _____

16. spider _____

17. elephant _____

18. ice cream _____

19. butter _____

20. cherries _____

21. squirrel _____   24. potato _____

22. orange _____   25. turtle _____

23. horse _____

L. For each of the following, write the appropriate IPA symbol for the description given.

Example:

dentalized /n/ _____[n̪]_____

1. aspirated /p/ _____   6. nasalized /o/ _____

2. raised /u/ _____   7. less rounded /w/ _____

3. devoiced /r/ _____   8. unreleased /k/ _____

4. labialized /g/ _____   9. denasalized /ŋ/ _____

5. lateralized /z/ _____   10. fronted /k/ _____

M. Select an English word in which you might find each of the following diacritics. Write the word in IPA using the appropriate transcription.

1. [t̚] _____   6. [n̩] _____

2. [m̃] _____   7. [d̪] _____

3. [bʲ] _____   8. [ɫ] _____

4. [ɛ̃] _____   9. [m̥] _____

5. [t̪] _____   10. [ʔ] _____

N. Circle the most accurate allophonic transcription for each of the following words.

1. clue   [kʰlu]   [k̥ɫu]   [kʰɫu]

2. lymph   [lɪɱf]   [ɫɪmf]   [lɪmpʰf]

3. money   [mʌni]   [mʌ̃nɪ]   [m̥ʌnɪ]

4. coop   [kʰupʰ]   [kʰupʰ]   [kʰup̚]

5. trial   [t̪ʰ̥ɹaɪɫ]   [t̪ʰɹaɪɫ]   [tʰɹaɪɫ]

6. skunk   [sk̚ʌŋkʰ]   [skʰʌŋkʰ]   [sk̚ʌ̃ŋkʰ]

7. menthol   [mɛ̃n̪θaɫ]   [mɛ̃nθal]   [mɛ̃nθaɫ]

8. sweet   [swit̚]   [swʷit̚]   [sʷw̥itʰ]

Study Questions

1. What is clinical phonetics?

2. What is the difference between an articulation disorder and a phonological disorder?

3. Define the terms *substitution, distortion, omission,* and *addition.*

4. Which manners of articulation appear first in typically developing children? Which places of articulation appear first?

5. What are the differences between syllable structure processes, assimilatory processes, and substitution processes?

6. Describe the following phonological processes:

   a. stopping
   b. fronting
   c. deaffrication
   d. gliding
   e. vocalization

   f. weak syllable deletion
   g. cluster reduction
   h. final consonant deletion
   i. reduplication
   j. labial assimilation

   k. alveolar assimilation
   l. velar assimilation
   m. prevocalic voicing
   n. devoicing

7. Which of the processes in question 6 disappear by the age of 3;0 in typically developing children?

8. What is an *idiosyncratic* phonological process? Describe four such processes.

9. Of what importance is being able to perform a *systematic allophonic transcription* of a speech sample?

10. What is meant by the terms *nasal emission* and *denasality*?

11. When do the following stop consonant allophones generally occur in English?

    a. unreleased   b. aspirated   c. unaspirated

12. What is meant by the following terms?

    a. labialization   b. dentalization   c. velarization

13. What is the extIPA? What is the VoQS? When would these diacritic sets be employed in transcription?

14. Why is it important to become familiar with non-English IPA symbols in transcription of speech sound disorders?

15. Describe several strategies you might employ when attempting to transcribe the speech patterns of a disordered client.

16. What would be the advantage of performing a *nonlinear phonological analysis* versus a *phonological process analysis* when examining the speech sound errors of a client?

Online Resource

Speech sound disorders: Articulation and phonological processes. American Speech-Language-Hearing Association (1997–2010). Retrieved from:
www.asha.org/public/speech/disorders/SpeechSoundDisorders.htm
(overview of speech sound disorders, causes, and treatment)

Assignment 7-1
Substitution Processes

Name _____

The productions of the following words all demonstrate one substitution process occurring. Indicate the phonemic alteration, describing the change in terms of place, manner, and/or voicing, and then label the process.

Example:

came → /teɪm/

___k → t___   voiceless, velar stop → voiceless, alveolar stop   fronting

1. catch → /kæʃ/

_____   _____   _____

2. dish → /dɪs/

_____   _____   _____

3. four → /pɔr/

_____   _____   _____

4. hurt → /hɔt/

_____   _____   _____

5. black→ /blæt/

_____   _____   _____

6. fairy → /fɛwɪ/

_____   _____   _____

7. seas → /tiz/

_____   _____   _____

8. fell → /fɛʊ/

_____   _____   _____

9. case → /teɪs/

_____   _____   _____

10. love → /jʌv/

_____   _____   _____

11. those → /doʊz/

_____   _____   _____

12. jam → /ʒæm/

_____   _____   _____

Assignment 7-2
Assimilation Processes

Name _____

The productions of the following words all demonstrate one assimilation process occurring. Indicate the phonemic alteration, describe the change, and then label the process.

Example:

bag →/bæk/

| g → k | voiced, velar stop → voiceless velar stop | devoicing |

1. bounce→/daʊns/

_____   _____   _____

2. ship →/pɪp/

_____   _____   _____

3. press →/brɛs/

_____   _____   _____

4. grade →/greɪg/

_____   _____   _____

5. moon→/nun/

_____   _____   _____

6. crab →/kræp/

_____   _____   _____

7. bean →/bim/

_____   _____   _____

8. pink →/kɪŋk/

_____   _____   _____

9. dad → /dæt/

_____   _____   _____

10. kind → /taɪnd/

_____   _____   _____

11. set → /zɛt/

_____   _____   _____

12. choose →/tʃus/

_____   _____   _____

Assignment 7-3   Name _____

1. Match the transcriptions with the process being demonstrated. Each item has only one correct answer.

_____ a. lake	→ /jeɪk/	_____ g. pitch	→ /pɪʃ/	A.	fronting
_____ b. with	→ /wɪt/	_____ h. dish	→ /dɪs/	B.	stopping
_____ c. very	→ /bɛrɪ/	_____ i. through	→ /tru/	C.	deaffrication
_____ d. camp	→ /tæmp/	_____ j. shop	→ /ʒɑp/	D.	prevocalic voicing
_____ e. chews	→ /ʃuz/	_____ k. dropped	→ /dwɑpt/	E.	gliding
_____ f. tree	→ /dri/	_____ l. song	→ /sɑn/		

2. Match the transcriptions with the process being demonstrated. Each item has only one correct answer.

_____ a. tickle	→ /dɪkl̩/	_____ g. case	→ /teɪs/	A.	labial assimilation
_____ b. feed	→ /fit/	_____ h. corn	→ /kɔrŋ/	B.	alveolar assimilation
_____ c. drop	→ /drɑt/	_____ i. was	→ /wʌs/	C.	velar assimilation
_____ d. bath	→ /bæf/	_____ j. camp	→ /pæmp/	D.	prevocalic voicing
_____ e. box	→ /gɔks/	_____ k. bring	→ /grɪŋ/	E.	devoicing
_____ f. pad	→ /pæb/	_____ l. share	→ /ʒɛr/		

3. For each of the following words, apply the phonological process given and transcribe the resulting production.

   Example:

lean	final consonant deletion	_____ /li/ _____
a. cost	prevocalic voicing	_____
b. flag	final consonant deletion	_____
c. tacky	velar assimilation	_____
d. spurt	cluster reduction	_____
e. wish	fronting	_____
f. than	alveolar assimilation	_____
g. glued	gliding	_____
h. cage	devoicing	_____
i. other	stopping	_____
j. chocolate	weak syllable deletion	_____
k. badge	deaffrication	_____
l. tough	labial assimilation	_____

Assignment 7-3 (cont.)

4. Circle the transcriptions that could be examples of the process given.

   a. fronting

   leash → /lis/   pack → /pæt/
   door → /tɔr/   juice → /zus/

   b. cluster reduction

   string → /rɪŋ/   lather → /læɾɚ/
   match → /mæs/   from → /rʌm/

   c. labial assimilation

   pig → /bɪg/   drink → /brɪŋk/
   money → /mʌmi/   cave → /peɪv/

   d. final consonant deletion

   obey → /oʊ/   cash → /kæs/
   nest → /nɛs/   both → /boʊt/

   e. velar assimilation

   bingo → /gɪŋgoʊ/   knee → /nik/
   singer → /nɪŋɚ/   class → /glæs/

   f. stopping

   puss → /pʊt/   math → /mæt/
   Vicki → /bɪkɪ/   badge → /bæd/

   g. gliding

   trust → /twʌst/   fly → /fwaɪ/
   turn → /tʊn/   lip → /jɪp/

   h. deaffrication

   Roger → /rɑʒɚ/   catch → /kæʃ/
   sheep → /sip/   measure → /mɛzɚ/

   i. alveolar assimilation

   make → /neɪk/   then → /zɛn/
   bunny → /dʌni/   sand → /tænd/

   j. vocalization

   like → /lɔk/   rain → /weɪn/
   tire → /taɪoʊ/   here → /hɪʊ/

Assignment 7-4

Name _____

 Transcribe the following sentences, as spoken by a 7-year-old female child. This child demonstrates both gliding and vocalization.

CD #3
Track 13

1. I put my right shoe on my left foot.

   _____

2. She'll have to wear a raincoat.

   _____

3. There was a hole in the roof.

   _____

4. My Grandma likes roses.

   _____

5. His sandwich fell apart.

   _____

6. I can't decide which I like best.

   _____

7. He pushed us on the merry-go-round.

   _____

8. Shannon was sick of school.

   _____

9. Grandpa fell asleep on the couch.

   _____

10. Jasmine hopes it'll stop raining soon.

    _____

11. My shirt is in the washing machine.

    _____

12. I had a seashell for show 'n' tell.

    _____

Assignment 7-5

Name _____

Transcribe the following utterances, as spoken by a 4-year-old male child. This child demonstrates the idiosyncratic processes of initial consonant deletion and glottal insertion.

CD #3
Track 14

1. black _____
2. pink _____
3. red _____
4. yellow _____
5. orange _____
6. white _____
7. blue _____
8. green _____
9. apple _____

10. pear _____
11. green beans _____
12. berries _____
13. icing _____
14. cheese _____
15. hotdog _____
16. cocoon _____
17. magic _____
18. caterpillar _____

19. What is these? _____

20. big tree and lake _____

21. See worm eat big leaf. _____

22. Me see egg right there. _____

23. Worm no hungry no more. _____

24. We have that movie. _____

25. I like long necks . . . him . . . er . . . Joshua likes sharp tooths. _____

26. Do you color dinosaurs with me? _____

Assignment 7-6

Name _____

1. For each of the following phonemes, provide two allophones. Then transcribe two words in which those allophones may be found.

   ***Example*:**

   /p/   i) [pʰ] push [pʰʊʃ]   ii) [p˭] spin [sp˭ɪn]

   a. /l/   i)   ii)

   b. /t/   i)   ii)

   c. /k/   i)   ii)

   d. /d/   i)   ii)

   e. /r/   i)   ii)

   f. /g/   i)   ii)

   g. /z/   i)   ii)

2. Transcribe each of the following words using the devoicing diacritic [̥].

   a. pew   _____   f. raise   _____

   b. leave   _____   g. fuse   _____

   c. plaque   _____   h. queen   _____

   d. phase   _____   i. live   _____

   e. crazy   _____   j. sweet   _____

3. Transcribe each of the following words using the diacritics for aspirated [ʰ] and for unaspirated [˭] where necessary.

   a. spank   _____   f. camera   _____

   b. treasure _____   g. table   _____

   c. skewed   _____   h. stared   _____

   d. peeked   _____   i. supposed _____

   e. clueless _____   j. retain   _____

4. Transcribe the following words using the diacritics for dental [̪] and labiodental [ɱ] articulations, where necessary.

   a. nineteenth _____   f. breadth   _____

   b. emphatic   _____   g. although _____

   c. enfold   _____   h. emphysema _____

   d. infrared   _____   i. healthier _____

   e. enthused   _____   j. inference _____

Assignment 7-7   Name _____

1. Explain the difference between the following allophones:

   Example:

       ε/ε̃   non-nasalized (oral) /ε/ versus nasalized /ε/

   a. z/ʐ

   b. pʰ/p˭

   c. l/ɬ

   d. ŋ/ŋ̃

   e. d̥/ḏ

   f. ɑ/ɑ̨

   g. t/ṱ

   h. u/uː

   i. s/sʷ

   j. ŋ/ɱ

   k. r/r̥

2. Indicate for each of the following whether the diacritic is used correctly by placing an "X" in the proper blank. If the diacritic is incorrect, explain the error.

a. plain	[plẽɪn]	_____ correct	_____ incorrect
b. licked	[l̥ɪkt]	_____ correct	_____ incorrect
c. freed	[friːd]	_____ correct	_____ incorrect
d. spread	[sp˭rɛd]	_____ correct	_____ incorrect
e. plaid	[p̥læd]	_____ correct	_____ incorrect
f. hark	[hɑrkʰ]	_____ correct	_____ incorrect
g. practice	[præk˺tɪs]	_____ correct	_____ incorrect
h. swirl	[sʷwɝl]	_____ correct	_____ incorrect
i. spry	[s̥pry]	_____ correct	_____ incorrect
j. clasp	[k̥læsp]	_____ correct	_____ incorrect

3. Each of the following non-English IPA symbols may serve as a substitution for a standard English phoneme when transcribing clients with speech sound disorders. Write the articulatory description for each of the IPA symbols, then give one example of a standard English phoneme it might replace.

Example:

    [β]   voiced, bilabial fricative   /v/

1. [ʤ̱] _____ _____

2. [ʕ] _____ _____

3. [ɣ] _____ _____

4. [ɸ] _____ _____

5. [ɠ] _____ _____

6. [ʋ] _____ _____

7. [ʕ] _____ _____

8. [ɬ] _____ _____

9. [k'] _____ _____

10. [x] _____ _____

CHAPTER

8

Dialectal Variation

Learning Objectives

After reading this chapter you will be able to:

1. Explain the difference between formal and informal Standard American English.
2. Explain the differences between General American English and regional dialects such as Southern and Eastern American English.
3. Describe ASHA's position concerning clinical treatment of individuals with dialectal variation.
4. Explain the ways in which chain shifts and mergers currently affect vowel pronunciation in the United States.
5. Explain the difference between a regional dialect and a social or ethnic dialect.
6. Explain the concept of language transfer in non-native speakers of English.
7. Describe the phonological characteristics consistent with African American English.
8. Describe the phonological characteristics consistent with Spanish-Influenced English, Asian/Pacific-Influenced English, Russian-Influenced English, and Arabic-Influenced English.

As college freshmen, many of you moved away from home for the first time. Once you arrived at college, you immediately found yourself thrust into new surroundings. You became a little fish in a big pond, the pond comprising people from various regions of the country. You also had the opportunity to meet people with quite varied social and cultural backgrounds. For the first time in your life, you may have realized the marked dialect in the speech and language patterns of people with backgrounds different from your own. The variations in the phonological patterns of your new college acquaintances may have been subtle, in the form of a slight accent. Or perhaps the differences were not so subtle, reflecting a difference in grammatical patterns, vocabulary, and even heavier accents. Prior to this time, the primary speech and language patterns to which you were exposed were probably those of your family and friends and from the newscasters you heard on the radio or saw on TV. Your exposure to varying dialects may have been limited to TV shows that took place in the South or in New York City.

The dialects of English spoken in the United States are quite variable in terms of syntax (grammatical rules), vocabulary, and phonology. The dialect you use in your daily life is the product of the region of the United States in which you grew up, your cultural background, your ethnic group membership and also the social class to which you belong. Social class in this sense refers to type of occupation (white collar, blue collar, etc.), socioeconomic class, level of education, and in which part of town you grew up. Factors such as age and gender also play important roles in determining the language patterns you will use on a day-to-day basis. In addition, as a speaker of a language you also possess an **idiolect,** an individual, idiosyncratic speech pattern, characteristic of your own personality.

Suppose you grew up in Cleveland and had to travel to New York City on business. You would immediately notice a sizable variation in the pronunciation patterns of the native New Yorkers. You would probably consider the native speakers to have an accent. This judgment would be made using your own, learned speaking habits as an internal yardstick or standard. Consider the fact that a New York City native would find your speech to have just as much of an accent as you do hers. Most likely, both of you would consider your own usage of English as the standard. This raises an interesting question, "Is there a standard form of American English?"

Standard American English (SAE) is a form of English that is relatively devoid of regional characteristics (Wolfram, 1991). SAE, which exists in both written and spoken forms, is sometimes referred to as General American English. In the United States, there is no *one* fixed standard of English. In several countries, including Spain, France, and Norway, there are academies that regulate the introduction of new words into the language as well as standardize allowable grammatical rules, especially for government publications and education. In the United States, there is no such formal academy that standardizes or regulates the rules of written and spoken English.

In the United States, SAE actually exists in two forms, **formal standard English** and **informal standard English** (Wolfram & Schilling-Estes, 2006). Formal standard English usually refers to the written form of the language; it is the English of dictionaries, grammar books, and most printed matter. As college students, you use formal standard English when writing a term paper. In spoken form, the standard may be observed in the speech of the national network newscasters who, for the most part, have limited regional accents that do not tie them to any particular geographic region. Formal standard English is the idealized form often adopted when teaching English.

In reality, most speakers in the United States do not speak formal standard English. Instead, we tend to speak some variety of informal standard English. Informal standard English is based on listener judgments of patterns of spoken English deemed to be acceptable or not. That is, societal judgment determines whether a particular speaker's dialect of English is acceptable or "standard" (Wolfram & Schilling-Estes, 2006).

Informal standard English actually consists on a continuum from "standard" to "nonstandard." Two people with different language and social backgrounds might judge a third speaker differently in terms of where that person might fall on the continuum. That is, one judge may place the speaker closer to "standard" on the continuum, and the other judge might place him closer to "nonstandard."

According to Wolfram and Schilling-Estes (2006), speakers of English do not tend to rate "standardness" on how well a particular person actually speaks the standard form. Instead, speakers tend to be judged in terms of the *absence* of "socially disfavored structures" that exist in their speech patterns. These judgments are not based so much on phonological patterns or "accent," but more on socially disfavored syntactic patterns. For instance, a speaker might be rated more substandard if he used sentences such as "I ain't goin' to the movies" or "We was in a hurry." An individual who is considered to be a nonstandard speaker of English is said to speak a **vernacular dialect** (Wolfram & Schilling-Estes, 2006). An individual would be judged to be using a vernacular dialect based on the *presence* of stigmatizing grammatical structures in spoken language patterns.

Formal standard English then, at least in a spoken form, is rarely achieved by speakers of American English. Virtually every speaker of American English belongs to some dialect group defined by region, ethnic group, or social class. For this reason, it is better to think of American English as having an informal standard that exists on a continuum as opposed to one fixed, formal standard. Several regional, social, and ethnic dialects will be discussed in the following sections. Because this is a phonetics book, the focus will be on the *phonological* aspects of dialect. Differences in dialects related to syntax and vocabulary will not be covered in this text.

EXERCISE 8.1

Which regional and social factors have influenced the particular dialect of English you speak? Do you have any particular idiosyncratic speech patterns that contribute to your idiolect?

As speech and hearing professionals, you often will be evaluating the speech and language capabilities of individuals from various regional, social, and cultural backgrounds. You will need to determine whether these individuals have a handicapping communicative problem, regardless of the particular dialect of English that they have acquired. It is important to realize that dialects of standard English should *not* be thought of as substandard versions of our language. That is, dialects should not be thought of automatically as "wrong," or in need of remediation. Instead, dialects should be considered strictly as a variety of standard English that reflects an individual's social class, ethnic group membership, or the region in which he or she grew up. In fact, dialects should be thought of as a communication *difference,* as opposed to a communication disorder, the difference being the variation in phonological rules, vocabulary, and syntax of any particular dialect.

In 2003, the American Speech-Language-Hearing Association (ASHA) published a technical report entitled "American English Dialects." This report promotes the idea that "no dialectal variety of American English is a disorder or a pathological form of speech or language" (ASHA, 2003). According to ASHA:

> Each dialect is adequate as a functional and effective variety of American English. Each serves a communication function as well as a social solidarity function. Each dialect maintains the communication network and the social construct of the community of speakers who use it. Furthermore, each is a symbolic representation of the geographic, historical, social, and cultural background of its speakers. (p. 45)

In some instances, speech-language pathologists are asked to assist nonnative English speakers (those learning English as a second language) in becoming more easily understood, that is, more intelligible, to the mainstream, standard English-speaking population. In this case, speech-language pathologists provide an elective service known as **accent modification.** The focus of these sessions is to help non-native speakers of English become more intelligible. Accent modification programs are becoming increasingly more common in university settings as the number of foreign instructors in the classroom increases. In fact, in Ohio, state law requires that all university teaching assistants must be proficient in the use of the English language. Therefore, mandatory accent modification programs have been set up in university speech and hearing clinics or in programs that teach English as a second language (ESL) to assist foreign-born instructors improve their pronunciation of English. Keep in mind that the focus of an elective accent modification program "is to assist in the acquisition of the desired competency in the second dialect without jeopardizing the integrity of the individual's first dialect" (ASHA, 2003, p. 46).

Regional Dialects

Several classification schemes have been used by researchers in an attempt to describe and categorize regional dialects in the United States. The regional use of certain vocabulary items have been studied to help define dialectal regions. For instance, in the eastern United States, many people refer to carbonated beverages as "soda," whereas people from the Midwest generally use the term "pop," and some people from the South use the term "coke." Likewise, the terms "pail" and "bucket" and "faucet" and "spigot" are used contrastively, depending on where a person lives. When using vocabulary items to demarcate regional dialects, research has shown conflicting evidence as to the actual number of dialectal regions present in the United States (Carver, 1987; Kurath, 1949). Some research indicates that the United States can be divided into three separate dialectal regions—North, Midland, and South (Kurath, 1949). Another approach divides the United States into two general dialect regions, North and South (Carver, 1987). Each of these regions is further divided into layers, in a hierarchical arrangement. The North dialect region is divided into three layers: Upper North (including New England), Lower North, and the West. The South dialect region has two layers: Upper South and Lower South.

Another approach to defining dialectal regions is to examine the phonological patterns of English speakers. The linguistics laboratory at the University of Pennsylvania has conducted extensive telephone surveys of over 700 speakers to determine how vowel pronunciation differs across the country. This investigation, the **Telsur Project,** systematically examined speakers from 145 urban centers. Most urban centers had populations greater than 200,000. However, several smaller cities were included in order to provide a better representative sample of dialects across the United States. The 145 urban centers account for 54 percent of the total United States population (Labov, Ash, & Boberg, 2006). The purpose of this investigation was (1) to identify the major dialectal regions in the country using phonological data instead of vocabulary data and (2) to determine the specific pronunciation patterns that are found in each of the dialect regions.

Results of the Telsur survey confirmed the well-known fact that vowel articulation in the United States is not static; the place of articulation of American English vowels is in an active state of change. The changes in place of vowel articulation can be categorized as *chain shifts* and *mergers* (Labov et al., 2006).

A **chain shift** occurs when the place of articulation of one vowel changes, causing the surrounding vowels in the quadrilateral to likewise shift in production. This causes a "chain reaction" in relation to the place of articulation for other vowels. Because chain shifting affects the production of several vowels at the same time, the articulation of a single vowel is not independent of the articulation of other vowels. Instead, vowel articulation is relative; place of articulation of one vowel is determined by the place of production of other vowels. A **vowel merger** occurs when vowels with separate articulations fuse into one similar place of articulation. For example, in many regions in the United States, the vowels /ɑ/ and /ɔ/ have merged so that their production and perception is the same—that is, /ɑ/. Another example involves the merger of /ɪ/ and /ɛ/ before nasals, so that the words "pin" and "pen" both are produced and perceived as "pin."

The Telsur Project has helped to demarcate several dialectal regions across the United States. However, three regions were identified *solely* on the basis of the chain shift and merger phonological data: (1) the Inland North, (2) the South, and (3) the West (Labov, 1991). Each of these regions will be discussed along with the major pronunciation patterns that help to define that region.

The Inland North

The Inland North is part of a larger dialect region Labov and colleagues (2006) have termed the North. Other regions of the North include the North Central Region, Eastern and Western New England, and New York City. The Inland North is composed of many large urban centers around the Great Lakes as well as in upper New York state. In cities such as Buffalo, Syracuse, Detroit, Chicago, and Milwaukee, people have begun to demonstrate a shift in the place of articulation of the six vowels /ɔ, ɑ, æ, ɪ, ɛ, and ʌ/ in what is known as the **Northern Cities Shift.** The Northern Cities Shift occurs in western New England, New York state, and the northern parts of Pennsylvania, Ohio, Indiana, Illinois, Michigan, and Wisconsin (Labov, 1991). A vowel quadrilateral demonstrating the Northern Cities Shift is presented in Figure 8.1. The shift reflects raising of /æ/, fronting of /ɑ/, lowering of /ɔ/, and backing of /ʌ, ɛ, and ɪ/. The shift occurs in a clockwise rotation so that the fronted production of /ɑ/ and the

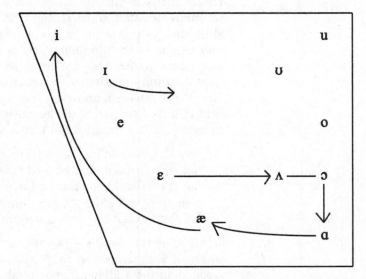

FIGURE 8.1 Vowel quadrilateral of the Northern Cities Shift (information from Labov, Ash, & Boberg, 2006).

backed production of /ɛ/ becomes quite similar; they both are produced more centrally in the oral cavity. To clarify vowel changes associated with the shift, the vowel /æ/ is produced higher and more forward in the mouth. This causes /ɑ/ to be produced more forward in the mouth (filling in the space that was previously occupied by /æ/), so that the word "hot" /hɑt/ would be produced similar to /hæt/. As a result, the vowel /ɔ/ is then produced lower in the mouth so that "caught" /kɔt/ would be produced more like /kɑt/. Further:

cut /kʌt/ would be produced more like /kɔt/
bet /bɛt/ would be produced more like /bʌt/
bit /bɪt/ would be produced more like /bɛt/

EXERCISE 8.2

Transcribe the following words, first in your own dialect, and then as they would be pronounced using the Northern Cities Shift dialect. Use the appropriate diacritics to indicate raising [˰], lowering [˯], advancement [₊], or retraction [˗] of the tongue. Refer to Figure 8.1 to help you complete this exercise.

Example:

dog	/dɑg/	[dɑ̠g]

1. lid   _____   _____
2. when   _____   _____
3. rub   _____   _____
4. caught   _____   _____
5. bag   _____   _____

The South

The South is defined geographically by the Southern, Middle Atlantic, and Southern Mountain states (Labov, 1991). A chain shift known as the **Southern Shift** affects the vowels /æ, ɛ, e, ɪ, i/ and the diphthong /aɪ/ (Figure 8.2). This shift begins as the diphthong /aɪ/ is simplified, and produced as the fronted monophthong /a/. Also, the vowel /e/ is lowered and centralized, produced in close proximity to where the monophthong /a/ is now produced. At the same time, /i/ is lowered, and /æ/, /ɛ/, and /ɪ/ are raised. Note that the Southern Shift reflects a tensing of the lax vowels /ɪ/ and /ɛ/, and a laxing of the vowels /i/ and /e/. The Southern Shift causes changes in vowel articulation so that:

buy /baɪ/ would be produced more like /ba/
bat /bæt/ would be produced more like /bɛt/
bet /bɛt/ would be produced more like /bėt/
beet /bit/ would be produced more like /bɪt/
bit /bɪt/ would be produced more like /bit/

Fronting of the vowels /u/ and /o/ was originally regarded as part of the Southern Shift. However, fronting of these back vowels has been observed by speakers in the Midland (Labov et al., 2006). As such, the shift in back vowel production is no longer a defining feature unique to the South.

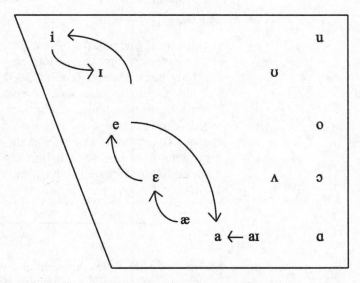

FIGURE 8.2 Vowel quadrilateral of the Southern Shift (adapted from Labov, Ash, & Boberg, 2006).

Southern dialect is also is marked by a second chain shift known as the **Back Upglide Shift** (Labov et al., 2006). This shift affects production of the vowel /ɔ/ and the diphthong /aʊ/. In this shift, the vowel /ɔ/ becomes unrounded and glides upward, becoming the diphthong /aʊ/. For example, the word "fraught" /frɔt/ would be pronounced as /fraʊt/. Additionally, the diphthong /aʊ/ would be produced as /æʊ/, causing the word "crown" to be produced (and heard) as "crayon" /kræʊn/ (Labov, n.d.). The Back Upglide Shift can be found in the Carolinas and in Tennessee, as well as in Arkansas, Texas, Missouri, and as far north as Kansas City (Labov et al., 2006).

EXERCISE 8.3

Transcribe the following words, first in your own dialect, and then as they would be pronounced using the Southern Shift dialect. Use the appropriate diacritical marking for raising, lowering, or advancement to indicate the appropriate transcription as predicted by the Southern Shift. Refer to Figure 8.2 to help you complete this exercise.

Examples:

red	/rɛd/	[rɛ̞d]
1. may	_____	_____
2. lick	_____	_____
3. cat	_____	_____
4. like	_____	_____
5. weed	_____	_____

The West

A third and somewhat different pattern of vowel articulation is currently being observed throughout various regions of the United States. This is known as the **Low Back Merger** (Labov, 1991). This change in pronunciation involves the merger of the low, back vowels /ɑ/ and /ɔ/. Speakers who merge these vowels show no phonemic contrast between them during the production of words. For instance, a speaker who merges these vowels would pronounce the names "Dawn" and "Don" the same—that is, /dɑn/. This merger occurs in a large section of the western United States as well as in eastern New England, southern Ohio, Pennsylvania (in the Pittsburgh area), northern Minnesota, and Wisconsin (Labov et al., 2006).

EXERCISE 8.4

Transcribe the following word pairs as you would pronounce them. Do you produce both /ɑ/ and /ɔ/ in your regional dialect of English? Or do you use the vowels /a/ or /ɒ/ (the rounded version of /ɑ/) in transcription of these words?

1. Lon   _____   lawn   _____

2. clod   _____   Claude   _____

3. caught   _____   cot   _____

4. taught   _____   tot   _____

The Midland and Western Pennsylvania

An additional dialect region, the Midland, was identified during the Telsur telephone project. Kurath (1949) also identified the Midland as a major dialectal area in the United States. According to the Telsur data, the Midland states extend westward from central Ohio and include parts of Indiana, Illinois, Iowa, Missouri, Nebraska, Kansas, and Oklahoma (Labov et al., 2006). The Midland is further divided into southern and northern regions. In terms of pronunciation, the main difference between the North and South Midland regions is the fronting of the diphthong /oʊ/, found by speakers in the South Midland. Further, the Midland dialect region as a whole (North and South) is resistant to the chain shifting associated with the North and the South. The Midland serves more as a demarcation that separates the dialectal patterns for speakers of the Inland North (Northern Cities Shift) and the South (Southern Shift). In addition, some cities of the Midland are in a transitional state in reference to the low back merger. Cities of the Midland, notably St. Louis, show their own unique dialectal patterns. According to Labov et al. (2006), "there is reason to believe that the Midland is becoming the default system of North American English" (p. 135).

Adjoining the Midland region is the western Pennsylvania dialect area. This region is distinct from the Midland because of its unique dialectal features associated with Pittsburgh and surrounding cities such as State College, Pennsylvania, and Youngstown, Ohio. The dialect spoken in Pittsburgh is often referred to as "Pittsburghese." Some examples of Pittsburghese include pronouncing "downtown" as /dantan/ and "meal" as /mɪl/.

Historically, phonetics books have described three major regional dialects specific to the United States: (1) Southern American English, (2) Eastern American

English, and (3) General American English (Edwards, 1992; Gray & Wise, 1959). In the next section of the book, we will continue with a more in-depth discussion on Southern and Eastern American English dialects. These two dialect patterns are undoubtedly the most recognized regional dialects. However, a word needs to be said concerning the term **General American English.** *General American English* traditionally has been used as a term to describe the dialect spoken in areas of the country other than the East or the South. As such, the term General American English is equated with the speech patterns of most of the western United States as well as most of the country east of the Mississippi and north of the Ohio River, not including the East Coast (Hartman, 1985). Because regional dialects do exist in the North and in the western half of the United States, the term General American English may not be the most accurate term in describing the dialectal patterns of so many Americans.

The term General American English has been used more recently to designate a "standard" dialect that lacks any regional pronunciation, such as that associated with the South or the East. In this manner, the use of the term is synonymous with the term Standard American English. As Wolfram and Schilling-Estes (2006) point out, the use of the term General American English is helpful when comparing regional or ethnic dialects to a national standard because any bias that might be inferred by use of the label "standard" would be avoided. That is, if a particular dialect varies from "standard" American English, it might be thought of incorrectly as being a "nonstandard" or vernacular dialect. Therefore, in this text, the term General American English only will be used when referencing regional or ethnic dialects.

Southern American English

Southern American English is the dialect of English spoken primarily in the southern states including all or part of Alabama, Arkansas, Florida, Georgia, Kentucky, Louisiana, Mississippi, North Carolina, Oklahoma, South Carolina, Tennessee, Texas, Virginia, and West Virginia. There are some general characteristics of southern speech that are fairly typical across the southern United States. However, not all of these characteristics would necessarily apply to the same speaker; there are regional variations of Southern American English.

It is important to consider the fact that dialects continually change over time. According to Hartman (1985), speakers shift their speech patterns to fit a particular audience or situation, and to sound more like their peers than their parents. He also states that younger speakers often adopt broader regional pronunciations in favor of more local ones. For instance, deleting post-vocalic /r/ has always been one noted characteristic of southern speech, e.g., pronouncing "car" as /kɑ:/ or "chord" as /kɔ:d/. Younger southern speakers have begun to restore final /r/ in words, so much so that deletion of post-vocalic /r/ is no longer a defining dialectal variation in the South (Labov et al., 2006). However, deletion of post-vocalic /r/ does still exist in the speech patterns of some older southern individuals. In addition to age, there appears to be a relationship between a person's educational level and production of /r/. That is, the more educated a person is, the more likely that person will produce final /r/ in words (Hartman, 1985; Labov et al., 2006).

Examples of the more common vowel, diphthong, and consonant features associated with Southern American English are described on the next few pages. They are also summarized in Table 8.1. Keep in mind that some of these features

TABLE 8.1   Common Features of Southern American English

English Word	Southern English Transcription	Phonological Pattern
fish	/fiʃ/	tensing of vowels
egg	/eɪg/	tensing of vowels
really	/rɪlɪ/	laxing of vowels
fire	/far/	monophthongization
foil	/fɔːl/	monophthongization
two	/tiu/	diphthongization
lettuce	/lɛrɪs/	/ɪ/ for /ə/ substitution, i.e., ɪ/ə
pen/pin	/pɪn/	vowel merger
Mary/merry	/mɛrɪ/	vowel merger
Harry	/hærɪ/	vowel lowering
fall	/fɔl/	lack of /ɔ/-/ɑ/ merger
terse	/tɜːs/	derhotacization
here	/hɪə/	derhotacization
far	/fɑː/	deletion of postvocalic /r/

Source: Information from Hartman, 1985; Labov et al., 2006.

are not necessarily limited only to speakers in the South; they may be found in other areas of the country as well.

Vowel and Consonant Characteristics

In Southern American English, diphthongs are produced as monophthongs by some speakers. This is called **diphthong simplification** or **monophthongization.** For instance, the diphthong /ɔɪ/ is simplified to /ɔ/ and is lengthened before /l/ as in "foil" /fɔːl/ and "spoil" /spɔːl/. Consistent with the Southern Shift, /aɪ / also is monophthongized to /a/, as in "fire" /far/ and "tired" /tard/. Other vowel productions reflective of the Southern Shift include tensing of /ɪ/ before /ʃ/, as in "fish" /fiʃ/; tensing of /ɛ/ when it precedes /g/, /ʃ/, or /ʒ/, as in "leg" /leɪg/ or "treasure" /treɪʒɚ/; and laxing of /i/when it precedes /l/, as in "really" /rɪlɪ/.

At one time, many speakers in the South (and the East) pronounced the vowel /u/ as the diphthong /ju/ (epenthesis of /j/) when it followed the alveolar consonants /t, d, or n/ as in "two" /tju/ or "new" /nju/. In time, the glide has, for the most part, disappeared in southern speech. In some portions of the South (mostly in North Carolina and in the southern regions of Mississippi, Alabama, and Georgia), what still occurs is the epenthesis of /i/ before /u/, resulting in a diphthong as in "too" /tiu/ or "new" /niu/ (Labov et al., 2006). There is also a tendency for some southern speakers to substitute /ɪ/ for /ə/ in the final syllable of words such as "pigeon" /pɪdʒɪn/ and "hopeless" /houplɪs/.

For some speakers, /ɛ/ may be raised and articulated as /ɪ/ when it precedes the nasal /n/. In this phonetic context, /ɪ/ and /ɛ/ merge so that the words "pen" and "pin" would both be produced and perceived as /pɪn/. Similarly, "sense" and "since" would both be produced and perceived as /sɪns/. Recall that the low-back vowel merger (merger of /ɔ/ and /ɑ/) is seen across much of the United States, especially in the West. In many areas of the South, the two vowels have *not* merged; production of /ɔ/ is found in words such as "haul," "gone," slaughter," and "caught."

In much of the country, the three vowels /eɪ/, /ɛ/, and /æ/ before intervocalic /r/ have merged so that the words /meɪrɪ/ "Mary," /mɛrɪ/ "merry," and /mærɪ/ "marry" are all pronounced the same, i.e., /mɛrɪ/. In the South, /eɪ/ and /ɛ/ have merged, however /æ/ remains distinct, that is:

Mary and merry → /mɛrɪ/   marry → /mærɪ/

This separation of /æ/ from the /eɪ/-/ɛ/ merger is seen in parts of Georgia, North Carolina, South Carolina, and Virginia (Labov et al., 2006). When "marry" is pronounced as /mærɪ/, the rhotic diphthong is lowered from /ɛr/ to /ær/. Other examples include "carry" /kærɪ/ and "Harry" /hærɪ/.

As mentioned earlier, deletion of postvocalic /r/ is not as prevalent in the South as it once was, even though some older southern speakers still delete postvocalic /r/. In words containing the rhotic diphthong /ɑr/, /r/ is deleted and /ɑ/ is lengthened, as in "car" /kɑ:/ and "farmer" /fɑ:mə/.

In words that contain the rhotic diphthongs /ɪr/, /ɛr/, /ɔr/, and /ʊr/, /r/ may lose its r-coloring, resulting in a substitution of the vowel /ə/ for /r/ as in "beer" /bɪə/, "door" /dɔə/ (or /doə/), "hair" /hɛə/, or "sure" /ʃʊə/. This loss of r-coloring is known as **derhotacization.** Southern speakers who delete postvocalic /r/ also tend to derhotacize the central vowels /ɝ/ and /ɚ/. When /ɝ/ is derhotacized, it tends to be lengthened as in "terse" /tɝ:s/ and "word" /wɝ:d/. Derhotacization of /ɚ/ results in production of /ə/ in postvocalic and word-final positions as in "others" /ʌðəz/ and "flour" /flaʊə/.

EXERCISE 8.5

Determine the phonological pattern(s) for each of Southern American English pronunciations given below. Write your answer in the blank.

Example:

ball	/bɔl/	lack of /ɔ/-/ɑ/merger
1. tunes	/tiunz/	
2. cautious	/kɔʃɪs/	
3. meal	/mɪl/	
4. bar	/bɑ:/	
5. trial	/tral/	
6. meant	/mɪnt/	
7. concern	/kənsɝ:n/	
8. spoiled	/spɔ:ld/	
9. precious	/preɪʃɪs/	
10. tear (noun)	/tɪə/	

Eastern American English

What is commonly recognized as **Eastern American English** is spoken predominantly by individuals in the New England states and by people from parts of New York, New Jersey, and eastern Pennsylvania. The dialectal patterns that will be introduced in the following section are speech patterns observed across several areas of the East. For instance, individuals in Boston may exhibit quite distinct articulation patterns when compared to individuals from other cities in Massachusetts and from other cities in New England. Similarly, some individuals in New York City have distinct dialectal characteristics. Due to the varied nature of Eastern regional dialects, only the more commonly shared dialectal patterns will be discussed below. Keep in mind that any one speaker of Eastern American English dialect will not demonstrate all of the examples given. A summary of the major characteristics of Eastern American dialect is displayed in Table 8.2.

Vowel and Consonant Characteristics

There are several *vowel* productions that differ from General American English. Recall that in the South, /eɪ/ and /ɛ/ have merged so that "Mary" and "merry" are pronounced the same (i.e., /mɛrɪ/). However, in southern New England, as well as in Philadelphia and New York City, they have *not* merged (Labov et al., 2006). In addition, the two vowels are distinct in production from /æ/, which involves the lowering of /ɛr/ to /ær/ (as in the South). An example of this pattern is:

Mary → /merɪ/   ferry → /fɛrɪ/   sparrow → /spæroʊ/

One of the more characteristic examples of New England dialect involves the substitution (backing) of either /ɑ/ or /a/ for /æ/ before the fricatives /f, v, s, θ, and ð/ or before the nasal /n/, as in "half" (/hɑf/ or /haf/) and "dance"

TABLE 8.2   Features of Eastern American Dialect

English Word	Eastern English Transcription	Phonological Pattern
Mary, merry, marry	/merɪ, mɛrɪ, mærɪ/	distinct /eɪ, ɛ, and æ/ (lack of merger)
sparrow	/spæroʊ/	lowering of /ɛ/
half	/hɑf/ or /haf/	backing of /æ/
moth	/maθ/	fronting of /ɑ/
room	/rʊm/	laxing of /u/
horses	/hɔrsɪz/	ɪ/ə substitution
here	/hɪə/	derhotacization
third	/θɜːd/	derhotacization
smart	/smɑːt/	deletion of postvocalic /r/
saw	/sɔɚ/	rhotacization

Source: Information from Hartman, 1985; Labov et al., 2006.

(/dɑns/ or /dans/). Another recognized characteristic involves the fronting of /ɑ/ to /a/ in areas of eastern New England, including Maine, New Hampshire, and eastern Massachusetts resulting in "spa" /spa/ and "moth" /maθ/ (Labov et al., 2006). Some older speakers may substitute /ʊ/ for /u/ (vowel laxing), as in "room" /rʊm/ and "hooves" /hʊvz/. Similar to Southern American English, there is a tendency to substitute /ɪ/ for /ə/ in the final syllable of words such as "hopeless" /hoʊplɪs/.

Deletion of postvocalic /r/ remains much more prevalent in the East than in the South. For words that contain the rhotic diphthong /ɑr/, speakers in northern New England (parts of Maine, New Hampshire, Vermont, and eastern Massachusetts) not only delete /r/ but also front the production of the vowel /ɑ/ to /a/ (Labov et al., 2006), as in "heart" /haːt/ and "tar" /taː/. This production of /ɑr/ is best exemplified in the classic phrase /paːk jə kaː ɪn haːvəd jaːd/. Speakers in eastern New England and in the New York City metropolitan area also derhotacize /r/ as in "chair" /tʃɛə/ and "here" /hɪə/ (Hartman, 1985; Labov et al., 2006). Individuals who derhotacize postvocalic /r/ also tend to derhotacize the central vowels /ɝ/ and /ɚ/ as in "word" /wɜːd/ and "letter" /lɛɾə/.

One last characteristic of Eastern American English involves the *rhotacization* of /ə/, resulting in /ɚ/. This occurs when a word that ends with /ə/ is followed by a word beginning with a vowel (Hartman, 1985). For example, "Cuba and America" would be pronounced as /kjubɚ ænd əmɛrɪkə/. In addition, /ɚ/ may be found to occur in words normally ending in /ə/ or /ɔ/, as in "Linda" /lɪndɚ/, "soda" /soʊdɚ/, "idea" /aɪdiɚ/, "saw" /sɔɚ/, and "McGraw" /məʔɡrɔɚ/.

EXERCISE 8.6

Determine the phonological pattern for each of the Eastern American English pronunciations given below. Write your answer in the blank.

Example:

hair	/hɛə/	derhotacization

1. roof	/rʊf /	_____
2. laugh	/laf/	_____
3. murder	/mɜːdə/	_____
4. ward	/wɔəd/	_____
5. can't	/kɑnt/	_____
6. marry	/mærɪ/	_____
7. Maria	/məriɚ/	_____
8. choir	/kwaɪə/	_____
9. pa	/pa/	_____
10. darker	/dɑːkə/	_____

Social and Ethnic Dialects

American English also has several dialects based upon social class and ethnic group membership. A dialect associated with a particular social class is referred to as a **sociolect,** whereas a dialect associated with a particular ethnic group is termed an **ethnolect.** In terms of social class, an individual's sociolect may be related to socioeconomic status, level of education, and/or vocation. It is not always easy to identify patterns of language variation or dialect based solely on social class membership or level of education. Other variables, such as age, gender, language background, and geographical region enter into the equation. In addition, people from the same social class may have the need to adopt different dialectal patterns based on their work environment. For individuals who hold positions in which communication is important to perform their jobs (e.g., teachers, lawyers, and health-care professionals), it becomes necessary to use a variety of language that would be deemed by the public as "standard" (Wolfram & Schilling-Estes, 2006). (Recall that informal standard English is based on speaker/listener judgment.) Individuals from the same social class who are not as much "in the public eye" may adopt a more local variety of language that might be judged as being less standard.

Similarly, the social network to which a person belongs will also dictate the variety of language an individual uses. For instance, individuals whose social situations place them in a smaller social network have different communication needs than individuals whose social networks are broader and make it necessary to interact with a wider variety of individuals on a daily basis. People who belong to larger social networks would avoid the use of socially unacceptable or stigmatizing language and speech patterns in order to avoid being identified as a speaker of a vernacular (nonstandard) dialect (Wolfram & Schilling-Estes, 2006).

Ethnolects, such as African American English and Chicano English are often identified as being associated with a particular ethnic group. According to the Merriam-Webster online dictionary, the word *ethnic* is defined as "of or relating to large groups of people classed according to common racial, national, tribal, religious, linguistic, or cultural origin or background" (Webster, 2010). Ethnic group membership is often related to social class, as well as language background and geographical region. Therefore, an ethnic dialect, such as African American English, is sometimes referred to in the literature as a social dialect (ASHA, 1983; Stockman, 2007) or even as a social *and* ethnic dialect (Pollock & Meredith, 2001). In this text, a dialect defined by association with a particular ethnic group, such as African American English, will be referred to as an *ethnic* dialect (ethnolect).

African American English

African American English (AAE) is probably the most noted dialect of English spoken in the United States. More is written about this ethnolect than any other. Not all African American people speak AAE, nor is this dialect limited solely to African Americans. The term AAE is the most recent term for this ethnolect. Previous terminology used by linguists, educators, and speech-language pathologists for this dialect have included *ebonics* (ASHA, 1983), *Black English* (Owens, 1991; Terrell & Terrell, 1993), *Vernacular Black English* (Wolfram, 1991; Wolfram & Fasold, 1974), *Black English Vernacular* (Iglesias & Anderson, 1993), and *African American Vernacular English* (Wolfram, 1994).

AAE has quite an interesting history. There are two widely believed historical accounts of its origin: the *Anglicist Hypothesis* and the *Creolist Hypothesis*. The Anglicist Hypothesis suggests that AAE can be traced back to the dialects of English spoken in Britain and brought to America by British settlers. After arriving in America, African slaves learned the regional and social varieties of English being spoken around them. Over several generations, only a vestige of their native African language remained. In this sense, their learning of English was no different than other immigrants coming to live in the United States who were learning English as a second language (Wolfram & Schilling-Estes, 2006). The Anglicist Hypothesis was popular in the 1960s and 1970s until the Creolist Hypothesis was proposed.

The Creolist Hypothesis suggests that AAE took root when Europeans traveled to Africa for reasons of business and commerce. A **pidgin** language developed between these two groups of people. A pidgin language develops when two different groups of people, with two distinct languages, attempt to communicate. The resulting pidgin language is typically characterized as having both a reduced vocabulary and grammar. The pidgin language that led to the development of AAE shared characteristics of both African and European languages. When slaves arrived in the United States, both the slaves' overseers as well as the owners of the plantations introduced new vocabulary items and grammatical structures to the pidgin. Children born to the slaves were taught this more fully developed pidgin language as their native language. Once a pidgin language is passed on to a new generation of users, the language is considered to be what is known as a **creole** language. According to the Creolist Hypothesis, AAE evolved from this creole, with characteristics of grammar and vocabulary from both African and European languages. The Creolist Hypothesis was in favor until the 1980s. Since then, research, including examination of written narratives from ex-slaves, has shown that the Anglicist Hypothesis better explains the origin of AAE.

AAE, as it is known today, has several regional variations. The form of AAE spoken in a northern city, such as Cleveland, differs from the version of AAE spoken in Atlanta. The phonological forms associated with AAE are quite variable among its speakers (Wolfram, 1994). According to Wolfram, the variability is constrained by social factors such as age, gender, and socioeconomic status, as well as by linguistic factors such as the position of sounds in words and the particular phoneme involved. Although AAE is characterized by several lexical, grammatical, and phonological features, we will focus only on the more noted phonological features common to AAE.

Consonant Characteristics

AAE can be characterized by several phonological processes that affect phoneme production, including syllable structure processes, substitution processes, and assimilatory processes. A summary of the major phonological traits associated with AAE consonants and vowels are presented in the next section and are also summarized in Table 8.3.

Syllable Structure Processes

Deletion of stops and nasals is common in AAE. Deletion of alveolar stops usually occurs in the word-final position as in "bat" /bæ/ or "would" /wʊ/. The voiced stop /d/ also may be deleted when it is followed by the morpheme /s/ as in "needs" /niz/ or "kids" /kɪz/. When final nasals are deleted, the preceding vowel becomes nasalized as in "pin" /pĩ/ or "home" /hõʊ̃/.

TABLE 8.3   Examples of AAE Phonology

Word	AAE Transcription	Phonological Process
Syllable Structure Processes		
hat; bad	/hæ/; /bæ/	final stop deletion
pin; home	/pĩ/; /hõũ/	final nasal deletion
through; more; story	/θu/; /moʊ/; /stoʊɪ/	/r/ deletion
chair; here	/tʃɛə/; /hɪə/	derhotacization
wolf; shelf	/wʊf/; /ʃɛf/	/l/ deletion
nickel; bell	/nɪkʊ/; /bɛʊ/	/l/vocalization
about; tomato	/baʊt/; /meɪroʊ/	deletion of unstressed initial syllable
haste; desk	/heɪs/; /dɛs/	cluster reduction
ghosts; desks	/goʊsəz/; /dɛsəz/	cluster reduction + plural
Substitution and Assimilatory Processes		
both; mother	/boʊf/; /mʌvə/	labialization
ask; grasp	/æks/; /græps/	metathesis
winning; running	/wɪnɪn/; /rʌnɪn/	fronting
isn't; hasn't	/ɪdn̩t/; /hædn̩t/	stopping
hit; bag	/hɪʔ/; /bæʔ/	glottal stop substitution
string; strong	/skrɪŋ/; /skraŋ/	backing
bid; bad	/bɪːt/; /bæːt/	devoicing of final stop
Vowel Characteristics		
pen; many	/pɪn/; /mɪnɪ/	/ɛ/-/ɪ/ merger
sister; doctor	/sɪstə/; /dɑktə/	derhotacization
tire; flour	/tar/; /flar/	monophthongization

Sources: Information from Pollock & Meredith, 2001; Terrell & Terrell, 1993; Wolfram, 1994; Wolfram & Fasold, 1974; Wolfram & Thomas, 2002.

Liquids also may be deleted or vocalized in AAE. /r/ may be deleted in prevocalic, intervocalic, and word-final positions, as in "through"/θu/, "story" /stoʊɪ/, and "door" /doʊ/. Postvocalic /r/ also may be derhotacized as in "cheer" /tʃɪə/ and "fair" /fɛə/. /l/ may be deleted when it occurs in the post-vocalic position of words, as in "wolf" /wʊf/ and "shelf" /ʃɛf/. /l/ also may be vocalized in word-final position, as in "nickel" /nɪkʊ/ or "bell" /bɛʊ/ (Pollock & Meredith, 2001).

Another AAE syllable structure process involves the elision of the un-stressed (weak) initial syllable of a word, as in "because" /kəz/ or "about" /baʊt/. Also, consonant clusters at the ends of words are often reduced when the final consonant is a stop. This simplification occurs when both consonants in the cluster share the same voicing pattern, that is, both voiced or both voiceless (Wolfram, 1994). Examples include "begged"/bɛg/, "desk" /dɛs/, and "ghost" /goʊs/. Words with a final cluster comprised of /s/ followed by a stop (e.g., "desk" or "ghost") will have an AAE plural form of /əz/ (Wolfram, 1994). Some examples in AAE include "desks" /dɛsəz/ and "ghosts" /goʊsəz/. This plural form is typical of General American English words ending in /s/, for example, /leɪs/ "lace" → /leɪsəz/ "laces."

Substitution and Assimilatory Processes

In AAE, *stopping* occurs when voiced fricatives precede a nasal (i.e., "isn't" /ɪdn̩t/ and "even" /ibm̩/). Stopping also occurs with the interdental fricatives /ð/ and /θ/, as in "these" /diz/ and "this" /dɪs/. In addition, glottal stops may replace final stops in some instances (e.g., "bag" /bæʔ/ and "bid" /bɪʔ/).

There are several other consonant substitutions observed in speakers of AAE: (1) the interdental fricatives /θ/ and /ð/ may be *labialized* and produced as /f/ and /v/, respectively, both in medial and word-final positions, as in "Ruth" /ruf/ and "brother" /brʌvə/; (2) /ŋ/ may be *fronted* to /n/ in words containing "ing" as in "hanging" /hæŋɪn/; (3) final clusters comprised of /s/ + stop may be reversed in certain words (metathesis), as in "ask" /æks/; and (4) /t/ in word-initial /str/ consonant clusters may be *backed* to /k/, as in "string" /skrɪŋ/ (Wolfram and Thomas, 2002).

One assimilatory process characteristic of AAE phonology is the *devoicing* of final voiced stops (e.g., "rag" /ræːk/ or "bad" /bæːt/). Note that the longer vowel length associated with voiced stops is maintained in this condition (Wolfram, 1994).

Vowel Characteristics

Similar to some speakers of Southern American English, the vowels /ɝ/ and /ɚ/ may become derhotacized, as in "third" /θɜːd/ or "mother" /mʌvə/. Also, in AAE some speakers merge /ɪ/ and /ɛ/ so that "many" and "Benny" would be produced and perceived as /bɪnɪ/. Finally, diphthongs are sometimes simplified in AAE, as in "tire" /tar/. Recall that this is a characteristic also observed in some southern speakers.

EXERCISE 8.7

Examine each of the words below. Then look at the AAE phonological pattern that should be applied to each word. Provide the appropriate transcription in the blank at the right.

Example:

east	cluster reduction	/is/

1.	ran	nasal deletion	_____
2.	with	labialization	_____
3.	Carol	/r/ deletion	_____
4.	weeds	stop deletion	_____
5.	wasn't	stopping	_____
6.	yelling	fronting	_____
7.	brother	derhotacization	_____
8.	behind	deletion of unstressed initial syllable	_____
9.	Denny	vowel merger	_____
10.	pickle	liquid vocalization	_____

Learning English as a Second Language

The demographic profile of the population of the United States has changed markedly over the last four decades. There has been a steady increase in the number of immigrants coming to the United States from other countries (especially from countries in the Eastern hemisphere) following the elimination of the national origins quota system when the Immigration Act of 1965 was signed into law by President Lyndon Johnson.

It is estimated that 38.1 million residents of the United States were foreign-born in 2007. According to the United States Census Bureau, foreign-born individuals are those who: (1) were not U.S. citizens or U.S. nationals at birth; or (2) were not U.S. citizens, or were naturalized U.S. citizens at the time the census was completed. The foreign-born population currently accounts for 12.6 percent of the total U.S. population, the largest percentage of foreign-born individuals living in the country since 1940 (Grieco, 2010; Schmidley, 2001). The total foreign-born population in the United States has increased by over 28 million since 1970, when the number of foreign-born individuals accounted for only 4.7 percent of the population (Schmidley, 2001).

In 2007, the largest number of foreign-born residents came from Latin America (54 percent), with the largest percentage coming from Mexico. Individuals from Asia accounted for 27 percent of the foreign-born population, whereas individuals from Europe accounted for only 13 percent (Grieco, 2010). It is interesting to contrast these statistics with the data from 1960, which shows that the largest number of foreign-born residents were from Europe (75 percent). In 1960, only 14 percent of the U.S. foreign-born population comprised individuals from Asia and Latin America, compared to 81 percent in 2007.

Nearly 20 percent of the U.S. population (age 5 or older) speaks a non-English language at home. This reflects an increase of 6 percent since 1990 (Shin & Bruno, 2003; U.S. Census Bureau, 2008b). Other than English, Spanish is the most spoken language in the United States. In the 55 million homes where a language other than English is spoken, 34 million families (62 percent) speak Spanish, 19 percent speak another Indo-European language, 15 percent speak an Asian/Pacific Islander Language, and 4 percent speak another language (U.S. Census Bureau, 2008b). Next to Spanish, Chinese is the most spoken language in the home (2.4 million speakers), followed by Tagalog (1.4 million), French (1.3 million), Vietnamese (1.2 million), German (1.1 million), and Korean (1 million) (U.S. Census Bureau, 2008a).

Approximately 39 percent of the residents of California, 37 percent of the residents of New Mexico, and 31 percent of the residents of Texas speak a non-English language. In addition, Arizona, Florida, Hawaii, New York, and New Jersey each report that more than 20 percent of their residents speak a second language. Close to one-half of all U.S. residents who speak a second language live in California, Texas, or New York (Shin & Bruno, 2003).

For someone learning a second language, the phonology of the person's native language (L_1), will influence the pronunciation of the second (target) language (L_2). The influence of one's native language on the learning of a new language is termed **language transfer.** Language transfer is the incorporation of L_1 language features (including phonology) into the L_2 as the second language is being learned.

Due to the influence of L_1 on L_2 as a new language is being learned, there often will be a mismatch between the two phonological systems. According to Yavaş (2006), this mismatch can take several forms, causing the L_2 learner to be perceived as having a "foreign accent." The first example of a phonological mismatch is the lack of a phoneme in the native (L_1) language that does exist in L_2. For example, the voiceless plosive /p/ is absent in Arabic. Arabic speakers learning English will typically substitute /b/ for /p/ (i.e., /bɑrtɪ/ for "party") since these two phonemes differ only in voicing, but share place and manner specifications. A second divergence in phonological systems occurs when phonemes in the L_2 exist only as allophones in the L_1. For instance, in Korean, /s/, /z/, and /ʃ/ are all allophones of /s/; they do not exist as separate phonemes. A third divergence occurs when a phoneme common to both L_1 and L_2 are pronounced differently. For instance, in some Asian languages, initial voiceless stops are unaspirated, whereas in English, they are aspirated. A fourth mismatch occurs when the allowable syllable structures of L_1 and L_2 differ. In Mandarin Chinese, the only final sounds allowed are /n/ and /ŋ/. A Mandarin speaker of English may then delete the final consonant in a word if the final sound is not /n/ or /ŋ/ (i.e., /fu/ for "food"). Another example involves production of the consonant clusters /sk/, /st/, and /sp/ by Spanish speakers learning English. These clusters do not occur in the initial position of Spanish words as they do in English. Either /ə/ or /ɛ/ is added prior to the cluster, splitting its components so that each element of the cluster will appear in two separate syllables, for example, /əspat/ or /ɛspat/ for "spot" or /əskul/ or /ɛskul/ for "school." Finally, suprasegmental differences between L_1 and L_2 often cause mismatches in pronunciation.

In addition to language transfer issues, the dialect of an individual's L_1 will have an impact on the pronunciation of the target language (L_2). As an example, a native, Spanish-speaking person originally from Mexico City would have a different English accent than would a native Spanish speaker originally from Chihuahua. This is because the dialects of Spanish spoken in those two Mexican cities vary. Additionally, the accent of an English second-language learner may reflect regional variations of English depending on where the person lives in the United States.

As practicing clinicians, you need to have a heightened awareness of the dialects and language practices of second-language learners, especially if you choose to work with children. You will need to learn what is considered to be normal phonological development and what is not, depending on an individual's L_1. The children you will be serving will have varied language backgrounds. That is, some will come from homes where only the L_2 is spoken, some will come from homes where only the L_1 is spoken, and others may rely more on one language than the other, or they may be completely bilingual.

An individual who is attempting to master English as a second language is said to be an **English Language Learner** (ELL). This term, adopted by the National Council of Teachers of English (NCTE), is similar to the term *Limited English Proficiency (LEP)* still in use by the U.S. Department of Education in reference to children who do not meet state standards in relation to English mastery. The term ELL underscores learning rather than focusing on deficiencies (NCTE, 2008).

As English develops, the ELL child may display a dialectal variation of English due to language transfer, factors associated with the child's environment and to familial language practice. If the child's language and speech performance are related to dialectal variation and not a communication disorder, therapeutic treatment is not necessarily indicated. However, it is possible for ELL children to have other communication deficits associated with hearing loss, cleft palate, fluency disorders, language disorders, or phonological disorders (not due to language transfer). In any of these instances, treatment might be indicated.

Adults who have learned English as a second language may elect to receive assistance in *accent modification* in order to improve overall speech intelligibility. This is especially important if an individual wishes to be more easily understood in the workplace, particularly in fields where good expressive communication skills are necessary.

Spanish-Influenced English

According to the 2007 *American Community Survey Reports* published by the U.S. Census Bureau, the Hispanic population in the United States numbered 45.4 million, or 15 percent of the total population. This makes the Hispanic population the largest minority group in the United States (Grieco, 2010).

The term *Hispanic* refers to an individual of Mexican, Puerto Rican, Cuban, or South or Central American descent, including individuals who indicated *ethnic origin* on their census report as "other Spanish culture or origin regardless of race" (U.S. Census Bureau, 2007a). Almost two-thirds of the Hispanic population in the United States comes from Mexico (64 percent), followed by Puerto Rico (9 percent), other Central American countries (8 percent), South America (5 percent), Cuba (4 percent), and "Other" (7 percent), which includes individuals who gave survey responses such as "Hispanic," "Spanish," or "Latino" (Grieco, 2010). Recall that Spanish is spoken in nearly 62 percent of the homes in the United States in which a second language is spoken. In addition, almost half of all Spanish speakers live in either Texas or California (U.S. Census Bureau, 2003).

Many Hispanic children in the United States are born into families in which Spanish is the primary language spoken, both by parents and by other family members. The extent to which a Hispanic child becomes masterful in the use of the English language depends on (1) the age when the child was first exposed to English, (2) the degree of acceptance of English by the immediate family members, (3) the degree of exposure to English in the child's daily environment, and (4) whether the child's family is monolingual or bilingual (Perez, 1994; Reed, 1994).

In relation to bilingualism, the family members may be fluent in both Spanish and English. However, not all bilingual individuals are skilled in both languages. Some bilingual individuals are more fluent in one language than the other. In some cases, there may be limited skill in both languages.

Phonological Characteristics of Spanish-Influenced English

Because some Hispanic children may be considered ELL when they enter school, speech-language pathologists should understand how Spanish may influence the further development of English. Otherwise, it would not be possible to tell whether a child's particular speech patterns were related to Spanish-Influenced English (SIE) or were reflective of a speech sound disorder.

The phonemic system of Spanish varies from that of English, both in terms of vowels and consonants. In English, there are 14 vowels (excluding the diphthongs). Spanish, on the other hand, has only five vowels: /i, e, a, o, and u/ (Iglesias & Goldstein, 1998; Perez, 1994). Therefore, knowledge of Spanish (L$_1$) may influence the production of English (L$_2$) vowels. Some vowel productions in SIE are predictable from a transfer point of view. That is, English words that contain vowels not typical of Spanish may be produced by substituting one of the five Spanish vowels located in close proximity to the English vowel in the vowel quadrilateral. Examples include a/ʌ, as in /sam/ for "some", and /i/ for /ɪ/, as in /sit/ for "sit." There are other vowel productions in SIE that are not predictable from a transfer view of speech sound production. In most cases, the substitution is for a vowel that shares a similar place of production. Examples include æ/ɛ, as in /mæn/ for "men" and ʊ/u as in /rʊm/ for "room" (Perez, 1994). More examples of SIE vowel productions are given in Table 8.4.

There are several consonants that are shared by both Spanish and English. These include the stops /p, t, k, b, d, and g/, the nasals /m/ and /n/, the fricatives /f/ and /s/, the affricate /tʃ/, and the approximants /w, l, and j/ (Iglesias & Goldstein, 1998). Spanish has several phonemes that are not found in English. These include the voiceless, velar fricative /x/, the voiced palatal nasal /ɲ/, and the trilled /r/ (Bleile & Goldstein, 1996). (Recall that the English approximant /r/ is not trilled and is officially represented by the IPA symbol /ɹ/.) Spanish also contains the voiced fricatives /β/ (bilabial) and /ɣ/ (velar), which are actually allophones of /b/ and /g/, respectively (Goldstein, 2001). In addition, English contains sounds that do not occur in Spanish. These include the aspirated stops [pʰ, tʰ, and kʰ]; the nasal /ŋ/, the obstruents /v, s, ʃ, θ, tʃ, and dʒ/; and the liquid /ɹ/. Some of these phonemes, however, exist in some Spanish dialects (Goldstein, 2001), and some exist as allophones (e.g., /ŋ/).

The differences in the English and Spanish consonant systems, and their affect on Spanish Influenced English, can be categorized in terms of syllable structure, substitution, and assimilatory processes (Perez, 1994). Some of the consonant productions can be explained in terms of transfer. For example, /θ/ does not exist in Spanish. A typical SIE substitution would be t/θ as in /tɪŋk/ for "think" (stopping). As mentioned earlier, the consonant clusters /sk/, /st/, or /sp/ do not occur in the initial position of words in Spanish. Therefore, a common SIE production involves the epenthesis of /ə/ to the initial portion of the cluster, creating two syllables, as in /əspat/ "spot." Examples of SIE consonant articulations are described in Table 8.5.

TABLE 8.4   Common Spanish-Influenced English Vowel Productions

English Word	SIE Transcription	Vowel Substitution
lid	/lid/	i/ɪ
need	/nɪd/	ɪ/i
late	/lɛt/	ɛ/eɪ
tennis	/teɪnɪs/	eɪ/ɛ
dead	/dæd/	æ/ɛ
bag	/bɑg/ or /bɛg/	ɑ or ɛ/æ
look	/luk/	u/ʊ
pool	/pʊl/	ʊ/u
bug	/bɑg/ or /bag/	ɑ or a/ʌ
word	/wɛrd/	ɛr/ɝ
boat	/bot/	monophthongization

Source: Information from Goldstein, 2001; Perez, 1994.

TABLE 8.5   Common Spanish-Influenced English Consonant Productions

English Word	SIE Transcription	Phonological Pattern
Syllable Structure Processes		
stand	/əstand/ or /ɛstand/	epenthesis of /ə or ɛ/ preceding initial /s/ + stop clusters
explain	/spleɪn/	unstressed syllable deletion
rest	/rɛs/	final consonant cluster reduction
hold	/hol/	final consonant cluster reduction
date	/deɪ/	final consonant deletion
Substitution Processes		
think	/tɪŋk/	stopping
vase	/bes/	stopping
you	/dʒu/	affrication of a glide
sheep	/tʃip/	affrication of a fricative
choose	/ʃuz/	deaffrication
Assimilation Processes		
zoo	/su/	devoicing (initial)
was	/wʌs/	devoicing (final)
tea	/t̪i/	dentalization

Sources: Information from Goldstein, 2001; Perez, 1994.

EXERCISE 8.8

Determine the phonological pattern being demonstrated in each of the following SIE pronunciations. Write your answer in the blank.

Examples:

need	/nɪd/	ɪ/i substitution
juice	/tʃus/	devoicing

1. last   /læs/   _____
2. much   /matʃ/   _____
3. check   /ʃɛk/   _____
4. yes   /dʒɛs/   _____
5. spoiled   /ɛspɔɪld/   _____
6. them   /dɛm/   _____
7. Cher   /tʃɛr/   _____
8. voice   /bɔɪs/   _____
9. mood   /mut/   _____
10. wound   /wun/   _____

Asian/Pacific-Influenced English

The 2004 U.S. Census Bureau's *American Community Survey Report* indicates that 13.5 million residents of the United States are Asian (almost 5 percent of the population). In addition, there are 743,000 Pacific Islanders living in the United States (less than one percent of the population) (U.S. Census Bureau, 2007b, 2007c). Almost one-half of these residents (7 million) speak either a Pacific Island or an Asian language; this reflects an increase of 2.5 million people since 1990. Approximately 35 percent of the Asian/Pacific Islands (API) population lives in California and approximately 10 percent live in New York State.

Sixty percent of the U.S. Asian population is either Chinese (2.8 million), Asian Indian (2.2 million), or Filipino (2.1 million). The most common API languages spoken in the United States are Chinese (over 2 million speakers), Filipino (the national language of the Philippines, often referred to as Tagalog; 1.2 million speakers), Vietnamese (1 million speakers), Korean (894,000 speakers), and Japanese (478,000 speakers). Forty percent of all Chinese speakers live in California (Reeves and Bennett, 2003).

The languages spoken in Asia and the Pacific Islands are quite diverse. There are over 1,200 languages spoken by the 5 million residents of the Pacific Islands alone (Cheng, 2001). As one might expect, Asian languages differ markedly from one another, both in terms of grammatical rules and phonology. Similarly, Asian languages vary greatly from the grammatical rules and phonology of English. For instance, in Chinese, each printed character is only one syllable in length. Therefore, when a Chinese person is learning English, there is a tendency to pronounce multisyllabic words syllable by syllable, in a telegraphic manner (Cheng, 2001).

Several Asian languages, such as Chinese and Vietnamese, are *tone languages*. In a tone language, a word's meaning may differ when pronounced with a varying tone or intonation pattern. For instance, in Mandarin, one of the major Chinese dialects spoken in the United States, the syllable /ba/ may mean "eight," "to pull," "handle," "to give up," or "okay," depending on the intonation produced as the word is articulated (Cheng, 1994). In a tone language, intonation is considered to be phonemic because each tone will convey a different meaning to the listener. As you know, in English, tone is not phonemic. Instead, tone generally indicates the speaker's mood or intent or signals whether the utterance is a statement or a question.

The speech patterns of Asian L_1 speakers as they produce English are, at least in part, due to transfer issues related to the speaker's native language. For instance, in Chinese and Vietnamese, consonant clusters do not exist. Vietnamese instead has vowel clusters, diphthongs, and triphthongs (Hwa-Froelich, Hodson, & Edwards, 2002). In Korean, consonant clusters do not exist in initial or final positions of words (Cheng, 1987b). Therefore, when an Asian/Pacific-Influenced English (APIE) speaker produces an English word containing a consonant cluster, there is a tendency to simplify the cluster. This results in deletion of consonants or insertion of a vowel between the consonants in the cluster, as in "glue" /gəlu/.

In English, voiceless initial stops are aspirated; this is not the case in Vietnamese and Tagalog. Initial voiceless stops are unaspirated and are perceived by English speakers as voiced, for example, [tʰ] would be perceived as /d/.

It is also quite common in English for words to end with a consonant; 21 of the English consonants occur at the ends of words. In Japanese, the only final consonant is /n/. In Mandarin, there are only two final consonants, /n/ and /ŋ/, and in Cantonese (the other major Chinese dialect spoken in the United States), there are seven final consonants, /m, n, ŋ, p, t, k, and ʔ/ (Cheng, 1987b). Mandarin, Cantonese, and Japanese speakers often delete final consonants of English words since it is not common for syllables and words to have a coda in their native languages.

Substitutions for final consonants do occur in some cases. For instance, in Cantonese, both voiceless and voiced stops may be unreleased; unreleased voiceless stops may be perceived by English speakers as voiced, for example, [pˈ] would be perceived as /b/ (Ball & Müller, 2005). In Vietnamese, a number of final consonant substitutions also are typical (Hwa-Froelich et al., 2002). Japanese speakers, on the other hand, will sometimes add a vowel to the ends of syllables and words in order to create an open syllable, such as "desk" /dɛskɚ/, since /n/ is the only consonant found in coda position (Cheng, 2001).

Table 8.6 displays several consonant substitutions that are associated with production of Asian/Pacific-influenced English. This table highlights English consonant substitutions by speakers of Cantonese Chinese, Mandarin Chinese,

TABLE 8.6 Common English Consonant Substitutions, as Spoken by Chinese, Vietnamese, Korean, Japanese, and Tagalog Speakers (Mandarin and Cantonese dialects of Chinese are shown separately)

Intended Phoneme		Observed Phoneme					
		Cantonese	Mandarin	Vietnamese	Korean	Japanese	Tagalog
Fricatives	θ	s, t, f	s	s, t	t	t, s, z, j	t
	ð	d, z	d, z	d, z	dz, d	d, z, j, t, s	d
	ʃ	s		s	s	s, tʃ	s
	ʒ			z, dʒ	z	dʒ	ds
	f			p	p	p, h	p
	v	f, w	f, w	j, b, p	b, p	b, f, w	b
	s			ʃ	ʃ	ʃ	
	z	s		s, ʃ	s, ts, dz	dz, dʒ, s	s
Affricates	tʃ		ʃ	s, ʃ	t	ts, t	ts
	dʒ	z		z, ʒ	tʃ	z, ʒ	ds
Stops	p	pˈ		b, f			
	pʰ			p⁼			p⁼
	t	tˈ		p			
	tʰ			t⁼		tʃ	t⁼
	k	kˈ					
	kʰ			k⁼			k⁼
	b	pˈ	p	p		p	
	d	tˈ		t		dʒ, t	
	g	kˈ		k			
Liquids	r	l	l	n	l	l
	l		r		r	r

Sources: Information from Bada, 2001; Ball & Müller, 2005; Cheng, 1987a, 1987b; Hwa-Froelich, Hodson, & Edwards, 2002; Shen, 1962; Yavaş, 2006.

Vietnamese, Korean, Japanese, and Tagalog. Remember that many consonants are deleted in *final* position.

L$_2$ English vowel production is challenging as well due to the differences between English and Asian vowel systems. Both Japanese and Tagalog have only five vowels. Transfer becomes an issue when trying to produce 14 English vowels with such a small set of native vowels. The vowel systems in Japanese, Korean, Tagalog, and Vietnamese do not maintain a tense/lax vowel distinction, as in English. For instance, in Korean, the vowel system is comprised of /i, e, ɛ, u, o, ʌ, and a/ as well as other vowels not typical of English (*Handbook of the International Phonetic Association,* 1999). Note the absence of /ɪ, ɛ, ʊ, and ɔ/, the lax counterparts of /i, e, u, and o/. Korean speakers therefore may substitute tense vowels when pronouncing English words, as in /sit/ for /sɪt/ or /buk/ for /bʊk/.

EXERCISE 8.9

Apply the given substitution to each transcription in order to produce an APIE pronunciation of each word. Provide both the APIE transcription and the English orthography.

English Transcription	*Substitution*	*APIE Transcription*	*English Orthography*
Example:			
/raɪs/	l/r	/laɪs/	rice
Cantonese			
1. /θɪŋk/	s/θ	_____	_____
2. /ʃuz/	s/ʃ	_____	_____
3. /vaɪn/	w/v	_____	_____
4. /bædz/	z/dʒ	_____	_____
Japanese			
5. /ðɪs/	z/ð	_____	_____
6. /fri/	h/f	_____	_____
7. /ʃɪp/	i/ɪ	_____	_____
Tagalog			
8. /faɪn/	p/f	_____	_____
9. /tʃɛk/	ts/tʃ	_____	_____
10. /vat/	b/v	_____	_____

Russian- and Arabic-Influenced English

Due to the large influx of individuals from Europe and Asia to the United States, it might be instructive to look at some other examples of phonological transfer from two vastly different languages, Arabic and Russian. Arabic is an Afroasiatic language, while Russian is a member of the Indo-European family of languages. Both Arabic and Russian have very different phonemic systems when compared to English, even though Russian (a Balto-Slavic language) and English (a Germanic language) are both Indo-European languages. Each language will be examined separately to help explain some of the mismatches between Arabic and Russian (L₁) and American English (L₂).

Russian-Influenced English

Russian has only five vowels, /i, e, a, u, and o/, and only one true diphthong, /aʊ/ (Berger, 1952). For this reason, Russian speakers learning English have difficulty with vowel production. In unstressed syllables, the five vowels are reduced to three: /i, a, and ə/, and similar to Asian languages, lax vowels are tensed as in the following substitutions: i/ɪ, e/ɛ, u/ʊ, and o/ɔ. The vowel /a/ is produced as a substitute for /æ, ɑ, and ʌ/ (Yavaş, 2006). See Table 8.7 for a summary of Russian-influenced English pronunciations.

The Russian consonant system also varies significantly when compared to English. For example, voiceless stop consonants in Russian tend to be unaspirated. Therefore, English words that begin with a voiceless stop may be unaspirated when spoken by a Russian individual learning English. An unaspirated voiceless stop at the beginning of a word will tend to sound voiced. For example, "came" [k⁼eɪm] will sound like "game" [geɪm] (Baker, 1982; Berger, 1952). Also, alveolar phonemes may be produced as dentalized consonants, e.g., [t̪, d̪, and n̪] (Yavaş, 2006).

TABLE 8.7   Common Russian-Influenced English Vowel and Consonant Productions

English Word	Russian-Influenced English Transcription	Substitution
Vowel Articulations		
sit	/sit/	i/ɪ
book	/buk/	u/ʊ
hat	/hat/	a/æ
caught	/kot/	o/ɔ
men	/men/	e/ɛ
Consonant Articulations		
pool	/p⁼ul/	unaspirated stop
tame	/t̪em/	dentalization
mood, bags	/mut/, /baks/	devoicing
this, thin	/dis/, /tin/	stopping
laughing	/lafɪŋk/	epenthesis
quota	/kvotə/	frication
vodka	/wodkə/	gliding
ham	/xam/	fronting
run (/ɹʌn/)	/ran/	r/ɹ substitution

Sources: Information from Berger, 1952; Power, 2003a; Yavaşş, 2006.

There are several consonants in English that do not exist in Russian: /ð, θ, dʒ, w, and r/; /ŋ/ exists only as an allophone of /n/. Because of phonological mismatch (transfer) between languages:

1. The interdental fricatives /ð and θ/ are often stopped, as in "them" /dɛm/ and "thin" /tɪn/.
2. The affricate /dʒ/ may be devoiced and produced as /tʃ/, as in "jam" /tʃam/.
3. The glide /w/ may be produced as /v/ (frication), as in "when" /vɛn/.
4. The approximant /ɹ / is pronounced as a trill, i.e., /r/.
5. The velar nasal /ŋ/ is produced *as an allophone of* /n/ when it occurs before velar stops.

Therefore, in words where /ŋ/ does not precede a velar stop, one is added (epenthesis), as in "running" /ranɪŋk/. In this context, the added velar is also devoiced: /rʌnɪŋg/→ /rʌnɪŋk/ (Power, 2003a; Yavaş, 2006).

Additionally, some Russian speakers front the production of the voiceless glottal /h/ and produce it as a voiceless velar fricative /x/ as in "hot" /xɑt/. Also, /v/ is produced either as the voiced bilabial fricative /β/, /w/, or /vw/ (Berger, 1952). For example, "vodka" could be produced as /βɔdkə/, /wɔdkə/, or /vwɔdkə/.

In Russian, voiced obstruents do not occur in word-final position resulting in devoicing of the final phoneme, such as "lag" /lak/ (Baker, 1982; Berger, 1952). Also, clusters comprised of voiced stops and fricatives do not occur together in the final position of a word. Therefore, the word "bags" would be pronounced as /bæks/ (/g/ and /z/ both being produced as their voiceless cognates /k/ and /s/). Finally, voiceless and voiced phonemes do not occur together at word boundaries (Berger, 1952). For example, "hit the ball," would be produced as /hɪdðəbal/. Note the effect of regressive assimilation in this case.

EXERCISE 8.10

For the following, fill in the blank with the correct phonological process being demonstrated. For some items, there will be more than one answer.

Example:

			Phonological Process
X	pack	/pˌak/	unaspirated stop, a/æ substitution
____ 1.	foot	/fut/	_____
____ 2.	very	/wɛri/	_____
____ 3.	badge	/batʃ/	_____
____ 4.	swim	/svɪm/	_____
____ 5.	those	/dos/	_____
____ 6.	eating	/it̪ɪŋk/	_____
____ 7.	rugs	/raks/	_____
____ 8.	kiss	/xis/	_____

Arabic-Influenced English

Arabic has only three vowels, /i/, /a/, and /u/ (all tense), which occur in both short and long forms. The vowels /i, ɪ, e/ are all produced as /i/, the vowels /æ, ɑ, and ʌ/ are produced as /a/, and /ʊ/ is produced as /u/; the vowel /ɛ/ may be produced as either /a/ or /i/ (Yavaş, 2006). Note that most of the substitutions reflect tensing of the vowels. The only diphthongs in Arabic are /eɪ/ and /aʊ/.

Several English obstruents do not exist in Arabic: /p, v, ʒ, and tʃ/ (Altaha, 1995; *Handbook of the International Phonetic Association,* 1999). Some of the obstruents do exist in some dialects of Arabic, however. Due to phonological transfer:

1. /p/ is voiced and produced as /b/, as in "peel" /bil/.
2. /v/ is devoiced and produced as /f/, as in "vote" /fot/.
3. /tʃ/ and /ʒ/ are often produced as /ʃ/ as in "choose" /ʃuz/ (deaffrication) and "measure" /mɛʃɚ/ (devoicing).

As in Russian, /ŋ/ exists as an allophone of /n/ before velar stops (Yavaş, 2006). Therefore, in words where /ŋ/ does not precede a velar stop, /g/ is added, as in "running" /ranɪŋg/ (epenthesis). Also, the English liquid /ɹ/ does not exist and is produced as the alveolar trill /r/. Phonemes of Arabic not found in English include the voiceless uvular plosive /q/, the velar fricatives /x/ (voiceless) and /ɣ/ (voiced), the voiceless pharyngeal fricative /ħ/, and several pharyngealized consonants including /tˤ, dˤ, sˤ, ðˤ, lˤ, and ʔˤ/ (*Handbook of the International Phonetic Association,* 1999).

In Arabic, it is not possible to have a cluster of two or three consonants at the beginning of a word. For this reason, vowels are added in production of clusters, as in /sikrim/ for "scream" and /sitrit/ for "street" (Altaha, 1995).

TABLE 8.8   Common Arabic-Influenced English Vowel and Consonant Productions

English Word	Arabic-Influenced English Transcription	Phonological Pattern
Vowel Articulations		
bit	/bit/	i/ɪ
cup	/kap/	a/ʌ
cap	/kap/	a/æ
set	/sit/ or /sat/	i or a/ɛ
look	/luk/	u/ʊ
Consonant Articulations		
put	/but/	voicing
love	/laf/	devoicing
lesion	/liʃən/	devoicing
watch	/waʃ/	deaffrication
reed (/ɹid/)	/rid/	r/ɹ
wing	/wɪŋg/	epenthesis
scream	/sikrim/	epenthesis

Sources: Information from Altaha, 1995; Baker, 1982; Power, 2003b; Yavaş, 2006.

Arabic speakers learning English will sometimes pronounce silent letters, since Arabic's alphabet is phonemic, as in "knot" /knat/, "could" /kuld/, and "lamb" /læmb/. Other difficulties that arise from English spelling intrusions include problems pronouncing words with the letter "c" as in "city" /kiti/ or "soccer" /sasɚ/. In a similar manner, since the letter "g" can be pronounced as either /dʒ/ or /g/, Arabic speakers may produce "gear" as /dʒir/ and "origin" as /arigin/. Also, the spelling "dg" may be pronounced as two separate phonemes, as in /badgit/ for "budget" (Altaha, 1995). Refer to Table 8.8 for a summary of Arabic-Influenced English productions.

EXERCISE 8.11

For the following, indicate (with an "X") the productions that are consistent with the phonological patterns associated with Arabic-Influenced English. For these words, fill in the blank with the correct description of the pattern. For some items, there will be more than one phonological pattern being demonstrated.

Example:			Phonological Process
__X__	luck	/luk/	u/ʊ substitution (vowel tensing)
_____	1. azure	/aʃɚ/	_____
_____	2. Paul	/bal/	_____
_____	3. hat	/xæt/	_____
_____	4. check	/ʃɛk/	_____
_____	5. did	/did/	_____
_____	6. vase	/fes/	_____
_____	7. hearing	/hiriŋ/	_____
_____	8. win	/vin/	_____

Review Exercises

A. Transcribe each of the following words as if they were pronounced by a Southern American English Speaker.

1. steal _____   6. fought _____
2. steer _____   7. coil _____
3. ferry _____   8. treasur _____
4. dew _____   9. lines _____
5. mesh _____   10. when _____

B. Provide English orthography for each of the following Southern American English pronunciations.

1. /lɪmɪn/ _____   7. /hɪl/ _____
2. /spoət/ _____   8. /wɜːðɪ/ _____
3. /preɪʃɪʃ/ _____   9. /tʃɛə/ _____
4. /pjuə/ _____   10. /stiu/ _____
5. /wiʃ/ _____   11. /kɑːt/ _____
6. /wɔtʃ/ _____   12. /kærɪ/ _____

C. Transcribe each of the following words as if they were pronounced by an Eastern American English speaker. All of these words involve some form of /r/ deletion or derhotacization.

1. beware _____   6. store _____
2. start _____   7. squirt _____
3. hanger _____   8. glare _____
4. severe _____   9. doctor _____
5. clergy _____   10. carbon _____

D. Provide English orthography for each of the following Eastern American English pronunciations.

1. /kɑnt/ _____   6. /ɛksploə/ _____
2. /brʊm/ _____   7. /tʃaːrə/ _____
3. /mæroʊ/ _____   8. /ladʒɪst/ _____
4. /baθ/ _____   9. /dɪmɑnd/ _____
5. /pærɪt/ _____   10. /kənspaɪə/ _____

E. Examine each of the words below. Then look at the AAE phonological pattern that should be applied to each word. Provide the appropriate transcription in the blank at the right.

Example:

| east | cluster reduction | /is/ |

1. moth   labialization   _____
2. because   deletion of unstressed initial syllable _____
3. then   /ɛ/-/ɪ/ merger   _____
4. can   nasal deletion   _____
5. Harold   /l/ vocalization   _____
6. them   stopping   _____
7. mind   monophthongization   _____
8. wastes   cluster reduction + plural   _____
9. eleven   stopping   _____
10. straight   backing   _____

F. For the following words, indicate (with an "X") the productions that are consistent with the phonological patterns associated with AAE. For those words, write the phonological pattern being demonstrated in the blank.

Example:

| east | /is/ | cluster reduction |

1. bread   /brɛ/   _____
2. broom   /brʊm/   _____
3. suppose /poʊz/   _____
4. raced   /reɪs/   _____
5. cat   /kæʔ/   _____
6. Ben   /bɪn/   _____
7. light   /lat/   _____
8. hold   /hoʊd/   _____
9. cola   /koʊlɚ/ _____

10. washing   /waʃɪn/   _____
11. carry   /kærɪ/   _____
12. men   /mẽː/   _____

G. **Spanish-Influenced English.** For the following words, write the description of the phonological pattern being displayed.

   Examples:

late	/lɛt/	ε/eɪ substitution
zebra	/sibrə/	devoicing

   1. bath   /bæt/   _____
   2. been   /bin/   _____
   3. chore   /ʃɔr/   _____
   4. oven   /avən/   _____
   5. young   /dʒaŋ/   _____
   6. told   /tol/   _____
   7. cushion /kuʃən/   _____
   8. Tom   /ṭam/   _____
   9. shallow /tʃælou/   _____
   10. vine   /baɪn/   _____
   11. them   /dɛm/   _____
   12. stood   /əstʊd/   _____

H. Examine the phonological pattern in the APIE pronunciation of each of the following words. From Table 8.6, determine the Asian language(s) in which the given pattern may occur. Write your answers in the blanks.

   Example:

them	/zɛm/	Vietnamese, Japanese, Mandarin, and Cantonese

   1. like   /raɪk/   _____
   2. very   /wɛrɪ/   _____
   3. vine   /baɪn/   _____
   4. shine   /saɪn/   _____
   5. joke   /tʃoʊk/   _____
   6. put   /p⁼ʊt/   _____
   7. thank   /fæŋk/   _____
   8. chant   /tsænt/   _____
   9. zoo   /dzu/   _____
   10. talk   /tʃɑk/   _____

I. Using Tables 8.7 and 8.8, determine whether the phonological process given is indicative of either Russian-Influenced English, Arabic-Influenced English, or both. Mark the appropriate blank with an "X." Then give the name of the process being demonstrated.

Example:

		Russian	Arabic	Both	Phonological Process
lesion	/liʃən/	___	X	___	devoicing
1. pass	/bæs/	___	___	___	_____
2. very	/wɛri/	___	___	___	_____
3. they	/deɪ/	___	___	___	_____
4. good	/gud/	___	___	___	_____
5. funny	/fani/	___	___	___	_____
6. happy	/xæpi/	___	___	___	_____
7. dogs	/daks/	___	___	___	_____
8. school	/sikul/	___	___	___	_____
9. yes mom	/jɛzmɑm/	___	___	___	_____
10. eating	/itɪŋg/	___	___	___	_____
11. roof (/ɹuf/)	/ruf/	___	___	___	_____
12. should	/ʃuld/	___	___	___	_____

J. Eastern American English Transcription Practice. Transcribe each of the following sentences as spoken by a female from New York City.

CD #3
Track 15

1. Ma, I gotta go to the store with Paul today.

_____

2. What are you talking about? Forget about it already.

_____

3. Carly, why do you have to ruin everything?

_____

4. I have a dentist appointment at 6:30.

_____

5. Robert needs to go to the barber, his hair is too long.

_____

6. I walked over to the mall yesterday afternoon to get a new pair of shoes.

_____

7. My dog likes to run all around the yard and bark.

_____

8. When I was playing basketball, I ran all over the court.

_____

9. I gotta go food shopping. I need watermelon, corn, and soda.

_____

10. My friend Mary is a weirdo. She don't want to leave me alone.

_____

K. Eastern American English Transcription Practice.

Transcribe each of the following sentences as spoken by a female from Massachusetts.

1. Park the car in the garage.

_____

2. I am going to the market in Boston.

_____

3. I love to shop Harvard Square.

_____

4. Have you guys been to the Cape or Martha's Vineyard for the summer?

_____

5. Don't forget to bring your pocketbook.

_____

6. Donna loves to drink tonic.

_____

7. Can you wear your dungarees and sneakers?

_____

8. Get a fork for that huge helping of pasta and gravy.

_____

9. Go ahead and give mommy some jimmies for her banana split.

_____

10. John Miller is a decent human being.

_____

L. Southern American English Transcription Practice.

Transcribe each of the following sentences as spoken by a female from Tennessee.

1. She's driving to Louisiana tomorrow morning.

_____

2. I'm going to boil a dozen eggs for Easter.

_____

3. Last night, I was talking to my friend Mary Lynn.

_____

4. I am fixing to have to buy some tires for my car.

_____

5. I am looking for my blue ballpoint pen.

_____

6. You better cover that broiling pan with aluminum foil.

_____

7. Wait a minute, Larry. I need another minute to make up my mind.

_____

8. I left the chicken out on the counter and it spoiled.

_____

9. The University of Tennessee is in Knoxville.

_____

10. Hurricanes and tornadoes are both large damaging wind storms.

_____

M. African American English Transcription Practice.

Transcribe each of the following sentences as spoken by a female from Ohio.

CD #3
Track 18

1. The boy needs more money.

_____

2. We fixin to go to the store.

_____

3. He be playing ball at the park.

_____

4. There four new kids in my class.

_____

5. My sister and brother was at that concert.

_____

6. My family go to church every Sunday.

_____

7. Your momma car in the middle of the street.

_____

8. She found five quarters in her purse.

_____

9. Kwanzaa got her hair done.

_____

10. The students helped themselves to breakfast.

_____

N. Spanish-Influenced English Transcription Practice.

Transcribe each of the following sentences as spoken by a female from Spain.

CD #3
Track 19

1. Please put the flowers in the vase.

_____

2. It was a very special occasion.

_____

3. You should quit yelling at your mother.

_____

4. I was not sure I would be able to help.

_____

5. My favorite teacher's name is Mister Jones.

_____

6. Don't let your dog play in my yard.

_____

7. Why don't you put these clothes in the garage?

_____

8. Yesterday, I went to the zoo with Doug.

_____

9. Shelley put the potato chips on the lower shelf.

_____

10. I was very excited about winning the football game.

_____

O. Asian-Influenced English Transcription Practice.

Transcribe each of the following sentences as spoken by a female from Japan.

1. I have one younger brother in my family.

CD #3
Track 20

_____

2. I would like a grilled cheese sandwich for lunch, please.

_____

3. It is supposed to rain heavily for much of the week.

_____

4. The river is heavily polluted.

_____

5. My sister Kyoko will be 23 years old next Thursday.

_____

6. Would you like to go shopping with me after I get off work?

_____

7. Would your other brother help me lift this? It's heavy.

_____

8. Thank you very much for the beautiful flowers.

_____

9. I have a hard time distinguishing between the singular and plural forms.

_____

10. The only connecting flight is through Portland, Oregon.

_____

P. Asian-Influenced English Transcription Practice.

Transcribe each of the following sentences as spoken by a male from Hong Kong. This male speaks the Cantonese dialect of Chinese.

CD #3
Track 21

1. Typing email helps me think in English.

   _____

2. I went to the zoo to see the new panda bears.

   _____

3. What do you think of the new television show?

   _____

4. I have two or three friends who are going to the soccer game.

   _____

5. Usually, she is not so forgetful.

   _____

6. I bet you that I will win the race.

   _____

7. My girlfriend sent me flowers last week for my birthday.

   _____

8. There are several people I need to get to know.

   _____

9. The layout of this city is not very convenient.

   _____

10. I plan to go to Purdue for my master's degree.

   _____

Q. Russian-Influenced English Transcription Practice.

Transcribe each of the following sentences as spoken by a male from Russia.

1. I would like a vodka and tonic, please.

CD #3
Track 22

   _____

2. Put the books over there on the table.

   _____

3. It was difficult for me to learn the correct pronunciation.

   _____

4. I have been living in the United States since last August.

   _____

5. He has many problems with his vocabulary.

   _____

6. The Russian economy depends on the current price of oil.

   _____

7. My younger brother Alexander is studying metallurgy at Moscow State University.

8. The author of the book was a famous writer.

9. I had several visitors from Virginia last month.

10. How many other people needed to take the class?

R. Arabic-Influenced English Transcription Practice.

Transcribe each of the following sentences as spoken by a male from Saudi Arabia.

1. Please use that word in a sentence.

2. I need sugar substitute for my coffee.

3. Dr. Cooper told me to make a copy of my homework assignment.

4. Their friend Robin got married to Victor, my next door neighbor.

5. I was depressed because we have had so much bad weather.

6. Pete got a prison sentence because he hit the policeman.

7. My favorite cotton shirt shrunk in the laundry.

8. Penny visited her fiancé on Friday.

9. I need to study English phonology to improve my pronunciation.

10. I grew a beard so that I would appear older.

Complete Assignment 8-1.

Study Questions

1. What is a dialect? What is the difference between a regional dialect and an ethnic dialect?
2. What is meant by the terms *Standard American English? General American English?*

3. What is chain shifting? How is chain shifting affecting English vowel production? Which areas of the country are associated with chain shifting?

4. Which features of Southern American English and Eastern American English are similar?

5. How does /r/ deletion and derhotacization affect pronunciation in Eastern, Southern, and AAE speech patterns?

6. What is African American English (AAE)? What are the two theories used to explain its origin?

7. Describe several vowel and consonant features of AAE that differ from General American English.

8. What is the basic difference between the type of dialect associated with AAE and the dialects associated with Spanish- and Asian/Pacific-influenced English?

9. What is meant by the term *language transfer*? How does transfer affect phoneme acquisition by an individual learning English as a second language?

10. Describe several consonant and vowel characteristics typical of Spanish-influenced English.

11. Describe some of the phonological characteristics typical of Asian/Pacific-influenced English.

12. Describe some general characteristics of Asian languages that add to the difficulty of learning English as a second language.

13. How does the Russian phonological system differ from General American English?

14. How does the Arabic phonological system differ from General American English?

15. Should individuals who speak with a dialect receive treatment in order to reduce their "accents"?

Online Resources

Second language acquisition (1997–2010). American Speech-Language-Hearing Association. Retrieved from: *www.asha.org/public/speech/development/second.htm*
(overview of issues involving second language acquisition)

Speech accent archive (2010). Administrator: Steven H. Weinberger, Program in Linguistics, Department of English, George Mason University, Fairfax, VA. Retrieved from: *http://accent.gmu.edu/howto.php*
(audio samples of non-native speakers of English from around the world)

University of Kansas (n.d.). International Dialects of English Archive (IDEA). Maintained by Paul Meier. Retrieved from: *http://web.ku.edu/~idea/*
(online archive of dialect and accent recordings; designed for the performing arts)

Assignment 8-1   Name _____

CD #3
Track 24

"The Grandfather Passage" (Darley, Aronson, and Brown, 1975) will be spoken by several individuals who demonstrate different regional and cultural dialects of American English. Transcribe the passage carefully for each speaker, using systematic phonemic transcription. In some instances, it may be necessary to use systematic narrow transcription. In addition to the phonological patterns produced by these speakers, pay attention to the suprasegmental patterns displayed.

You wish to know all about my grandfather. Well, he is nearly 93 years old, yet he still thinks as swiftly as ever. He dresses himself in an old black frock coat, usually several buttons missing. A long beard clings to his chin, giving those who observe him a pronounced feeling of the utmost respect. When he speaks, his voice is just a bit cracked and quivers a bit. Twice each day he plays skillfully and with zest upon a small organ. Except in the winter when the snow or ice prevents, he slowly takes a short walk in the open air each day. We have often urged him to walk more and smoke less, but he always answers, "Banana oil!" Grandfather likes to be modern in his language.

CD #3
Track 25

1. African American English (Ohio)

_____

_____

_____

_____

_____

_____

_____

_____

CD #3
Track 26

2. Eastern American English (Massachusetts)

_____

_____

_____

_____

_____

_____

_____

_____

Assignment 8-1 (cont.)

CD #3
Track 27

3. Asian/Pacific-Influenced English (China–Cantonese)

_____
_____
_____
_____
_____
_____
_____
_____

CD #3
Track 28

4. Spanish-Influenced English (Spain)

_____
_____
_____
_____
_____
_____
_____
_____

CD #3
Track 29

5. Southern American English (Tennessee)

_____
_____
_____
_____
_____
_____
_____
_____

Assignment 8-1 (cont.)   Name _____

CD #3
Track 30

6. Asian/Pacific-Influenced English (Japan)

_____
_____
_____
_____
_____
_____
_____
_____

CD #3
Track 31

7. Eastern American English (New York City)

_____
_____
_____
_____
_____
_____
_____
_____

CD #3
Track 32

8. Russian-Influenced English

_____
_____
_____
_____
_____
_____
_____
_____

Assignment 8-1 (cont.)

CD #3
Track 33

9. Arabic-Influenced English

_____

_____

_____

_____

_____

_____

_____

_____

References

Altaha, F. M. (1995). Pronunciation errors made by Saudi University students learning English: Analysis and remedy. *I.T.L. Review of Applied Linguistics, 109–110*, 110–123.

American Speech-Language-Hearing Association. (1983). Social dialects. *ASHA, 25*(9), 23–27.

American Speech-Language-Hearing Association. (2003). *Technical report: American English dialects.* (ASHA Supplement 23), 45–46.

Bada, E. (2001). Native language influence on the production of English sounds by Japanese learners. *The Reading Matrix, 1*(2). Retrieved April 7, 2010, from www.readingmatrix.com/articles/bada/article.pdf

Baker, A. (1982). *Introducing English pronunciation: A teacher's guide to tree or three? and ship or sheep?* Cambridge, UK: Cambridge University Press.

Ball, M. J. (2008). Transcribing disordered speech: By target or by production? *Clinical Linguistics & Phonetics, 22,* 864–870.

Ball, M. J., Esling, J., & Dickson, J. (1995). The VoQS system for the transcription of voice quality. *Journal of the International Phonetics Association, 25*(2), 71–80.

Ball, M., & Müller, N. (2005). *Phonetics for communication disorders.* Mahwah, NJ: Lawrence Erlbaum.

Ball, M. J., & Müller, N. (2007). Non-pulmonic-egressive speech in clinical data: A brief review. *Clinical Linguistics & Phonetics, 21,* 869–874.

Bauman-Waengler, J. (2008). *Articulatory and phonological impairments: A clinical focus* (3rd ed.). Boston: Pearson.

Berger, M. D. (1952). The American English pronunciation of Russian immigrants. Unpublished doctoral dissertation, Columbia University, New York.

Bleile, K., & Goldstein, B. (1996). Dialect. In K. Bleile, *Articulation and phonological disorders: A book of exercises* (pp. 73–82). San Diego: Singular Publishing Group.

Boone, D., & McFarlane, S. (1994). *The voice and voice therapy* (5th ed.). Boston: Allyn and Bacon.

Borden, G., Harris, K., & Raphael, L. (1994). *Speech science primer* (3rd ed.). Baltimore: Williams and Wilkins.

Calvert, D. (1986). *Descriptive phonetics.* New York: Thieme.

Carrell, J., & Tiffany, W. (1960). *Phonetics: Theory and application to speech improvement.* New York: McGraw-Hill.

Carver, C. (1987). *American regional dialects: A word geography.* Ann Arbor: University of Michigan Press.

Cheng, L. (1987a). Cross-cultural and linguistic considerations in working with Asian populations, *ASHA, 29*(6), 33–38.

Cheng, L. (1987b). *Assessing Asian language performance.* Rockville, MD: Aspen.

Cheng, L. (1994). Asian/Pacific students and the learning of English. In J. Bernthal & N. Bankson (Eds.), *Child phonology: Characteristics, assessment and intervention with special populations* (pp. 255–274). New York: Thieme.

Cheng, L. (2001). Transcription of English influenced by selected Asian languages. *Communication Disorders Quarterly, 23*:1, 40–46.

Chomsky, N., & Halle, M. (1968). *The sound pattern of English.* Cambridge, MA: MIT Press.

Cruttenden, A. (2001). *Gimson's pronunciation of English* (6th ed.). London: Edward Arnold.

Crystal, D. (1987). *The Cambridge encyclopedia of language.* Cambridge, UK: Cambridge University Press.

Daniloff, R., Schuckers, G., & Feth, L. (1980). *The physiology of speech and hearing.* Englewood Cliffs, NJ: Prentice-Hall.

Darley, F., Aronson, F., & Brown, J. (1975). *Motor speech disorders.* Philadelphia: W.B. Saunders Co.

Duckworth, M., Allen, G., Hardcastle, W., & Ball, M. (1990). Extensions to the International Phonetic Alphabet for the transcription of atypical speech. *Clinical Linguistics and Phonetics, 4*(4), 273–280.

Edwards, H. (1992). *Applied phonetics.* San Diego, CA: Singular Publishing Group.

Elbert, M., & Gierut, J. (1986). *Handbook of clinical phonology: Approaches to assessment and treatment.* San Diego: College-Hill Press.

Erber, N. (1983). Speech perception and speech development in hearing-impaired children. In I. Hochberg, H. Levitt, & M. Osberger (Eds.), *Speech of the hearing impaired: Research, training and personnel preparation* (pp. 131–145). Baltimore: University Park Press.

Fletcher, H. (1953). *Speech and hearing in communication.* Princeton, NJ: Van Nostrand Company.

Fudge, E. (1984). *English word-stress.* London: George Allen & Unwin Publishers.

Goldstein, B. (2001). Transcription of Spanish and Spanish-Influenced English. *Communication Disorders Quarterly, 23*:1, 54–60.

Gray, G., & Wise, C. (1959). *The bases of speech* (3rd ed.). New York: Harper and Row.

Grieco, E. M. (2010). *Race and Hispanic origin of the foreign-born population in the United States: 2007.* American Community Survey Reports, ACS-11, U.S. Census Bureau, Washington, DC. Retrieved March 22, 2010, from www.census.gov/prod/2010pubs/acs-11/pdf

Grunwell, P. (1987). *Clinical phonology* (2nd ed.). Baltimore: Williams and Wilkins.

Grunwell, P., & Harding, A. (1996). A note on describing types of nasality. *Clinical Linguistics and Phonetics, 10,* 157–161.

Handbook of the International Phonetic Association. (1999). Cambridge, UK: Cambridge University Press.

Hartman, J. (1985). Guide to pronunciation. In F. Cassidy (Ed.), *Dictionary of American regional English: Volume I, introduction and A-C* (pp. xli–lx). Cambridge, MA: Belknap Press of Harvard University Press.

Higgins, M. B., Carney, A. E., McCleary, E., & Rogers, S. (1996). Negative intraoral air pressures of deaf children with cochlear implants: Physiology, phonology, and treatment. *Journal of Speech and Hearing Research, 39,* 957–967.

Hodson, B. W., & Paden, E. P. (1991). *Targeting intelligible speech: A phonological approach to remediation* (2nd ed.). Austin, TX: Pro-Ed.

Hwa-Froelich, D., Hodson, B. W., & Edwards, H. E. (2002). Characteristics of Vietnamese phonology. *American Journal of Speech-Language Pathology, 11,* 264–273.

Iglesias, A., & Anderson, N. (1993). Dialectal variation. In J. Bernthal & N. Bankson (Eds.), *Articulation and phonological disorders* (3rd ed., pp. 147–161). Englewood Cliffs, NJ: Prentice-Hall.

Iglesias, A., & Goldstein, B. (1998). Language and dialectal variations. In J. Bernthal & N. Bankson (Eds.), *Articulation and phonological disorders* (4th ed., pp. 148–171). Boston: Allyn and Bacon.

Ingram, D. (1976). *Phonological disability in children.* London: Edward Arnold.

Jones, D. (1963). *The pronunciation of English.* Cambridge, UK: Cambridge University Press.

Jones, D. (1967). *An outline of English phonetics*. Cambridge, UK: W. Heffner and Sons.

Kent, R. (1997). *The speech sciences*. San Diego: Singular Publishing Group.

Kurath, H. (1949). *Word geography of the eastern United States*. Ann Arbor: University of Michigan Press.

Labov, W. (1991). The three dialects of English. In P. Eckert (Ed.), *New ways of analyzing sound change* (pp. 1–44). San Diego: Academic Press.

Labov, W. (n.d.). Natural misunderstandings. In *Principles of linguistic change, Volume 3: Cognitive and cultural factors*. Retrieved from www.ling.upenn.edu/phonoatlas/PLC3/Ch2.pdf

Labov, W., Ash, S., & Boberg, C. (2006). *The atlas of North American English: Phonetics, phonology and sound change*. Berlin: Mouton de Gruyter.

Ladefoged, P. (2001). *A course in phonetics* (4th ed.). Fort Worth, TX: Harcourt Brace.

Lehiste, I. (1970). *Suprasegmentals*. Cambridge, MA: MIT Press.

Levitt, H., & Stromberg, L. (1983). Segmental characteristics of the speech of hearing-impaired children: Factors affecting intelligibility. In I. Hochberg, H. Levitt, & M. J. Osberger (Eds.), *Speech of the hearing impaired: Research, training, and personnel preparation* (pp. 53–73). Baltimore: University Park Press.

Louko, L. J., & Edwards, M. L. (2001). Issues in collecting and transcribing speech samples. *Topics in Language Disorders, 21*(4), 1–11.

Lowe, R. (1996). *Workbook for the identification of phonological processes*. Austin, TX: Pro-Ed.

MacKay, I. (1987). *Phonetics: The science of speech production* (2nd ed.). Boston: College-Hill Press.

Monsen, R. B. (1983). General effects of deafness on phonation and articulation. In I. Hochberg, H. Levitt, & M. J. Osberger (Eds.), *Speech of the hearing impaired: Research, training, and personnel preparation* (pp. 23–34). Baltimore: University Park Press.

NCTE. (2008). *English language learners: A policy research brief*. National Council of Teachers of English, Urbana, Illinois. Retrieved from www.ncte.org/library/NCTEFiles/Resources/PolicyResearch/ELLResearchBrief.pdf

Ohde, R., & Sharf, D. (1992). *Phonetic analysis of normal and abnormal speech*. New York: Merrill.

Owens, R. (1991). *Language disorders: A functional approach to assessment and intervention* (2nd ed.). Boston: Allyn and Bacon.

Perez, E. (1994). Phonological differences among speakers of Spanish-influenced English. In J. Bernthal & N. Bankson (Eds.), *Child phonology: Characteristics, assessment and intervention with special populations* (pp. 245–254). New York: Thieme.

Peterson, G. E., & Barney, H. L. (1952). Control methods used in a study of the vowels. *Journal of the Acoustical Society of America, 24,* 175–184.

Pike, K. L. (1945). *The intonation of American English*. Ann Arbor: University of Michigan Press.

Pollock, K. E., & Meredith, L. H. (2001). Phonetic transcription of African American Vernacular English. *Communication Disorders Quarterly*, 23:1, 47–53.

Poole, I. (1934). Genetic development of articulation of consonant sounds in speech. *Elementary English Review, 11,* 159–161.

Powell, T. W. (2001). Phonetic transcription of disordered speech. *Topics in Language Disorders, 21*(4), 52–72.

Power, T. (2003a). *Practice for Russian language backgrounds*. Retrieved from www.btinternet.com/~ted.power/l1russian.html

Power, T. (2003b). *Practice for Arabic language backgrounds*. Retrieved from www.btinternet.com/~ted.power/l1arabic.html

Prather, E. D., Hedrick, D. L., & Kern, C. A. (1975). Articulation development in children aged two to four years. *Journal of Speech and Hearing Disorders, 40,* 179–191.

Pullum, G. K., & Ladusaw, W. A. (1996). *Phonetic symbol guide* (2nd ed.). Chicago: University of Chicago Press.

Reed, V. (1994). *An introduction to children with language disorders* (2nd ed.). New York: Merrill.

Reeves, T., & Bennett, C. (2003). *The Asian and Pacific Islander population in the United States: March 2002*. (U.S. Census Bureau, Current Population Reports, Series P20-540.) Washington, DC: U.S. Government Printing Office.

Sander, E. (1972). When are speech sounds learned? *Journal of Speech and Hearing Disorders, 37,* 55–63.

Schmidley, A. D. (2001). *Profile of the foreign-born population in the United States 2000* (U.S. Census Bureau, Current Population Reports, Series P23-206). Washington, DC: U.S. Government Printing Office. Retrieved from www.census.gov/prod/2002pubs/p23-206.pdf

Shen, Y. (1962). *English phonetics: (Especially for teachers of English as a Foreign Language).* Ann Arbor: University of Michigan Press.

Shin, H. B., & Bruno, R. (2003). *Language use and English-speaking ability: 2000.* Census 2000 Brief, C2KBR-29, U.S. Census Bureau, Washington, DC. Retrieved from www.census.gov/prod/2003pubs/c2kbr-29.pdf

Shriberg, L., & Kent, R. (2003). *Clinical phonetics* (3rd ed.). Boston: Allyn and Bacon.

Singh, S., & Singh, K. (2006). *Phonetics: Principles and practices* (3rd ed.). San Diego, CA: Plural Publishing.

Smit, A., Hand, L., Freilinger, J., Bernthal, J., & Bird, A. (1990). The Iowa articulation norms project and its Nebraska replication. *Journal of Speech and Hearing Disorders, 55,* 779–798.

Stampe, D. (1969). *The acquisition of phonetic representation.* Paper presented at the Fifth Regional Meeting of the Chicago Linguistic Society.

Stevick, R. D. (1968). *English and its history.* Boston: Allyn and Bacon.

Stockman, I. J. (2007). African American English speech acquisition. In S. McLeod (Ed.), *The international guide to speech acquisition* (pp. 148–160). Clifton Park, NY: Thomson Delmar Learning.

Stoel-Gammon, C. (1983). The acquisition of segmental phonology by normal and hearing-impaired children. In I. Hochberg, H. Levitt, & M. J. Osberger (Eds.), *Speech of the hearing impaired: Research, training, and personnel preparation* (pp. 267–280). Baltimore: University Park Press.

Stoel-Gammon, C. (1996). Phonological assessment using a hierarchical framework. In K. N. Cole, P. S. Dale, & D. J. Thal (Eds.), *Communication and language intervention series: Vol. 6. Assessment of communication and language* (pp. 77–95). Baltimore: Brookes.

Stoel-Gammon, C. (2001). Transcribing the speech of young children. *Topics in Language Disorders, 21*(4), 12–21.

Stoel-Gammon, C., & Dunn, C. (1985). *Normal and disordered phonology in children.* Austin, TX: Pro-Ed.

Templin, M. C. (1957). *Certain language skills in children.* Minneapolis: The University of Minnesota Press.

Teoh, A. P., & Chin, S. B. (2009). Transcribing the speech of children with cochlear implants: Clinical application of narrow phonetic transcriptions. *American Journal of Speech-Language Pathology, 18,* 388–401.

Terrell, S., & Terrell, F. (1993). African American cultures. In D. Battle (Ed.), *Communication disorders in multicultural populations* (pp. 3–37). Boston: Andover Medical Publishers.

Trost-Cardamone, J. E. (2009). Articulation and phonologic assessment procedures and treatment decisions. In K. T. Moller & L. E. Glaze (Eds.), *Cleft lip and palate: Interdisciplinary issues and treatment* (3rd ed., pp. 377–413). Austin, TX: Pro-Ed.

Trost-Cardamone, J. E., & Bernthal, J. E. (1993). Articulation assessment procedures and treatment decisions. In K. T. Moller & C. D. Starr (Eds.), *Cleft palate: Interdisciplinary issues and treatment* (pp. 307–336). Austin, TX: Pro-Ed.

U.S. Census Bureau. (2003). *Table 5. Detailed list of languages spoken at home for the population 5 years and over by state: 2000.* Retrieved from www.census.gov/population/cen2000/phc-t20/tab05.pdf

U.S. Census Bureau. (2007a). *The American community—Hispanics: 2004.* American Community Survey Reports, U.S. Census Bureau, Washington, DC. Retrieved from www.census.gov/prod/2007pubs/acs-03.pdf

U.S. Census Bureau. (2007b). *The American community—Pacific Islanders: 2004.* American Community Survey Reports, U.S. Census Bureau, Washington, DC. Retrieved from www.census.gov/prod/2007pubs/acs-06.pdf

U.S. Census Bureau. (2007c). *The American community—Asians: 2004.* American Community Survey Reports, U.S. Census Bureau, Washington, DC. Retrieved from www.census.gov/prod/2007pubs/acs-05.pdf

U.S. Census Bureau. (2008a). *B16001. Language spoken at home by ability to speak English for the population 5 years and over.* 2006–2008 American Community Survey 3-year Estimates, Detailed Tables, U.S. Census Bureau, Washington, DC. Retrieved from: www.factfinder.census.gov/servlet/DTTable?_bm=y&-geo_id=01000US&-ds_name=ACS_2008_3YR_G00_&-_lang=en&-redoLog=false&-mt_name=ACS_2008_3YR_G2000_B16001&-format=&-CONTEXT=dt

U.S. Census Bureau. (2008b). *Selected social characteristics in the United States: 2006–2008.* 2006–2008 American Community Survey 3-year estimates, U.S. Census Bureau, Washington, DC. Retrieved from: www.factfinder.census.gov/servlet/ADPTable?_bm=y&-lang=en&-caller=geoselect&-qr_name=ACS_2008_3YR_G00_DP3YR2&-ds_name=ACS_2008_3YR_G00_&-geo_id=01000US&-ds%20name=ACS20083YRG00&-_sse=on&-%20redoLog=false&-_lang=en&-geo%20id=01000US

Webster. (2010). Definition of "ethnic." Retrieved March 22, 2010, from www.merriam-webster.com/dictionary/ethnic.

Wellman, B., Case, M., Mengert, E., & Bradbury, D. (1931). *Speech sounds of young children* (University of Iowa studies in Child Welfare, 5). Iowa City: University of Iowa Press.

Wolfram, W. (1991). *Dialects and American English.* Englewood Cliffs, NJ: Prentice-Hall.

Wolfram, W. (1994). The phonology of a sociocultural variety: The case of African American Vernacular English. In J. Bernthal & N. Bankson (Eds.), *Child phonology: Characteristics, assessment and intervention with special populations* (pp. 227–244). New York: Thieme.

Wolfram, W., & Fasold, R. W. (1974). *The study of social dialects in American English.* Englewood Cliffs, NJ: Prentice-Hall.

Wolfram, W., & Schilling-Estes, N. (2006). *American English: Dialects and variation* (2nd ed.). Malden, MA: Blackwell Publishing.

Wolfram, W., & Thomas, E. R. (2002). *The development of African American English.* Malden, MA: Blackwell.

Yavaş, M. (2006). *Applied English phonology.* Malden, MA: Blackwell.

Answers to Questions

Chapter 1

Chapter Exercises

1.1 1. are you → ya; going to → gonna
    2. can't you → cantcha; see her → see 'er
    3. did you → ja

1.2 1. d   2. f   3. e   4. b   5. a   6. c

1.3 1. ə   2. θ   3. ʊ   4. ŋ   5. ɹ

Chapter 2

Chapter Exercises

2.1

4	lazy	4	smooth	3	cough
5	spilled	6	driven	1	oh
3	comb	2	why	5	raisin
4	thrill	3	judge	3	away

2.2 1. measure   2. rag   3. though   4. wood   5. was

2.3 Possible answers include:

1. deduct	4. scrutinize	7. dishonest 10. magnetize
2. protection	5. laborious	8. indecent
3. potential	6. greatly	9. later

2.4

1	caution	2	running	2	lived	3	relistened
2	warmly	1	finger	2	talker	1	kangaroo
3	prorated	2	clarinetist	2	sharply	2	swarming

2.5 1. lend   ɛ   4. should   ʊ
     2. man   æ   5. rude   u
     3. flick   ɪ   6. week   i

2.6 1. ram   m   4. sung   ŋ
     2. laugh   f   5. bath   θ
     3. wish   ʃ   6. leave   v

2.7
1. ʃ   5. ʊ   9. dʒ
2. ð   6. f   10. k
3. tʃ   7. t   11. ʒ
4. ɪ   8. ŋ   12. ɚ

2.8 Sample minimal pairs include:

1. lame, came   4. wood, hood   7. toad, toes   10. rug, rush
2. rate, sate   5. coil, toil   8. well, wedge
3. doll, hall   6. harm, hard   9. cheat, cheese

2.10 ouch   **crab**   **hoe**   oats   elm   **your**
     re act   **car go**   **be ware**   a **tone**   **cour** age   eat ing

2.11 shrine   scold   plea   produce   schism   **away**
     elope   selfish   **auto**   biceps   flight   truce

2.12 through   spa   **rough**   bough   row   spray
     law **ful**   **fun** ny   cre **ate**   **in verse**   **can** dy   re ply

2.13   O pliant   C comply   O coerced   C minutes
     O decree   C encase   C flatly   O preface

2.14   C pliant   O comply   C coerced   C minutes
     O decree   C encase   O flatly   C preface

2.15
1. shampoo   4. Marie
2. careful   5. injure
3. okay

2.16 propose   **contest**   **protest**   congress   **research**
     project   consume   **compress**   reasoned   confines

2.17 decoy   thesis   **derail**   **suspend**   **provide**
     stipend   planted   circus   **cassette**   **platoon**
     timid   **parade**   **devoid**   **regret**   **Maureen**
     transcend   **cajole**   puzzle   falter   peon
     lucid   **pastel**   reason   **restricts**   shoulder
     mirage   **undo**   virtue   movie   merchant

2.18 **pondering**   **asterisk**   **caribou**   contended   **Philistine**
    plentiful   December   **telephoned**   umbrella   **ebony**
    surrounded   hydrangea   courageous   **calendar**   example
    terrified   **skeletal**   **misery**   distinctive   lasagna
    musical   **consequent**   persona   Barbados   **India**
    edited   pharyngeal   **underling**   perfected   perusal

2.19 **stupendous**   answering   murderer   **discover**   muscular
    corporal   clarinet   integer   **immoral**   magical
    plantation   violin   expertise   elevate   **bananas**
    heroic   **subscription**   carefully   **placenta**   horribly
    daffodil   **creative**   **presumption**   **decorum**   **majestic**
    pliable   spectacle   predisposed   clavicle   **Hawaii**

2.20 <u>1, 3, 5</u> phonemic
      <u>2, 4, 5</u> allophonic
      <u>2, 4</u> impressionistic

Review Exercises

A. 1. bread   <u>4</u>   4. news   <u>3</u>   7. **fluid**   <u>5</u>   10. tomb   <u>3</u>
   2. coughs   <u>4</u>   5. **plot**   <u>4</u>   8. **spew**   <u>4</u>   11. walked   <u>4</u>
   3. throw   <u>3</u>   6. stroke   <u>5</u>   9. **fat**   <u>3</u>   12. **last**   <u>4</u>

B. 1. clueless   <u>2</u>   6. rewrite   <u>2</u>
   2. tomato   <u>1</u>   7. winterized   <u>3</u>
   3. pumpkin   <u>1</u>   8. edits   <u>2</u>
   4. likable   <u>2</u>   9. thoughtlessness   <u>3</u>
   5. cheddar   <u>1</u>   10. coexisting   <u>3</u>

C. 1. puss   6. flew
   2. dogs   7. limb
   3. league   8. wheeze
   4. pant   9. giraffe
   5. beau   10. cloth

D. 1. ten   6. name
   2. less   7. nip
   3. stop   8. nab
   4. tan   9. cat
   5. dean   10. newt

E. 1. chef   6. song
   2. cut   7. gnat
   3. think   8. chore
   4. came   9. goat
   5. please   10. their

F. Possible answers include:

1. slit
2. band
3. sink
4. win
5. paid

6. fun
7. rink
8. hid
9. cook
10. rib

G. 1. **maybe, baby**
2. plaid, prod
3. **looks, lacks**
4. mail, snail
5. **prance, prince**

6. **bribe, tribe**
7. smart, dart
8. dinner, runner
9. window, minnow
10. **lumpy, bumpy**

H. 1. mar<u>ble</u>   C
2. <u>pre</u>vious   O
3. pa<u>tron</u>   C
4. <u>tri</u>fle   O
5. <u>so</u>dium   O

6. <u>awe</u>some   O
7. mis<u>take</u>   C
8. luck<u>y</u>   O
9. prof<u>it</u>   C
10. <u>sys</u>tem   C

I.

| | Onset | | Coda | |
	Yes	No	Yes	No
1. mentions	X		X	
2. icon		X		X
3. camper	X		X	
4. instinct		X	X	
5. able		X		X
6. lotion	X			X
7. charming	X		X	
8. asterisk		X	X	
9. Japan	X			X
10. aloof		X		X

J. 1 1. loser
2 2. unsure
1 3. anxious
2 4. disturb
1 5. Grecian

2 6. provoke
1 7. stagnant
2 8. beside
2 9. germane
2 10. gourmet

1 11. plastic
2 12. divorce
1 13. western
1 14. language
2 15. defer

K. 2 1. provincial
1 2. sorceress
1 3. indigent
2 4. commander
3 5. arabesque

1 6. hypocrite
3 7. indisposed
2 8. uncertain
2 9. magenta
1 10. platypus

3 11. picturesque
1 12. relegate
2 13. foundation
2 14. contagious
1 15. constable

L. __3__ 1. problematic __3__ 6. correlation __3__ 11. protozoan
   __1__ 2. mercenary __1__ 7. catamaran __1__ 12. contradiction
   __2__ 3. statistical __2__ 8. continuant __1__ 13. protoplasm
   __1__ 4. ecosystem __1__ 9. allegory __1__ 14. Argentina
   __2__ 5. gregarious __2__ 10. carnivorous __2__ 15. obstructionist

Chapter 3

Chapter Exercises

3.1 Possible answers include:
  voiced   /r/, /l/, /d/
  voiceless /p/, /t/, /h/

3.2 The phoneme /p/ is produced by closing the lips.
   The phoneme /w/ is produced by rounding the lips; the lips do not close.

3.3 The phoneme in the word <u>th</u>ink is voiceless: /θ/
   The phoneme in the word <u>th</u>at is voiced: /ð/

3.4 1. soft palate or velum   5. hard palate
   2. alveolar ridge   6. glottis
   3. tongue   7. teeth
   4. lips

Review Exercises

A. 1. b   2. c   3. d   4. a

B. 1. fundamental frequency   4. diaphragm
   2. mandible   5. subglottal
   3. a. in front of   6. habitual
      b. below   7. eustachian tubes
      c. above   8. blade, apex
      d. to the rear   9. front, back

C. 1. c   5. c   9. a
   2. a   6. d   10. d
   3. b   7. c
   4. b   8. b

D. 1. T   5. T   9. F
   2. F   6. F   10. T
   3. F   7. T
   4. T   8. T

Chapter 4

Preliminary Exercise 1

U	1.		R	6.
R	2.		U	7.
R	3.		U	8.
U	4.		U	9.
R	5.		R	10.

Preliminary Exercise 2

T	1.		T	5.
L	2.		T	6.
L	3.		L	7.
L	4.		T	8.

Preliminary Exercise 3

270	/i/	300	/u/	2290	/i/	870	/u/
390	/ɪ/	440	/ʊ/	1990	/ɪ/	1020	/ʊ/
530	/ɛ/	570	/ɔ/	1840	/ɛ/	840	/ɔ/
660	/æ/	730	/ɑ/	1720	/æ/	1090	/ɑ/

As the tongue lowers, the frequency of F_1 increases. As the tongue moves from front to back, the frequency of F_2 decreases.

Chapter Exercises

4.1—The Vowel /i/

A. paper   train   **Cleveland**   **seaside**
    please   picture   trip   trail
    tribal   **machine** labor   **trees**
    settle   **screen**   **Toledo**   lip
    nice   foreign   **Levi**   **jeans**

B. **/ist/**   /flip/   **/min/**   **/hid/**
    /iv/   /hig/   /lim/   /wins/
    /rift/   /if/   **/trit/**   **/lik/**

C. /lip/ leap _____ /it/ eat _____ /brizd/ breezed _____

    /pip/ peep _____ /hip/ heap _____ /spik/ speak _____

    /mit/ meat, meet _____ /sip/ seep _____ /klin/ clean _____

    /rid/ reed, read _____ /did/ deed _____ /krist/ creased _____

D.
___	dream	drip		X	east	eaves
X	seek	wheel		___	chief	vein
___	same	land		___	base	lease
X	creek	steam		___	need	pain
X	bean	heed		X	creed	cream

4.2—The Vowel /ɪ/

B.
peace	friend	enthrall	**bitter**
mythical	**silver**	woman	**tryst**
click	**ingest**	**build**	**fear**
thread	**pink**	**bowling**	tried
pride	**clear**	**sporty**	**synchronize**

C.
/vɪl/	/sɪst/	/fɪld/	/wɪns/
/izɪ/	/klip/	/spid/	/hik/
/hɪr/	/ɪl/	/sɪg/	**/pɪgɪ/**

D.
/stip/	steep		/pɪk/	pick
/pliz/	please		/kɪst/	kissed
/mɪt/	mitt		/bik/	beak
/dɪd/	did		/pɪp/	pip
/fɪr/	fear		/mɪstɪ/	misty
/rilɪ/	really		/ɪndid/	indeed

E.
X	feel	teach		X	win	king
___	lip	thread		X	mint	inch
X	been	drink		X	deed	flea
___	vent	list		X	dish	ill
___	tied	pig		X	kick	mill

F.
1. ___ flirt		5. X smeared		9. ___ stirred
2. X peerless		6. ___ worried		10. ___ stared
3. ___ bird		7. X steered		11. X earring
4. ___ shrill		8. ___ harder		12. ___ cursor

4.3—The Vowel /e/ - /eɪ/

B.
trail	**rage**	wheel	**palatial**
vice	**razor**	manage	green
transit	machine	**whale**	**potato**
lazy	bread	football	temperate
dale	tackle	**daily**	bright

C. /**freɪd**/   /deɪs/   /dɪnt/   /**deɪlɪ**/
   /**kreɪt**/   /**biz**/   /**spid**/   /**deɪm**/
   /**neɪp**/   /trips/   /**treɪ**/   /fril/
   /pɪln/   /**blid**/   /feɪlm/   /streɪp/

D. /bleɪz/   blaze   /pleɪket/   placate

   /pleɪd/   played   /rimeɪn/   remain

   /beɪn/   bane   /ɪnmeɪt/   inmate

   /iveɪd/   evade   /ribet/   rebate

   /krɪmp/   crimp   /steɪnd/   stained

   /rikt/   reeked   /deɪzɪ/   daisy

E. _O_ crayon   _C_ unmade
   _O_ prepay   _O_ stay
   _C_ baking   _O_ tailor
   _O_ masonry   _C_ betrayed

F. ___ braid   hid   _X_ state   rain
   ___ feed   hate   ___ fist   flea
   _X_ lane   aim   _X_ cringe hid
   _X_ fill   kissed   ___ deal   will
   ___ treat   sling   _X_ wheel   meat

G. _eɪ_ neighbor   _e_   Crayola
   _eɪ_ crate   _eɪ_ basin
   _e_   donate   _eɪ_ stay
   _eɪ_ hooray   _e_   prostrate
   _eɪ_ saber   _e_   incubate

4.4—The Vowel /ɛ/

B. pimple   jeep   **thread**   build   **contend**
   syrup   trip   pistol   **prepare**   **pretzel**
   pencil   **caring**   **ensure**   **unscented** tried
   thing   butter   women   tryst   **remember**

C. /**mɛrɪ**/   /hint/   /split/   /istɛr/
   /**slɛpt**/   /**fɛr**/   /ɪrk/   /**meɪd**/
   /sɪsɪ/   /kleɪ/   /**wɛl**/   /**krip**/

D. /reɪk/   rake   /stɛr/   stare

/fɪz/   fizz   /treɪl/   trail

/smɛl/   smell   /pritɛnd/   pretend

/sid/   seed   /hɛvɪ/   heavy

/kreɪn/   crane   /friz/   freeze

/breɪzd/   braised   /blɛst/   blessed

E.

X	fill	fear		X	step	edge
X	made	cage		___	bread	breathe
___	wind	best		___	flit	red
___	trade	peel		X	sill	kit
X	rid	sing		X	care	meant

F.

C	1.	trail	O	6.	spree
O	2.	repay	C	7.	arouse
C	3.	strike	C	8.	rough
O	4.	plea	O	9.	undo
C	5.	late	O	10.	chow

G.

1.	X	share	6.	X	careful
2.	___	early	7.	X	sparrow
3.	___	dearly	8.	___	third
4.	X	compare	9.	___	corridor
5.	___	fluoride	10.	___	certain

4.5—The Vowel /æ/

B.

straddle	**practice**	**lapse**	**revamp**
pale	**panther**	**repast**	straight
Lester	pacific	**pacify**	farmer
baseball	**hanged**	**chances**	cards
jazz	pistol	tamed	**bombastic**

C.

/**klæd**/	/prid/	/strɪv/	/wæd/
/**slæpt**/	/**bɪrd**/	/bæz/	/**trækt**/
/web/	/steɪp/	/**sprɪg**/	/læzɪ/

D.

/klæn/	clan	/spɪr/	spear
/sprɪnt/	sprint	/hɛrɪ/	hairy, Harry
/rɛk/	wreck	/pækt/	packed
/teɪstɪ/	tasty	/dræg/	drag
/præns/	prance	/bɛrɪ/	berry
/læft/	laughed	/tinz/	teens

E. ___   badge   rage   <u>X</u>   hair   bend

___   seed   shade   <u>X</u>   lick   beer

___   cab   blonde   ___   beak   bless

<u>X</u>   tray   whale   ___   trap   bake

<u>X</u>   crank   shag   <u>X</u>   lapse   crag

4.6—The Vowel /u/

A. **ghoul**   oboe   **crew**   plural
butter   stuck   **Lucifer**   must
should   luck   lusty   shook
fuchsia   look   molding   **stupor**
loosely   **glue**   blouse   **choose**

B. /ust/   **/krud/**   /prus/   **/tul/**
/suv/   /tug/   /pus/   **/wund/**
/pul/   /rup/   **/lus/**   /slug/

C.
/spun/	spoon	/sup/	soup
/tun/	tune	/lud/	lewd
/rut/	root	/stru/	strew
/mud/	mood	/flu/	flew, flue, flu
/klu/	clue	/grum/	groom
/ruf/	roof	/snut/	snoot

D. ___ 1. could   showed   ___ 6. brood   hood

<u>X</u> 2. suit   loon   <u>X</u> 7. stood   could

___ 3. lute   book   ___ 8. hoops   poor

<u>X</u> 4. crew   scoot   <u>X</u> 9. feud   moose

<u>X</u> 5. push   foot   ___ 10. muse   cook

E. ___ 1. oozing   ___ 4. ruined   ___ 7. Pluto   ___ 10. spooky

<u>X</u> 2. cute   ___ 5. sloop   <u>X</u> 8. useful

<u>X</u> 3. huge   <u>X</u> 6. fuming   <u>X</u> 9. viewing

4.7—The Vowel /ʊ/

B. hole   **wooden**   snooze   stunned
shut   punched   luscious   spook
hood   **couldn't**   **pulled**   **shook**
flushed   **mistook**   beauty   person
rudely   **cooker**   brood   **stood**

C. /**buk**/   /stʊ/   /**rul**/   /sul/
   /lʊv/   /**lum**/   /**rʊk**/   /**frut**/
   /**trups**/   /stʊr/   /**buts**/   /slʊg/

D. /pʊs/   puss   /tʊr/   tour
   /tru/   true   /hʊk/   hook
   /stʊd/   stood   /lum/   loom
   /dum/   doom   /fluk/   fluke
   /gru/   grew   /prun/   prune
   /good/   good   /krʊk/   crook

E. ___ 1. loot   foot   ___ 6. what   look
   X 2. tune   mute   X 7. nook   stood
   X 3. coupe   soon   ___ 8. rust   rook
   ___ 4. flood   cute   X 9. goof   cruise
   X 5. would   soot   ___ 10. mutt   look

4.8—The Vowel /o/ - /oʊ/

B. **mope**   aloof   root   **toll**
   noose   **slowed**   pond   push
   soda   lost   **loaded**   **lasso**
   nosy   book   sugar   **remote**
   dole   **spoke**   doily   **wholly**

C. /**toʊ**/   /**boʊn**/   /**stup**/   /prʊb/
   /bʊt/   /**floʊd**/   /**boʊd**/   /**krud**/
   /stub/   /**stud**/   /flʊk/   /**woʊnt**/

D. /moʊld/   mold   /tupeɪ/   toupee
   /kupt/   cooped   /bruzd/   bruised
   /boʊnɪ/   bony   /bændeɪd/   Band-Aid
   /ivoʊk/   evoke   /kʊkɪ/   cookie
   /stoʊd/   stowed   /koʊɛd/   coed
   /doʊpɪ/   dopey   /rizum/   resume

E. o Romania   oʊ snowman   oʊ bowling
   oʊ corroded   o location   oʊ though
   oʊ stolen   oʊ jello   o notation
   oʊ magnolia   o coagulate   o potential

4.9—The Vowel /ɔ/
  A. **/bɔt/**   /drʊm/   /stɔn/   **/brɔn/**
      /koʊt/   /grɔn/   /tɔk/   /pʊl/
      /lʊps/   **/fɔrt/**   /flʌm/   /ɔrn/

  B. /spɔrt/   sport___   /sprɔl/   sprawl___

      /kʊd/   could___   /stʊd/   stood___

      /proʊb/   probe___   /frɔt/   fraught___

      /pruv/   prove___   /kɔrps/   corpse___

      /stɔrd/   stored___   /hʊkt/   hooked___

      /ɔfʊl/   awful___   /doʊnet/   donate___

  C. 1. ___ farm   4. X storm   7. ___ lured

      2. ___ third   5. ___ worm   8. ___ worth

      3. X horrid   6. X thorn   9. ___ spar

4.10—The Vowel /a/
  B. /wond/   /tɔb/   **/harm/**   **/blab/**
      /koʊd/   /sɔt/   /blad/   **/armɪ/**
      /frɔd/   /pʊnt/   /ad/   **/kad/**

  C. /frast/   frost___   /zar/   czar___

      /lʊkt/   looked___   /prund/   pruned___

      /bɔrd/   board, bored___   /blɔnd/   blonde___

      /kroʊm/   chrome___   /ansɛt/   onset___

      /want/   want___   /krɔdæd/   crawdad___

      /starvd/   starved___   /ardvark/   aardvark___

  D. 1. ___ war   7. ___ orchard

      2. ___ cleared   8. X March

      3. ___ quartz   9. ___ poorly

      4. ___ flare   10. X smarter

      5. X starred   11. X carbon

      6. ___ dirt   12. ___ spore

4.11—The Vowel /ə/
  A. rowing   injure   **motion**   **fuchsia**
      lasagna   poorly   holding   laundry
      wooded   ruled   **untamed**   petunia
      Laverne   **control**   **opera**   cockroach
      decision   glamour   puppy   **lotion**

B. /sətɪn/   /zəbrɑ/   /əbeɪt/   /əluf/
  /drɑmə/   /ləpʊr/   **/bəlun/**   /rədæn/
  /səpoʊz/   /rəpik/   **/brəzɪl/**   /əndu/

C. /pinət/   peanut   /kənteɪn/   contain
  /əkrɑs/   across   /lɛmən/   lemon
  /vəlɔr/   velour   /bətɑn/   baton
  /səpɔrt/   support   /əwɔrd/   award
  /kɔfɪn/   coffin   /eɪprəl/   April
  /plətun/   platoon   /kəsɛt/   cassette

4.12—The Vowel /ʌ/

B. awful   **blunder**   laundry   Hoover
  custard   laborious   **Sunday**   lawyer
  pushy   cushion   **hundred**   **trumpet**
  cologne   **abundant**   plural   shouldn't
  charades   mundane   wander   conducive

C. 1. hooked   /hʌkt/   X   6. rookie   /rʌkɪ/   X
  2. bond   /bʊnd/   X   7. mistook   /mɪstʊk/   ___
  3. bluff   /blʌf/   ___   8. lucky   /lʌkɪ/   ___
  4. hood   /hud/   X   9. rubbing   /rʊbɪŋ/   X
  5. cluck   /klʌk/   ___   10. crooked   /krɔkəd/   X

D. /klʊstɪ/   /əpʌft/   /dʊkɪ/   /sʌntæn/
  /rizən/   /krɑmd/   **/pʊlɪ/**   /vɪstʌ/
  /mʌstɪ/   /əndʌn/   **/plʌmət/**   **/plæzə/**

E. /pɛrəs/   Paris   /robʌst/   robust
  /hʌnɪ/   honey   /sʌdən/   sudden
  /əlɑt/   allot; a lot   /kəbus/   caboose
  /kənvɪns/   convince   /tʌndrə/   tundra
  /gɑrdəd/   guarded   /kəlæps/   collapse
  /flʌbd/   flubbed   /bəfun/   buffoon

F. lumber   /ʌ/   suspend /ə/
  abort   /ə/   suppose /ə/
  shaken   /ə/   induct   /ʌ/
  contain /ə/   serpent /ə/
  thunder /ʌ/   rusty   /ʌ/

G. ____ 1. nuts   could   ____ 6. crook   fund
    ____ 2. foot   stoop   _X_ 7. blood   crust
    _X_ 3. done   rubbed   _X_ 8. runs   floods
    _X_ 4. crumb   rust   _X_ 9. loom   food
    _X_ 5. cook   should   ____ 10. rush   look

4.13—The Vowel /ɚ/

B. **clover**   rebel   barley   dearly
    fearless   endear   **perjure** **fester**
    carbon   torment   **harbor**   electric
    tremor   written   poorly   breezy
    laundered   **perhaps** torpedo   **surprise**

C. /kɑnvɚt/   **/pɚteɪn/**   **/pɚsɛnt/**   /lɛpɚd/
    /rabɚ/   /tɚoʊd/   **/drimɚ/**   /fɚəst/
    /sɚvɛs/   /ɚdɪ/   /ʌnfɛr/   **/hɪndɚ/**

D. /drɛsɚ/   dresser   /kəntɔrt/   contort
    /kæmrə/   camera   /pɚɑnə/   piranha
    /rʌbɚ/   rubber   /pɚu/   Peru
    /mɑrbəl/   marble   /sɪmɚ/   simmer
    /tɚeɪn/   terrain   /kɛrosin/   kerosene
    /flʌstɚd/ flustered   /əweɪtəd/   awaited

4.14—The Vowel /ɝ/

B. forward   pretend   January   barren
    disturbed   **turban** **stirrup** morale
    terrible   arid   steered   persistent
    conversion warship   distort   choir
    muster   **wordy**   **conserve** fearless

C. /kʌstɚd/   /lɝdɪ/   /kərɪr/   /vɝsəz/
    /pɝsən/   **/hɝdəd/**   /fɝmɚ/   /dɝsənt/
    /plædʒɝ/   /fɔrən/   /ɝbɔrt/   **/kɝsɚ/**

D. /smɝkt/   smirked   /kənvɚt/   convert
    /ovɝt/   overt   /wɪspɚ/   whisper
    /kɛrət/   carrot   /bɝbən/   bourbon
    /sʌbɚb/   suburb   /skwɝts/   squirts
    /supɝb/   superb   /səhɛrə/   Sahara

E.
erasure	/ɚ/	ermine	/ɝ/
surprise	/ɚ/	color	/ɚ/
furnace	/ɝ/	infer	/ɝ/
curtail	/ɚ/	terror	/ɚ/
immerse	/ɝ/	duster	/ɚ/

F. ____ 1. herd   cheered   ____ 6. hair   queer

    ____ 2. cord   word   __X__ 7. birch   lurk

    ____ 3. lured   stored   __X__ 8. hoard   lord

    __X__ 4. ark   smart   ____ 9. pear   heard

    __X__ 5. fears   cheer   ____ 10. term   peered

G.
ɝ	1. myrth		ɪr	11. appearance
ɛr	2. flared		ɛr	12. Carol
ɪr	3. cirrus		ɝ	13. furtive
ɛr	4. serenade		ɛr	14. larynx
ɝ	5. Merlin		ɪr	15. experience
ɛr	6. cherub		ɝ	16. disturbing
ɔr	7. portion		ɪr	17. clearance
ɑr	8. farming		ɝ	18. nervous
ɛr	9. sparrow		ɝ, ʊr	19. furious
ɝ	10. nervous		ɛr	20. clairvoyant

4.15—The Diphthong /aɪ/

B.
power	spacious	machine	replaced
slice	delicious	**formica**	traded
contrite	**spider**	maybe	**piped**
lever	**Cairo**	**cider**	**supplied**
rivalry	razor	piano	spigot

C.
/fraɪdeɪ/	/braɪmɚ/	/taɪfraɪn/	/rəvaɪz/
/məbaɪ/	**/naɪlɔn/**	/prədaɪt/	**/traɪdɛnt/**
/traɪd/	/laɪɚ/	**/haɪəst/**	**/straɪpt/**

D.
/sɚpraɪz/	surprise	/klaɪmaks/	climax
/kəlaɪd/	collide	/preɪlɪn/	praline
/treɪlɚ/	trailer	/baɪsɛps/	biceps
/praɪmeɪt/	primate	/waɪɚd/	wired
/vaɪrəs/	virus	/taɪred/	tirade
/deɪlaɪt/	daylight	/daɪmənd/	diamond

4.16—The Diphthong /ɔɪ/

B.
repay	**hoisted**	**voiceless**	reward
loiter	crowded	fiery	tiled
straight	feisty	**coy**	**cloying**
crime	**broiler**	stoic	**destroy**
goiter	razor	**avoid**	supplied

C.
/kwaɪət/	/sprɔɪdɪn/	/dɔɪəz/	/plɔɪdənt/
/mɝdɚ/	/blaɪndlɪ/	/ənstraɪt/	/taɪpsɛt/
/pɔɪzən/	/vɔɪdəd/	/rikɔɪld/	/taɪwɑn/

D.
/ɔɪlɪ/	oily	/ændrɔɪd/	android
/maɪstroʊ/	maestro	/laɪvlɪ/	lively
/taɪfɔɪd/	typhoid	/ɪnvɔɪs/	invoice
/parbɔɪl/	parboil	/ɔɪstɚ/	oyster
/haɪndsaɪt/	hindsight	/haɪɔɪd/	hyoid
/baɪaʊt/	buyout	/deɪlaɪt/	daylight

4.17—The Diphthong /aʊ/

B.
toilet	**dowdy**	**frown**	**bounty**
mousy	**allowed**	loaded	probate
beauty	explode	soils	**proud**
astound	toil	**chowder**	crowbar
hello	toad	chastise	scrolled

C.
/taɪɚd/	/laʊzɪ/	/aɪvrɪ/	/hoʊmbɔɪ/
/rɪbaʊ/	/blaʊkɚ/	/rɔɪdɪ/	/kaʊtaʊ/
/waʊntɪd/	/roʊgbɪ/	/pauzɚ/	/aʊɚlɪ/

D.
/bɔɪfrɛnd/	boyfriend	/roʊboʊt/	rowboat
/klɑndaɪk/	Klondike	/pispaɪp/	peace pipe
/daʊntaʊn/	downtown	/sɚaʊnd/	surround
/sloʊɚ/	slower	/doʊnʌt/	doughnut
/faʊndəd/	founded	/klaɪənt/	client
/vaɪzɚ/	visor	/braʊzɚ/	browser

Review Exercises

A.
ʊ	high	back	yes	lax
ɝ	mid	central	yes	tense
ə	mid	central	no	lax
o	high-mid	back	yes	tense
u	high	back	yes	tense
ɛ	low-mid	front	no	lax

ɚ	mid	central	yes	lax
ʌ	low-mid	back-central	no	lax
e	high-mid	front	no	tense
ɪ	high	front	no	lax
ɑ	low	back	no	tense
ɔ	low-mid	back	yes	tense
æ	low	front	no	lax

B.
1. æ, bad
2. ʌ, sun
3. ɛ, slept
4. u, soup
5. ɔ, cord
6. ʊ, foot
7. ɪ, fizz
8. ɑ, park
9. ɝ, word
10. oʊ, crows

C.
1. Sunday   L   T
2. bashful   L   L
3. laundry   T   L
4. confused   L   T
5. fender   L   L
6. concern   L   T
7. regroup   T   T
8. obese   T   T
9. layette   T   L
10. abrupt   L   L

D.
1. foolish   R   U
2. curfew   R   R
3. decade   U   U
4. collate   R   U
5. football   R   U/R*
6. Pluto   R   R
7. person   R   U
8. pursuit   R   R
9. rugby   U   U
10. lower   R   U

*(depending on pronunciation, i.e., /ɑ/ or /ɔ/)

E.
/eɪ/ 1. straight
/i/ 2. bees
/ɛ/ 3. bread
/æ/ 4. can
/ɪ/ 5. filled
/ɪ/ 6. bring
/æ/ 7. lapse
/æ/ 8. sang
/ɛ/ 9. fair
/i/ 10. mean
/ɛ/ /ɪ/ 11. empty
/eɪ/ /ɪ/ 12. rabies
/ɪ/ /ɛ/ 13. instead
/æ/ /i/ 14. stampede
/eɪ/ /e/ 15. vacate
/i/ /ɪ/ 16. pleasing
/æ/ /ɪ/ 17. transit
/i/ /æ/ 18. beer can
/ɪ/ /æ/ 19. implant
/ɛr/ /ɪ/ 20. barely

F.

/oʊ/	1. moat	/ɔ/	/ʊ/	11. awful	
/ʊ/	2. push	/ɔr/	/ɑ/	12. Clorox	
/ɑ/	3. laud	/oʊ/	/oʊ/	13. loco	
/ɑ/	4. locks	/oʊ/	/oʊ/	14. oboe	
/u/	5. crude	/ɑ/	/oʊ/	15. taco	
/oʊ/	6. chose	/ɑ/	/ɑr/	16. monarch	
/ɑ /	7. raw	/ɑ/	/ɔr/	17. popcorn	
/ʊr/	8. lure	/u/	/ʊ/	18. truthful	
/ɔr/	9. sword	/ɑ/	/u/	19. costume	
/ɑr/	10. card	/u/	/ɑ/	20. crouton	

G.

/ɝ/	/ə/(ɪ)	1. certain	/ɝ/	/ə/	11. purpose
/ʌ/	/ə/	2. rusted	/ʌ/	/ə/(ɪ)	12. sudden
/ɚ/	/ɝ/	3. perturb	/ʌ/	/ɚ/	13. luster
/ə/	/ɝ/	4. assert	/ɝ/	/ə/	14. purchase
/ʌ/	/ɚ/	5. upper	/ɝ/	/ɚ/	15. sherbet
/ɝ/	/ɚ/	6. merger	/ʌ/	/ɚ/	16. mother
/ʌ/	/ɚ/	7. clutter	/ə/	/ɝ/	17. converge
/ɝ/	/ə/	8. verbal	/ɝ/	/ɚ/	18. herder
/ə/	/ɝ/	9. traverse	/ɝ/	/ə/	19. worded
/ɝ/	/ɚ/	10. learner	/ʌ/	/ɚ/	20. mustard

H.

1. word	/wɝd/		16. maestro	/maɪstroʊ/	
2. lard	/lɔrd/	/ɑr/	17. flour	/floʊɚ/	/aʊ/
3. carp	/kɝp/	/ɑr/	18. pouring	/pɔrɪŋ/	
4. war	/wɑr/	/ɔr/	19. liar	/laɪɚ/	
5. mere	/mɪr/		20. appear	/əpɛr/	/ɪr/
6. wide	/weɪd/	/aɪ/	21. tighter	/taɪtɝ/	/ɚ/
7. curd	/kʊrd/	/ɝ/	22. parrot	/pɝət/	/ɛr/
8. stay	/steɪ/		23. corner	/kɔrnɚ/	
9. pray	/praɪ/	/eɪ/	24. oyster	/ɔɪstɛr/	/ɚ/
10. crow	/kraʊ/	/oʊ/	25. squarely	/skwɛrlɪ/	
11. coin	/kɔɪn/		26. silence	/sɪləns/	/aɪ/
12. pride	/praɪd/		27. smarter	/smɔrtɚ/	/ɑr/
13. firm	/fɪrm/	/ɝ/	28. avoid	/əvaɪd/	/ɔɪ/
14. tour	/tʊr/		29. prowess	/proəs/	/aʊ/
15. fair	/fɛr/		30. license	/leɪsəns/	/aɪ/

I. 1. p___   pier (peer), pour (poor), pore, par, pear (pair), purr

   2. r___   rear, roar, rare

   3. d___t   dart, dirt

   4. w___d   weird, ward, word

   5. k___d   cord, card, cared, curd

J. 1. ___d   id, aid, Ed, add, oohed, owed, awed, odd

   2. ___n   in, an (Ann), own, on, urn (earn)

   3. l___st   least, list, laced, lest, last, lost, lust

   4. sk___n   skin, skein, scan, scone

   5. st___d   steed, stayed (staid), stead, stewed, stood, stowed, stirred, stud

   6. b___rd   beard, bared, board (bored), bard, bird

   7. t___nt   tint, taint, tent, taunt

   8. s___t   seat, sit, sate, set, sat, suit, soot, sought, sot

   9. r___t   writ, rate, ret, rat, root, wrought, rote, rot, rut

   10. r___bd   ribbed, robed, robbed, rubbed

   11. sp___t   spit, spate, spat, spot, spurt

   12. w___d   weed, wade, wed, wooed, wood (would), wad, word

K. 1. customs   11. sirens   21. wonderful   31. Mexico

   2. abound   12. cloistered   22. calendar   32. quagmire

   3. toward   13. Ohio   23. remorseful   33. orderly

   4. slender   14. radio   24. stupendous   34. herbicide

   5. carefree   15. corrosive   25. laxative   35. repulsive

   6. vacant   16. platonic   26. sincerely   36. character

   7. bunted   17. resonate   27. colander   37. sassafras

   8. cloudy   18. digress   28. Raisinettes   38. xylophone

   9. stapler   19. siphoned   29. baritone   39. quarterback

   10. contort   20. Arkansas   30. December   40. embarrassed

L. /ɛ/ /ɪ/   1. epic   /æ/ /ə/   10. palace

   /æ/ /ɚ/   2. faster   /ɛr/ /ɪ/   11. barely

   /ʌ/ /ɚ/   3. wonder   /eɪ/ /ə/   12. nation

   /ɑ/ /ɛ/   4. octet   /i/ /ə/   13. genius

   /ʊ/ /ə/   5. woolen   /ʌ/ /ɚ/   14. cupboard

   /i/ /oʊ/   6. depot   /ɑr/ /u/   15. cartoon

   /oʊ/ /ɚ/   7. soldier   /æ/ /ɪ/   16. nasty

   /ɪ/ /ɪ/   8. itchy   /ɪr/ /ə/   17. fearless

   /ɝ/ /ɪ/   9. worship   /ʌ/ /ɚ/   18. number

/æ/ /ə/ 19. sanction

/oʊ/ /ə/ 20. ocean

/ɪ/ /ɪ/ 21. inkling

/ɛr/ /æ/ 22. Fairbanks

/ɑr/ /u/ 23. car pool

/ə/ /i/ 24. machine

/æ/ /ə/ 25. Athens

/ɑ/ /ə/ 26. autumn

/i/ /ə/ 27. rebus

/ɔr/ /ɛ/ 28. torment

/ʌ/ /ɚ/ 29. utter

/ʊ/ /ə/ 30. bushel

/ɔr/ /ɚ/ 31. corner

/ɑ/ /ɪ/ 32. quandary

/æ/ /ɚ/ 33. aster

/oʊ/ /u/ 34. phone booth

/ɝ/ /ə/ 35. turban

/i/ /eɪ/ 36. key case

/ɔr/ /ɚ/ 37. boarder

/ɛr/ /ɪ/ 38. blaring

/æ/ /ə/ 39. strangle

/ɔ/ /ə/ 40. awesome

M. /ɔɪ/ /ɚ/ 1. broiler

/aʊ/ /æ/ 2. mousetrap

/ɔr/ /ɑ/ 3. boardwalk

/oʊ/ /ɚ/ 4. closure

/aɪ/ /ɑ/ 5. nylons

/ɛr/ /ɔɪ/ 6. steroid

/ɑr/ /ʌ/ 7. starstruck

/ə/ /i/ 8. regime

/æ/ /ʊ/ 9. bashful

/ɝ/ /ɚ/ 10. perjure

/ɪr/ /ɪ/ 11. spearmint

/aɪ/ /ʌ/ 12. lightbulb

/i/ /ɔɪ/ 13. destroy

/æ/ /ə/(ɪ) 14. banquet

/aɪ/ /ɔr/ 15. eyesore

/ɛ/ /ɚ/ 16. gender

/aɪ/ /ə/ 17. China

/ɔ/ /ɪ/ 18. jaundiced

/ɝ/ /ɔɪ/ 19. turquoise

/ɪ/ /ɔɪ/ 20. invoice

/aɪ/ /æ/ 21. financed

/ɝ/ /ə/ 22. merchant

/o/ /eɪ/ 23. proclaim

/oʊ/ /e/ 24. probate

/ə/ /aɪ/ 25. July

/ɑr/ /ə/ 26. martian

/u/ /ɚ/ 27. future

/ɑ/ /ɛ/ 28. prospect

/ɑ/ /ə/ 29. product

/o/ /u/ 30. tofu

N. 1. rises

2. lowers

3. rises

4. lowers

5. F_1 lowers; F_2 lowers

Chapter 5

Preliminary Exercise 1

<u>a</u> 1. s<u>ee</u>m   <u>b</u> 6. oi<u>l</u>y

<u>c</u> 2. tra<u>d</u>e   <u>a</u> 7. hot<u>d</u>og

<u>b</u> 3. a<u>w</u>ay   <u>b</u> 8. ha<u>s</u>ten

<u>a</u> 4. <u>c</u>ruise   <u>b</u> 9. o<u>p</u>en

<u>c</u> 5. oa<u>f</u>   <u>c</u> 10. foo<u>t</u>ball

Preliminary Exercise 2

<u>f</u> 1. /r/   <u>b</u> 4. /f/

<u>a</u> 2. /d/   <u>d</u> 5. /n/

<u>e</u> 3. /w/   <u>c</u> 6. /tʃ/

Preliminary Exercise 3

____ 1. me, we   ____ 6. shoot, suit

<u>X</u> 2. seal, zeal   ____ 7. flame, blame

____ 3. plan, clan   <u>X</u> 8. dram, tram

____ 4. lice, rice   ____ 9. yes, chess

<u>X</u> 5. grain, crane   <u>X</u> 10. vender, fender

Chapter Exercises

5.1—The Stop Consonants

A. ____ 1. wish   ____ 6. runs   ____ 11. church   <u>X</u> 16. think

   <u>X</u> 2. spring   <u>X</u> 7. whisper   <u>X</u> 12. tomb   ____ 17. rummage

   ____ 3. loom   <u>X</u> 8. question   <u>X</u> 13. logical   ____ 18. realm

   <u>X</u> 4. brush   <u>X</u> 9. system   ____ 14. jeans   <u>X</u> 19. guess

   <u>X</u> 5. window   ____ 10. phase   <u>X</u> 15. Stephen   <u>X</u> 20. fox

B. 1. *Contains a high front vowel*   perky, green

   2. *Contains a voiceless alveolar stop*   about

   3. *Contains no stops*   man

   4. *Contains a velar stop*   perky, could, plaque, green

   5. *Contains a central vowel*   about, perky

   6. *Ends with a voiceless sound*   about, plaque

   7. *Begins with a voiced sound*   man, about, green

8. *Contains a back vowel and a voiced stop* — could

9. *Begins with a voiceless sound* — perky, could, plaque

10. *Contains a front vowel and a voiceless stop* — perky, plaque

C.
___	1. table	___	6. uncle	___	11. pushin'	___	16. talkin'
T	2. better	G	7. written	T	12. splatter	G	17. bitten
___	3. errand	G	8. beaten	T	13. rotted	T	18. wedded
___	4. listen	___	9. walked	G	14. sweatin'	G	19. rotten
G	5. quittin'	___	10. Lincoln	T	15. bottle	T	20. fodder

D.
t	1. wished	t	6. danced	d	11. sailed	d	16. crabbed
d	2. loaded	t	7. wrapped	t	12. leased	t	17. placed
t	3. endorsed	d	8. hanged	t	13. reached	t	18. meshed
d	4. endangered	t	9. hoped	d	14. toted	d	19. burned
d	5. robbed	d	10. traded	t	15. wrecked	d	20. carved

E.
1. /kɪpɚt/
2. /təkɪd/
3. /ədɛbt/
4. /paʊrɚ/
5. /pɝˈkt/
6. /pækət/
7. /tɛpɪd/
8. /taɪrɚ/
9. /pɝˈpət/
10. /pɪkɪ/
11. /ətæk/
12. /tɔrkot/
13. /tʊkɪ/
14. /gækət/
15. /dɛrbɪ/
16. /pipʔd/

F.
1. pottery
2. puckered
3. potato
4. doctor
5. target
6. puppet
7. guppy
8. packing
9. diapered
10. paperboy
11. daiquiri
12. dieted

G.
1. direct — no error
2. tighter — no error
3. petted — no error
4. corker — no error
5. Carter — /karrɚ/
6. partake — /parteɪk/
7. repeat — /ripit/ or /rəpit/
8. poet — no error
9. oboe — no error
10. paper — /peɪpɚ/

H.
1. /kɪd/ — kid
2. /igɚ/ — eager
3. /tɛpɪd/ — tepid
4. /əbʌt/ — abut
5. /dakt/ — docked
6. /gɔdɪ/ — gaudy

I.
1. /keɪp/
2. /pɛrd/
3. /dɔg/ or /dag/
4. /taɪd/
5. /kɛpt/
6. /dɛt/
7. /beɪk/
8. /pɔr/
9. /bɔrd/
10. /pɔrk/
11. /pit/
12. /toʊp/
13. /tʊk/
14. /pʌt/
15. /koʊt/
16. /əpart/
17. /gardəd/ or /garrəd/
18. /boʊrɚ/

19. /bɑbɪ/	27. /pɝkɪ/	35. /taɪəd/
20. /bɑrrɚ/	28. /gɪrd/	36. /bægbɔɪ/
21. /bɪgɚ/	29. /dægɚ/	37. /dəbeɪt/ or /dibeɪt/
22. /bikɚ/	30. /gɪdɪ/ or /gɪɾɪ/	38. /tɔrɪd/
23. /tubə/	31. /kɑrpət/	39. /pɛrət/
24. /kæbɪ/	32. /dɑktɚ/	40. /dɝɪ/
25. /pɪrd/	33. /tɪkət/	
26. /bækt/	34. /dɛkt/	

5.2—The Nasal Consonants

A.
X 1. ring	X 6. jasmine	X 11. moan	X 16. ripen
X 2. bomb	___ 7. crease	X 12. spanking	X 17. unfair
___ 3. pet	X 8. inside	___ 13. possible	X 18. monkey
___ 4. stop	___ 9. trait	X 14. trench	___ 19. lure
X 5. tomb	X 10. loaner	X 15. lung	___ 20. failure

B.
X 1. **angle**	___ 8. singe	X 15. banging
___ 2. angel	___ 9. ginger	X 16. manx
X 3. brink	___ 10. danger	___ 17. ingest
X 4. **mango**	X 11. blinker	X 18. singer
___ 5. Angie	X 12. **hanger**	X 19. **hunger**
X 6. **single**	X 13. ringing	X 20. **jangle**
___ 7. conjure	X 14. **mingle**	___ 21. congeal

C. See Exercise B directly above (**bold words**).

D.
___ 1. hinge	___ 7. ring	X 13. tango
X 2. bangle	___ 8. drank	___ 14. flange
___ 3. wings	___ 9. onyx	___ 15. engine
X 4. single	X 10. tingle	X 16. English
___ 5. wrong	___ 11. bungee	___ 17. tongue
X 6. mangle	X 12. kangaroo	___ 18. dangerous

E.
___ 1. pharynx	X 7. engine	X 13. ginger
X 2. England	___ 8. flank	___ 14. blanket
X 3. bungee	___ 9. tingle	___ 15. tongue
___ 4. length	X 10. lunge	X 16. danger
___ 5. lungs	___ 11. strength	X 17. vengeance
___ 6. jungle	___ 12. tango	X 18. ranges

F. 1. *Contains an initial labial sound* — mutton, bank

2. *Contains a voiced initial sound* — good, mutton, bank, napped

3. *Ends with a stop* — good, bank, napped, code

4. *Contains a central vowel* — mutton, curving, taken, carton

5. *Ends with a voiceless sound* — bank, napped

6. *Contains a velar nasal* — curving, bank

7. *Contains a syllabic consonant* — mutton, carton

8. *Contains no nasals* — good, code

9. *Contains a low front vowel and a labial consonant* — bank, napped

10. *Contains a velar consonant and a back vowel* — good, carton, code

G.
1. /kæmp/
2. /neɪm/
3. /mɛlɪ/
4. /pɪnt/
5. /tɪŋgə/
6. /nɪŋgɪd/
7. /kræŋkɪ/
8. /kɔrn/
9. /dænk/
10. /bʌmpɪ/
11. /pɪntoʊ/
12. /pɑrmɔɪ/

H.
1. nab
2. conned
3. amass
4. anger
5. morning
6. bending
7. candy
8. appoint
9. cooking
10. tumor
11. tighten
12. minded

I.
1. camper — no error
2. adorn — no error
3. duffer — /dʌfɚ/
4. bunting — no error
5. bingo — /bɪŋgoʊ/
6. pecking — /pɛkɪŋ/
7. Dayton — /deɪʔn̩/
8. batter — /bærɚ/
9. baking — /beɪkɪŋ/
10. doorknob — /dɔrnɑb/

J.
1. /kænd/ — canned
2. /mʌnɪ/ — money
3. /əteɪn/ — attain
4. /kɑŋgoʊ/ — congo
5. /bɝpt/ — burped

K.
1. /mɪŋk/
2. /pɝt/
3. /tæn/
4. /kɪŋ/
5. /dʌn/
6. /nɪd/
7. /bæŋ/
8. /noʊm/
9. /mʌŋk/
10. /kɔɪn/
11. /ɝn/
12. /nut/
13. /taʊn/
14. /mud/
15. /naɪt/
16. /dʌm/
17. /kʊd/
18. /tɔrn/
19. /tʌŋ/
20. /gɔn/

21. /ʌndɚ/
22. /tæŋkɚd/
23. /pinʌt/ or /pinət/
24. /dændɪ/
25. /partɛik/
26. /mʌndeɪ/
27. /noʊmæd/
28. /bɑŋgoʊ/
29. /mædəm/
30. /gændɚ/

31. /omɪt/
32. /nəgeɪt/
33. /tunɪk/
34. /dɑŋkɪ/
35. /kəmænd/
36. /mɪrɚ/
37. /kaʊnʔn̩/ or /kaʊntɪn/
38. /dɛrɪŋ/
39. /ɛmpaɪɚ/
40. /kaʊɚd/

5.3—The Fricative Consonants

A.
X	1. push	X	6. brazen		11. Montana		16. hombre
X	2. thesis	X	7. cares	X	12. pleasure	X	17. leaks
	3. loom		8. burlap	X	13. leather	X	18. worthy
X	4. happy	X	9. croissant		14. marrow		19. crouton
X	5. caution	X	10. vender	X	15. other	X	20. rajah

B.
	1. mishap	ʃ	7. election	ʃ	13. friction	ʒ	19. allusion
ʒ	2. usually		8. badge		14. juice		20. inject
ʒ	3. decision	ʒ	9. lesion	ʃ	15. Sean	ʒ	21. Persia
	4. cheese	ʃ	10. lotion	ʃ	16. passion		
	5. largest	ʒ	11. corsage	ʃ	17. ricochet		
	6. reason		12. changed		18. college		

C.
ð	1. smoothly	ð	8. writhe	θ	15. oath	θ	21. author
θ	2. method	ð	9. lathe	ð	16. scathing	ð	22. smother
ð	3. other	θ	10. thought	ð	17. another	ð	23. bothers
ð	4. those	ð	11. clothes	θ	18. anything	θ	24. atheist
θ	5. moth	ð	12. weather	θ	19. withstand		
ð	6. gather	θ	13. thimble	ð	20. wither		
θ	7. wrath	θ	14. booth				

D.
1. /mu___/	v, s, z	move, moose, moos
2. /wɪ___/	f, θ or ð, z, ʃ	whiff, with (θ or ð), whiz, wish
3. /ʌ___ɚ/	ð, ʃ	other, usher
4. /lɛ___ɚ/	v, ð, s, ʒ	lever, leather, lesser, leisure
5. /___ɛrɪ/	f, v, ʃ, h	fairy (ferry), very, sherry, hairy
6. /ru___/	f, θ, z, ʒ	roof, Ruth, ruse, rouge
7. /___aɪ/	f, v, θ, ð, s, ʃ, h	fie, vie, thigh, thy, sigh, shy, high (hi)
8. /___ɪr/	f, v, s, ʃ, h	fear, veer, seer (sear), shear, here (hear)

E. 1. *Begins with a voiceless fricative*   hug, soon

    2. *Begins with a voiced obstruent*   them, beige, vend

    3. *Ends with a voiceless obstruent*   wreath, tape, cash

    4. *Contains a front vowel and a voiceless fricative*   wreath, cash

    5. *Contains an alveolar sound*   tape, soon, vend

    6. *Contains all voiced phonemes*   them, beige, vend

    7. *Contains a stop and a fricative*   beige, hug, cash, vend

    8. *Contains a nasal and a fricative*   them, soon, vend

    9. *Contains a fricative and a central vowel*   hug

    10. *Contains no fricatives*   tape

F. z 1. babes   z 7. bananas   z 13. dramas

    s 2. chafes   s 8. drinks   s 14. croaks

    z 3. cars   z 9. passes   s 15. meats

    s 4. books   z 10. throws   z 16. affairs

    s 5. carpets   z 11. loaves   s 17. loafs

    z 6. pushes   s 12. roasts   z 18. birds

G. 1. /ʃʊk/   5. /vɛrɪ/   9. /pɝs/   13. /feɪvɚ/

    2. /ʒɪŋ/   6. /ðaɪ/   10. /ʃark/   14. /kreɪzd/

    3. /zɔrt/   7. /θrʊ/   11. /ɪrðu/   15. /bɪʒɚ/

    4. /θɝd/   8. /vɔɪnz/   12. /ʃæku/   16. /hoʊðɚ/

H. 1. Asian   5. spared   9. serviced   13. fatten

    2. vortex   6. thanks   10. others   14. horror

    3. varnish   7. hearsay   11. frozen   15. gazebo

    4. bother   8. urban   12. shivered   16. birthdays

I. 1. bijou   /biʒu/   8. favored   /feɪvɚd/

    2. neither   /niðɚ/   9. shining   /ʃaɪnɪŋ/

    3. verify   /vɛrɪfaɪ/   10. earthy   /ɝθɪ/

    4. hosed   /hoʊzd/   11. amnesia   no error

    5. Hoosier   no error   12. unthinking   /ənθɪŋkɪŋ/

    6. panther   /pænθɚ/

    7. assure   no error; (or /əʃɝ/)

J. 1. /gɑrθ/   8. /θɔrnz/

    2. /fɛns/   9. /ðoʊz/

    3. /ʃɝ/, /ʃɔr/, or /ʃʊr/   10. /heɪst/

    4. /doʊzd/   11. /pɚhæps/

    5. /sɔrd/   12. /ʃɔrtɚ/, /ʃɔrɾɚ/

    6. /haɪvz/   13. /pɚuzd/

    7. /ʃaʊt/   14. /ənvɝst/

15. /mʌðɚ/
16. /kənsumd/
17. /məraʒ/ or /mɚɑʒ/
18. /pouʃənz/
19. /ovɜt/
20. /tɑrzæn/
21. /θʌndɚ/
22. /hɛðɚ/
23. /sæʔn̩/
24. /ʃipɪʃ/
25. /sɚaʊndz/
26. /hɔrʔn̩/
27. /θɜɾɪ/

28. /vɪʒən/
29. /fɛrɪŋks/
30. /θɜˑd beɪs/
31. /gɔɪɾɚ/
32. /tɛɾɚ/
33. /θaʊzənd/
34. /kɑ(ɔ)ntɔ(ʊ)r/
35. /ʃɔrtkek/
36. /vɛrid/
37. /də(i)faɪz/
38. /dɪ(ə)skʌst/
39. /ʃɔrthænd/
40. /mʌɾɚd/

5.4—The Affricate Consonants

A.

___	bon voyage	___	fantasia	dʒ	cabbage	
___	barrage	tʃ	touches	___	exertion	
dʒ	arrange	tʃ	pasture	___	sabotage	
tʃ	charming	dʒ	nitrogen	dʒ	gender	
tʃ	vulture	tʃ	riches	___	glacier	
___	mushroom	___	charade	dʒ	eject	
dʒ	gerbil	dʒ	rigid	tʃ	unchained	

B.
1. /___ɛr/   f, ð, ʃ, h, tʃ   fair, there, share, hair, chair
2. /___æt/   f, v, ð, s, h, tʃ   fat, vat, that, sat, hat, chat
3. /___oʊ/   f, ð, s, ʃ, h, dʒ   foe, though, sew (so), show, hoe, Joe
4. /___ɑrm/   f, h, tʃ   farm, harm, charm
5. /___ɪn/   f, θ, s, ʃ, tʃ, dʒ   fin, thin, sin, shin, chin, gin
6. /ri___/   f, θ, tʃ   reef, wreath, reach
7. /bæ___/   θ, s, ʃ, tʃ, dʒ   bath, bass, bash, batch, badge
8. /bi___/   f, z, tʃ   beef, bees, beach

C.
1. *Contains an initial voiced phoneme*   other, none, jeans, measure
2. *Contains a fricative*   other, shrunk, jeans, hedge, measure
3. *Contains affricate and front vowel*   jeans, hedge
4. *Contains an affricate and a nasal*   jeans, churned
5. *Contains a palatal obstruent*   shrunk, jeans, hedge, churned, measure
6. *Contains an obstruent and a central vowel*   other, shrunk, churned, measure
7. *Contains a stop, nasal, and affricate*   churned
8. *Contains all voiced sounds*   other, none, jeans, measure

D. 1. /skrʌntʃ/   5. /muʒd/   9. /ouðən/   13. /fæʃtɚ/
    2. /pʊdʒɪ/   6. /kɪtʃən/   10. /dʒeɪd/   14. /gaʊtʃt/
    3. /tʃɔrz/   7. /moʊtʃ/   11. /hʌdʒ/   15. /dʒʌmpɪ/
    4. /harʃɚ/   8. /ʃarm/   12. /tʃɝn/   16. /partʃt/

E. 1. chirped   5. adjoined   9. surely   13. mature
    2. junk   6. macho   10. jersey   14. chummy
    3. chit chat   7. garage   11. purchase   15. agitate
    4. wishbone   8. pasture   12. chocolate   16. jezebel

F. 1. major   /meɪdʒɚ/   6. usher   no error
    2. March   no error   7. sergeant   /sardʒənt/
    3. jumped   no error   8. massage   no error
    4. Wichita no error   9. gorge   /gɔrdʒ/
    5. wedged   /wɛdʒd/   10. manger   /meɪndʒɚ/

G. 1. /ʃakt/   11. /vɪvɪ(ə)d/   21. /kæʒmɪr/   31. /ɛ(ə)gzɪsts/
    2. /steɪʃən/   12. /ʃʌrɚ/   22. /tʃapɪŋ/   32. /dʒɪndʒɚ/
    3. /bʊtʃɚ/   13. /ə(ɛ)ksaɪt/   23. /kæʃbaks/   33. /θɔrnɪ/
    4. /nɪkəz/   14. /æksan/   24. /dʒɛndɚz/   34. /idʒɪ(ə)pt/
    5. /ɛkstrə/   15. /skaʊəd/   25. /tʃarmɪŋ/   35. /tʃaʊmeɪn/
    6. /tændʒənt/   16. /karvd/   26. /ʃarpənd/   36. /pɚvɝs/
    7. /sʌðən/   17. /aʊtʃaɪm/   27. /kæʃɪr/   37. /dʌtʃə(ɪ)s/
    8. /nɛktaɪ/   18. /dʒɛndɚ/   28. /garbədʒ/   38. /æŋkʃə(ɪ)s/
    9. /kɔrsaʒ/   19. /kɛrləs/   29. /ɔrkə(ɪ)dz/   39. /mɪstʃə(ɪ)f/
    10. /spɪrɪ(ə)ts/ 20. /nɝtʃɚ/   30. /stræŋ(k)θən/   40. /kæp(t)ʃɚ/

5.5—The Approximant Consonants

A. _w_ awkward   _r_ reasoned   _w_   suede   _w, l_ jonquil
    _l_ bellow   ___ towered   _j_   fewer   _r_ screaming
    _w_ quick   ___ Jupiter   _r, l_ peril   _r, l_ barley
    ___ today   _l_ lazy   _w_   swiped   _j_ puny
    _r_ torpedo   _r_ repaid   _j_   yawned   ___ fired

B. ___ tune   ___ hood   ___   choosy
    ___ jealous   ___ piano   _X_   compute
    _X_ putrid   ___ maybe   _X_   usual
    ___ loop   ___ jar   _X_   yours
    _X_ fuel   ___ adjourn   ___   daisy
    ___ keynote   _X_ Cupid   ___   boysenberry

C.   ___   awesome   X   why   X   warrior

    X   well   ___   awry   X   swept

    X   stalwart   ___   wrath   X   quirk

    ___   how   ___   rowboat   ___   borrowed

    ___   showed   X   reward   ___   wrist

    ___   lower   ___   Howard   X   wayward

D.   ___   lurk   ___   surround   ___   purchase

    X   barter   X   rewritten   ___   perfected

    ___   burgundy   ___   tires   X   scorpion

    X   unreal   X   fourth   ___   flirtatious

    X   guarded   X   spirited   X   grandiose

    X   grasp   ___   curvature   ___   divert

E. 1. /**dʒɛloʊ**/   6. /**sɚklz**/   11. /**spjud**/   16. /fjunts/

   2. /**blaɪð** /   7. /fjɜt/   12. /walʃat/   17. /jɛlɪ/

   3. /riljə/   8. /**kwɔrl̩d**/   13. /**swɪlz**/   18. /**skjud**/

   4. /ɚoʊlɚ/   9. /**wʊln̩**/   14. /**riwɜd**/   19. /ɑkwɚd/

   5. /**dʒɑr**/   10. /pjaɪd/   15. /poʊləs/   20. /riɚən/

F. 1. yellow   9. liquid

   2. robust   10. tiled

   3. warrior   11. curtailed

   4. yearned   12. quarrel

   5. beetles   13. luckily

   6. grouched   14. Latin

   7. repute   15. fuchsia

   8. guava   16. question

G. 1. bowling   /boʊlɪŋ/   7. lawyer   /lɔɪɚ/ or /lɔjɚ/

   2. wrongful   /raŋfʊl/   8. flurries   /flɜɪz/

   3. warbled   no error   9. fuming   no error

   4. pewter   /pjurɚ/   10. baloney   /bəloʊnɪ/

   5. quandary   /kwandrɪ/   11. relish   /rɛlɪʃ/

   6. regional   no error   12. confusion   /kənfjuʒən/

H. 1. /kwɪksænd/   8. /skjuɚ/

   2. /slaʊtʃt/   9. /kɔrdʒəl/

   3. /dʒɜɪ/ or /dʒʊrɪ/   10. /jusfʊl/

   4. /əkweɪnt/   11. /wɪθdru/

   5. /ʃoʊldɚ/   12. /wɜʃɪp/

   6. /slɪðɚ/   13. /ɛ(ə)nʃraɪnd/

   7. /sɑrdʒənt/   14. /fjumd/

15. /lʌn(t)ʃən/
16. /dʒunjɚ/
17. /ənskeɪðd/
18. /ʃrɪvl̩/
19. /jæŋkiz/
20. /kwɔrrɚ/
21. /bjugl̩/
22. /tʃɪzl̩/
23. /junə(ɪ)k/
24. /tʃɑrl̩z/
25. /bəlɑŋ(g)ɪŋ/
26. /rubrɪ(ə)k/
27. /junik/
28. /bi(ə)kwɪðd(θt)/
29. /kaɪæk/
30. /bɪljɚdz/
31. /aɪwɑ(ɔ)ʃ/
32. /lɪŋgwəl/
33. /kwɔrl̩d/
34. /æŋgwɪ(ə)ʃt/
35. /aʊtwɚd/
36. /rʌp(t)ʃɚ/
37. /ʃu wæks/
38. /kwoʊʃənt/
39. /stræŋglɚ/
40. /əlʊr/

Review Exercises

A. ?   1. writin'   ?   6. certain
    ɾ   2. rudder   ɾ   7. crater
    ?* 3. about   ___ 8. winter
    ɾ   4. nutty   ?   9. Martin
    np 5. harden   np 10. sudden

   *possibly in coda position

B. ___ 1. wheel   ___ 6. pull
     X   2. written   ___ 7. contagious
     X   3. regal   X   8. that'll
     X   4. Seton Hall   X   9. grab 'em by the neck
     X   5. candles   ___ 10. hold 'er by the tail

C. /k/   stop   velar   voiceless
    /r/   liquid   palatal   voiced
    /θ/   fricative   interdental   voiceless
    /ŋ/   nasal   velar   voiced
    /dʒ/ affricate   palatal   voiced
    /b/   stop   bilabial   voiced
    /ʃ/   fricative   palatal   voiceless
    /j/   glide   palatal   voiced
    /f/   fricative   labiodental   voiceless
    /n/   nasal   alveolar   voiced

D. Possible answers include:

1. deed, need
2. cone, cove
3. hum, thumb
4. hip, ship
5. rag, lag, nag

E.
1.	sin-sing	place
2.	jaw-raw	manner
3.	sue-shoe	place
4.	tin-tip	voice, manner, place
5.	clue-crew	place
6.	cop-mop	voice, manner, place
7.	choke-joke	voice
8.	pet-met	voice, manner
9.	done-gun	place
10.	even-Eden	manner, place
11.	Yale-rail	manner
12.	late-lake	place
13.	fame-shame	place
14.	cat-cad	voice
15.	pass-pad	voice, manner

F.
1.	jester	/dʒ/	voiced	prevocalic
2.	version			
3.	itchy	/tʃ/	voiceless	intervocalic
4.	cash			
5.	switched	/tʃ/	voiceless	postvocalic
6.	January	/dʒ/	voiced	prevocalic
7.	regime			
8.	mashing			
9.	crush			
10.	urgent	/dʒ/	voiced	intervocalic

G.
1.	<u>c</u>elery	/s/	voiceless	alveolar	fricative
2.	bree<u>ch</u>	/tʃ/	voiceless	palatal	affricate
3.	<u>ph</u>ase	/f/	voiceless	labiodental	fricative
4.	w<u>r</u>eck	/r/	voiced	palatal	liquid
5.	ca<u>ll</u>	/l/	voiced	alveolar	liquid
6.	me<u>th</u>od	/θ/	voiceless	interdental	fricative
7.	<u>y</u>es	/j/	voiced	palatal	glide

8. cru<u>d</u>e	/d/	voiced	alveolar	stop
9. <u>ch</u>asm	/k/	voiceless	velar	stop
10. e<u>dge</u>	/dʒ/	voiced	palatal	affricate
11. <u>w</u>alk	/w/	voiced	labiovelar	glide
12. cohe<u>s</u>ion	/ʒ/	voiced	palatal	fricative

H.
1. /bɝθmɑrks/
2. /kandʒɚɪŋ/
3. /bitʃkomɚ/
4. /ʌðɚwaɪz/
5. /dʒɔrdʒ bʊʃ/
6. /værɪkən/
7. /zɪŋk aksaɪd/
8. /hæŋkɚtʃɪf/
9. /ɛkspədaɪt/
10. /faʊndeɪʃən/
11. /ædmɪrəd/
12. /ðɛræftɚ/
13. /ɪndʒʌŋkʃən/
14. /kənvɝdʒəns/
15. /sæbətɑʒ/
16. /fəzɪʃən/
17. /bʌʔn̩ hol/
18. /dɪskɝədʒd/
19. /ivɑlvd/
20. /ɪndɪdʒənt/
21. /kazmos/
22. /tʃɪmpænziz/
23. /dɪskɑrdəd/
24. /prɛstidʒəs/
25. /tʃɑrmɪŋ/
26. /tɝkɪʃ bæθ/
27. /bɑðɚsəm/
28. /dʒæk naɪf/
29. /ɛnzaɪm/
30. /tuθ fɛrɪ/
31. /tʃɛrɪ paɪ/
32. /koɑθɚ/
33. /haɪəsɪnθ/
34. /ɛndʒɔɪmənt/
35. /fɑrməsɪst/
36. /ənwɝðɪ/
37. /wən hʌndrətθ/
38. /pæstʃɚaɪzd/
39. /fɪdʒɪrɪ/
40. /fɑðɚz deɪ/

I.
1. /eɔrrə/
2. /ɛrlaɪnɚ/
3. /kəndʒild/
4. /kɔkeɪʒən/
5. /vokeɪʃən/
6. /fjunəl̩/
7. /rɛdʒɪstɚd/
8. /jɛstɚdeɪ/
9. /novɛmbɚ/
10. /trʌbl̩səm/
11. /əphoʊlstɚd/
12. /ɪmpjudɪnt/
13. /tɔrɛntʃəl/
14. /dɪstrɪbjut/
15. /daɪəfræm/
16. /æpətaɪt/
17. /pɚsəvɪr/
18. /kɚeɪdʒəs/
19. /mʌskjulɚ/
20. /pəpaɪrəs/
21. /sikwɛnʃəl/
22. /pɔrtreɪl/
23. /θæŋksgɪvɪŋ/
24. /zaɪləfon/
25. /ɑrrɪtʃok/
26. /pɪdʒənhol/
27. /wɪljəmzbɚg/
28. /ʌndɚgroθ/
29. /hjumɚəs/
30. /wɪrɪnəs/
31. /junɪ(ə)vɚs/
32. /əngæðɚd/
33. /mænjuskrɪpt/
34. /əbskjɝlɪ/
35. /nuklɪəs/
36. /kwɑdræŋgl̩/
37. /hɑrmənaɪz/
38. /rɛdʒɪstrɑr/
39. /par bɔɪld/
40. /strʌkʃɚl̩/

J. 1. A. "mad"—nasal murmur can be seen prior to onset of vowel
   B. "bad"—no aspiration on release of /b/
   C. "pad"—aspiration visible on release of /p/

2. A. "song"
   B. "thong"
   The friction noise for the initial fricative in spectrogram A is much greater in intensity than that in spectrogram B.

3.

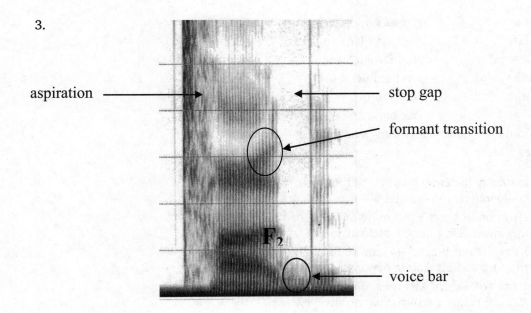

aspiration ⟶   ⟵ stop gap

⟵ formant transition

F₂

⟵ voice bar

Chapter 6

Chapter Exercises

6.1 1. /θ/
   2. /d/
   3. /t/
   4. /d/

   5. /t/
   6. /h/
   7. /v/
   8. /h/

6.2			
1.	noon	/nuən/	X
2.	pants	/pænts/	___
3.	choose	/tʃjuz/	X
4.	friends	/frɛndz/	___
5.	lamb	/læm/	___
6.	straw	/strɔr/	X
7.	rinse	/rɪns/	___
8.	milk	/mɛlk/	___
9.	clam	/kəlæm/	X
10.	Wednesday	/wænzdeɪ/	___

6.3 1. [mɪrəkl̩]
       [məæ̃kjələs]

   2. [əkjuz]
       [ækjəzeɪʃən]

   3. [ɑ(ɔ)θɚaɪz]
       [əθɔrəɾɪ]

   4. [dəmɑləʃ]
       [dɛməlɪʃən]

   5. [məkænɪkl̩]
       [mɛkənɪstɪk]

6.4 1. your mother   /jɔr mʌðɚ/   /jəmʌðɚ/
    2. right and left   /raɪt ænd lɛft/   /raɪʔn̩lɛft/
    3. food for thought   /fud fɔr θɑt/   /fudfɚθɑt/
    4. What will they do?   /wʌt wɪl ðeɪ du/   /wərl̩ðedu/
    5. Thank him.   /θæŋk hɪm/   /θæŋkəm/
    6. as big as   /æz bɪg æz/   /æzbɪgəz/
    7. of mice and men   /ʌv maɪs ænd mɛn/   /əvmaɪsn̩mɛn/
    8. What is her name?   /wʌt ɪz hɚ neɪm/   /wʌtsəneɪm/

6.5 1. /aɪ bɛt ju aɪ kæn hɛlp ðɛm gɛt aʊt əv ðæt mɛs ‖/
      /aɪbɛtʃuaɪkənhɛlpm̩gɛtaʊrəðætmɛs ‖/
    2. /aɪ kɑt ju tʃirɪŋ an ðæt tɛst ‖ aɪ æm goʊɪŋ tu tɛl ðə titʃɚ ‖/
      /aɪkɑtʃutʃirɪŋanðæt tɛst ‖ aɪmgunətɛlðətitʃɚ ‖/
    3. /wʌt ɪz hɪz rizn̩ fɔr nɑt biŋ eɪbl̩tə kʌm tu ðə pɑrɪ ‖/
      /wətsɪzrizn̩fɚnɑtbiəneɪbl̩təkəmtə ðəpɑrɪ ‖/
    4. /wʌts ðə mærɚ wɪθ θɛlmə ‖ lɛt mi si ɪf aɪ kæn tʃir hɚʌp ‖/
      /wətsðəmærəwɪθ θɛlmə ‖ lɛmɪsiəfaɪkəntʃirəəp ‖/
    5. /wʌt dɪd ju du tu jɚ kar ‖ aɪ ʃud bi eɪbl̩tu gɛt ɪt goʊɪŋ ‖/
      /wədʒədurəjɚkar ‖ aɪʃədbieɪbl̩rəgɛtɪtgoən ‖/

6.6 1. ˌinˈtense   5. ˈteaˌbag   9. eˈrode
    2. ˈfalseˌhood   6. ˈfrostˌbite   10. ˈhandˌshake
    3. ˈLuˌcite   7. ˌoˈbese   11. ˌreˈact
    4. ˌroˈsette   8. ˈenˌtree   12. ˈhouseˌhold

6.7 1. ˈleopard   5. ˈmurky   9. ˈscary
    2. ˈsweater   6. aˈnoint   10. ˈnaked
    3. ˈrhythm   7. ˈmagnet   11. exˈtreme
    4. conˈtend   8. beˈlief   12. paˈrade

6.8 1. ˈmeasuring   5. couˈrageous   9. soˈrority
    2. staˈtistics   6. ˈGermany   10. fraˈternity
    3. laˈryngeal   7. unˈbearable   11. ˈAlbuquerque
    4. ˈwarranted   8. Caˈnadian   12. dysˈphonia

6.9 1. ˌmyˈopic   5. ˌciˈtation   9. ˈaliˌmony
    2. ˈcyberˌspace   6. ˈcircumˌstance   10. comˈmuniˌcate
    3. ˈarchiˌtect   7. ˌbacˈteria   11. ˈeleˌvator
    4. ˌiˈdea   8. ˌefferˈvescent   12. ˌIndiˈana

6.10 The underlined words should be:
    1. matinee   4. uncle
    2. East   5. Mr.
    3. Flo

6.11 1. The girl's name was <u>Chris</u>.
Her name wasn't Pat.

2. Jared only forgot to get the <u>toothpaste</u> at the store.
Jared remembered to get everything else.

3. Why did they <u>walk</u> to the playground?
Why didn't they drive?

4. Why did they walk to the <u>playground</u>?
Why didn't they walk to the zoo?

5. <u>Mark</u> got a new blue bike for his birthday.
Louise didn't get a new bike.

6. Mark got a new blue <u>bike</u> for his birthday.
He did not get a blue baseball cap.

7. Mark got a new <u>blue</u> bike for his birthday.
The bike wasn't green.

6.12 The answers are in bold.

Waitress: Would you like something to **drink**?

Customer: **Lemonade**, please. I would also like to **order**.

Waitress: Would you like an **appetizer**?

Customer: **No, thank you.**

Waitress: Would you like to hear about our **specials**?

Customer: **Please.**

Waitress: We have **grilled salmon** and **fettuccine alfredo**.

Customer: I'll have the **fettuccine**.

Waitress: Would you like our **house dressing** on your **salad**? It's **Italian**.

Customer: I would like to have **blue cheese**, please.

Waitress: I'll also bring out some **fresh rolls**.

Customer: **Thank you.**

Waitress: **You're welcome.**

6.13 1. a. ˌSteve's ˈroommate is from ˌMinneapolis.
b. ˌSteve's ˌroommate is from Minneˈapolis.

2. a. ˌTim went ˌskydiving on ˈSaturday.
b. ˈTim went ˌskydiving on ˌSaturday.

3. a. The ˈanswer on the ˌexam was "false."
b. The ˌanswer on the ˌexam was ˈ"false."

4. a. ˌMary's ˌbirthday is next ˈTuesday.
b. ˌMary's ˈbirthday is next ˌTuesday.

5. a. ˈI'd like a ˌsteak for ˌdinner.
b. ˌI'd like a ˈsteak for ˌdinner.

6. a. ˌI went to New York ˈCity to see some ˌplays.
b. ˌI went to ˌNew York City to see some ˈplays.

7. a. ˌMy ˌprofessor ˌshaved his ˈmustache.
b. ˌMy ˈprofessor ˌshaved his ˌmustache.

8. a. ˌI need poˈtatoes from the ˌstore.
b. ˈI need ˌpotatoes from the ˌstore.

6.14 The answers are in bold.

1.	When will you leave?	Rising	**Falling**
2.	Is your brother home?	**Rising**	Falling
3.	I need to go the library.	Rising	**Falling**
4.	What's your favorite season?	Rising	**Falling**
5.	Did you get paid yet?	**Rising**	Falling
6.	The dog ran away.	Rising	**Falling**
7.	Sophie is my oldest friend.	Rising	**Falling**
8.	How did you know about that?	Rising	**Falling**
9.	Honest?!?	**Rising**	Falling
10.	I'm sure!!!	Rising	**Falling**

6.15 1. [piːz]   4. [spɑː]
2. [liːv]   5. [læːg]
3. [ruːd]   6. [tuː]

6.16 1. [raɪsːup]   5. [kɑ(l)mːɔrnɪŋ]
2. [kaʔn̩ːɛɾɪŋ]   6. [bɑrːum]
3. [bɪgːʌnz]   7. [lifːaɪɚ]
4. [teɪlːaɪt]   8. [puʃːɛɾɪ]

6.17 1. [I want hot dogs | ice cream | and cotton candy ‖]
2. [They left | didn't they ‖]
3. [The family | who lived next door | moved away ‖]
4. [What is her problem ‖]
5. [My uncle | the dentist | is 34 years old ‖]

Review Exercises

A.

1.	[kæm meɪk]	m/n	bilabial
2.	[haʊʒɚ mʌðɚ]	ʒ/z+j	palatal
3.	[dʒɪŋ geɪm]	ŋ/n	velar
4.	[lɛb paɪp]	b/d	bilabial
5.	[hæʒ ʃeɪkn̩]	ʒ/z	palatal
6.	[rɛg gaʊn]	g/d	velar

B. 1. /bɛnz/   5. /kaʊnɚ/
2. /wɪnɚ/   6. /twɛlfs/
3. /lænmaɪn/   7. /wɑts ɚ prɑbləm/
4. /kæn ə wɝmz/   8. /wɛp laʊdlɪ/

C. 1. /aɪ wɑnt tu goʊ hoʊm/
/aɪwɑnəgohom/

2. /lɛt mi si jɔr bʊk/
/lɛmɪsijɚbʊk/

3. /kʊd ju muv eɪ lɪtl̩ tu ðə raɪt/
/kʊdʒəmuvəlɪɾl̩təðɚaɪt/

4. /dɪd dʒan ɛvɚ gɛt peɪd/
   /dɪdʒanɛvɚgɛtpeɪd/

5. /waɪ dɪd ʃi liv soʊ ɝli
   /waɪdʃilivsoɝli

6. /ɪt ɪz reɪnɪŋ kæts ænd dagz/
   /ɪtsreɪnɪŋkætsn̩dagz/

7. /wɛn ɑr ju goʊɪŋ tu liv/
   /wɛnɚjəgʊnəliv/

8. /ju hæv gat tu bi kɪdɪŋ/
   /juvgarəbikɪdɪŋ/

9. /hu ɪz goʊɪŋ tu reɪk ðʌ livz tunaɪt/
   /huzgʊnərekðəlivztənaɪt/

10. /aɪ want tu wæks maɪ trʌk tumaroʊ mɔrnɪŋ/
    /aɪwanəwæksmaɪtrəktəmaromɔrnɪŋ/

D. 1. Did you ever go to the circus?
   2. When did she leave Georgia?
   3. My sister got a new boyfriend.
   4. Give me a day or two to decide.
   5. I am going to have to say "no" for now.
   6. I think it is going to rain either today or tomorrow.
   7. Would you ever think of doing that for me?
   8. Do you think that Susan took enough of them?
   9. I am sure that they are going to tell you what you need to do it.
   10. Try as he might, he just could not do what she wanted.

E. 1. cour'ageous   11. ˌcompu'tation
    2. 'terri ˌfied   12. 'cran ˌberry
    3. ma'jestic   13. 'bulletin
    4. ˌasth'matic   14. sur'rendered
    5. 'Plexi ˌglas   15. se'mantics
    6. plur'ality   16. co'lonial
    7. 'manda ˌtory   17. 'mercen ˌary
    8. ˌclan'destine   18. inde'pendent
    9. flam'boyant   19. ˌOc'tober
    10. ˌcre'ation   20. ˌballer'ina

F.

		Reduced	Full
1. /ˈɔrɪdʒɪn/	/əˈrɪdʒɪnˌet/	X	
2. /ˈmaɪkrəˌskop/	/ˌmaɪˈkraskəpɪ/	—	X
3. /əˈrɪstəˌkræt/	/ˌɛrɪsˈtakrəsɪ/	—	X
4. /ˈstrærədʒɪ/	/strəˈtidʒɪk/	—	X
5. /ˈmeɪnɪˌæk/	/məˈnaɪəkl̩/	X	
6. /ˌhoˈmadʒənəs/	/ˌhoməˈdʒinɪəs/	—	X

		Rising	Falling
7. /ˈpɛrəˌlaɪz/	/pəˈræləsɪs/	—	X
8. /ˈfɛlənɪ/	/fəˈloʊnɪəs/	—	X
9. /pɚˈspaɪɚ/	/pɚspəˈeɪʃn̩/	X	—
10. /ˌriˈpit/	/ˌrɛpəˈtɪʃəs/	X	—

G.

		Rising	Falling
1. I got a sweater for my birthday.		—	X
2. Are you happy?		X	—
3. The girls had spaghetti for supper.		—	X
4. Are you positive?		X	—
5. When you're finished, go to bed.		—	X
6. Were you late for work today?		X	—
7. Let me get back to you.		—	X
8. Did you buy a new CD?		X	—
9. What do you mean?		—	X
10. Is that your idea of a joke?		X	—

H. 1. If I want your help | you'll be the first to know ‖
   2. Maybe I will | maybe I won't ‖
   3. They bought a new house | didn't they ‖
   4. The girls | who went swimming | all got a cold ‖
   5. I can't really make up my mind ‖
   6. I scream | you scream | we all scream | for ice cream ‖
   7. When are you leaving on vacation ‖
   8. Are your cousins coming for a visit | or not ‖
   9. Do you have ants in your pants ‖
  10. I quit my job | but only when I was sure I could get another ‖

I. 1. [aɪkɔtmaɪkæt:ɑmbaɪðəteɪl ‖]
   2. [wɪtʃ:æmpudɪðʒubaɪætðəstɔr ‖]
   3. [wʊdʒupʊtðəwaɪt:ebl̩klɑθɑnðəteɪbl̩pliz ‖]
   4. [mɑm:aɪt:ekmiʃɑpɪŋɪfaɪgɛtgʊdgredz ‖]
   5. [hævjufɪnɪʃt:epɪŋðətivispɛʃl̩jɛt ‖]
   6. [wɪθ:ɛm | ɪtshɑrdtətɛlwətðɛrθɪŋkɪŋ ‖]
   7. [plizgɪmijɚfon:ʌmbɚbifɔrjuliv ‖]
   8. [klɛm:erə hoʊmrʌnætðəbɪg:emlæst:uzdeɪ ‖]
   9. [tɛrɪŋferl̩:ʌvtupleaʊtsaɪdwɪð:əwɑrɚsprɪŋklɚ ‖]
  10. [aɪwont:ekɛnɪmɔrəvðədʒʌŋk:ɛnhænzaʊt ‖]

J. 1. /waɪkæntʃuɛvɚæktʃɚeɪdʒ ‖/
    /waɪkæntʃuɛvɚæktjɚeɪdʒ ‖/

2. /waɪ owaɪ | dɪdaɪɛvɚlivaɪowə ‖/
  /waɪowaɪdɪdaɪɛvɚlivaɪowə ‖/

3. /wɛndðeseðɛrflaɪtwəz ‖/
  /wɛndɪdðeseðɛrflaɪtwəz ‖/

4. /ɑlprɑbligohomtəmɑrou ɔrðədeæftɚ ‖/
  /aɪwɪlprɑbligohoumtəmɑrou ɚ ɔrðədeæftɚ ‖/

5. /wɛrdʃiɛvɚgeʔn̩ aɪdiəlaɪkðæt ‖/
  /wɛrdɪdʃiɛvɚgetænaɪdiəlaɪkðæt ‖/

6. /jugɑrəbipulmmaɪlɛg ‖/
  /juvgatːəbipulŋmaɪlɛg ‖/

7. /maɪfrɛnz | ɛsbɪnd̩eɪl | ɑrgunəpɪkmiəpətθri ‖/
  /maɪfrɛnz | ɛsbɪnd̩eɪl | ɑrgouɪntəpɪkmiəpætθri ‖/

8. /waɪdʒuripentðəbɑrnalrɛɪ ‖/
  /waɪdɪdʒuripentðəbɑrnalrɛɪ ‖/

9. /ðɛrgunətɛljuwətʃənid ‖/
  /ðɛrgouɪntətɛljuwətjunid ‖/

10. /dɪdʃitektuəvəm ‖ næʃitukfɔr ‖/
   /dɪdʃitektuəvðəm ‖ nɑːʃitukfɔr ‖/

Chapter 7

Chapter Exercises

7.1 1. nasals and stops
   2. labial, alveolar, and velar
   3. liquids, some fricatives, and affricates
   4. stops

7.2

___	1. yes	___	6. milk
X	2. baby	X	7. mitten
X	3. banana	___	8. lady
___	4. mama	X	9. scissors
X	5. today	___	10. juice

7.3

away	1.	___	___	say	6.	___	___
cup	2.	X	/kʌ/	phone	7.	X	/fou/
through	3.	___	___	black	8.	X	/blæ/
clown	4.	X	/klaʊ/	stop	9.	X	/stɑ/
bread	5.	X	/brɛ/	go	10.	___	___

7.4 ___ 1. wagon

    _X_ 2. children

    ___ 3. jacket

    _X_ 4. pencil

    _X_ 5. water

    ___ 6. yellow

7.5 _X_ 1. blue

    ___ 2. spot

    _X_ 3. stripe

    ___ 4. path

    _X_ 5. spring

    _X_ 6. stop

    _X_ 7. crayon

    _X_ 8. milk

    ___ 9. wish

    _X_ 10. grape

7.6 ___ 1. shoe

    _X_ 2. thank

    ___ 3. raisin

    _X_ 4. march

    ___ 5. shave

    ___ 6. comb

    _X_ 7. summer

    ___ 8. yellow

    _X_ 9. bath

    _X_ 10. shop

7.7 ___ 1. candy

    _X_ 2. rake

    _X_ 3. bring

    ___ 4. clown

    _X_ 5. brush

    _X_ 6. ridge

    ___ 7. fishing

    ___ 8. paper

    _X_ 9. goose

    ___ 10. sing

7.8 ___ 1. shake

    ___ 2. choose

    ___ 3. brush

    _X_ 4. Jack

    ___ 5. mesh

    ___ 6. gem

    _X_ 7. witch

    _X_ 8. chalk

    _X_ 9. chase

    ___ 10. bridge

7.9 ___ 1. soap

    _X_ 2. leaf

    _X_ 3. ring

    _X_ 4. lazy

    ___ 5. rice

    ___ 6. yes

    _X_ 7. loop

    _X_ 8. grow

    _X_ 9. laugh

    ___ 10. free

7.10 _X_ 1. middle

    ___ 2. lamp

    _X_ 3. answer

    _X_ 4. Kirk

    ___ 5. could

    _X_ 6. belt

    ___ 7. telephone

    _X_ 8. curtain

    ___ 9. bark

    ___ 10. fire

7.11 ___ 1. pie   _X_ 6. boat
    _X_ 2. tap   ___ 7. train
    ___ 3. frog   _X_ 8. peg
    ___ 4. lip   ___ 9. cause
    _X_ 5. numb   _X_ 10. big

7.12 ___ 1. pig   _X_ 6. knife
    _X_ 2. pat   _X_ 7. that
    _X_ 3. short   _X_ 8. phone
    ___ 4. Tom   ___ 9. vat
    ___ 5. tune   ___ 10. hard

7.13 _X_ 1. turkey   ___ 6. ring
    ___ 2. kill   _X_ 7. bang
    ___ 3. mouse   ___ 8. shook
    ___ 4. grass   _X_ 9. cap
    _X_ 5. fake   _X_ 10. brag

7.14 _P_ 1. pear   ___ 6. gone
    _D_ 2. led   _P_ 7. train
    _P_ 3. fair   _D_ 8. flag
    _D_ 4. card   _P_ 9. shoe
    ___ 5. high   ___ 10. chair

7.15
1. chairs   initial consonant deletion
2. letter   fricative replacing a stop
3. witch   stop replacing a glide
4. tape   backing
5. bunny   initial consonant deletion; glottal replacement
6. bad   backing; glottal replacement

7.16

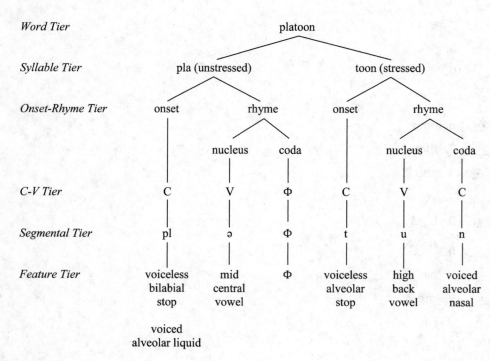

Word Tier	platoon
Syllable Tier	pla (unstressed) toon (stressed)
Onset-Rhyme Tier	onset rhyme onset rhyme
	nucleus coda nucleus coda
C-V Tier	C V Φ C V C
Segmental Tier	pl ə Φ t u n
Feature Tier	voiceless bilabial stop mid central vowel Φ voiceless alveolar stop high back vowel voiced alveolar nasal
	voiced alveolar liquid	

7.17 1. ___ could   3. _X_ drop   5. _X_ keep

      2. _X_ kiss   4. ___ clam   6. ___ comb

7.18 1. /ɔ/   5. /ʊ/
      2. /ɛ/   6. /æ/
      3. /ɔ/   7. /ʊ/
      4. /e/   8. /i/

7.19 1. [hʷʊd]   5.
      2.   6.
      3. [rʷuf]   7. [sʷwit]
      4.   8. [dʷun]

7.20 1. ɔ   4. ɔ
      2. c   5. c
      3. c   6. ɔ

7.21 1. ɤ   4. ɯ
      2. œ   5. ø
      3. ɒ   6. ʌ

7.22 1. [æn̪θ̪əm]   5. [mæθ̪taɪm]
      2.   6. [wɛl̪θ̪]
      3.   7.
      4.   8. [pæn̪θ̪ɚ]

7.23 1. [ɪɱfɚɛntʃəl] 6. [kæɱfɚ]
2. 7. [sʌɱflaʊɚ]
3. [mɛɱfəs] 8.
4. 9.
5. [əɱfrɛndlɪ] 10. [kɪɱfo(l)k]

7.24 1. _X_ lake 6. _X_ liked
2. ___ mingle 7. ___ hilly
3. _X_ loop 8. ___ Elton
4. ___ beagle 9. _X_ lady
5. ___ balding 10. _X_ alone

7.25 1. ___ slack 5. _X_ excuse
2. ___ praised 6. ___ surprise
3. _X_ scorn 7. _X_ stripe
4. _X_ despite 8. ___ smooth

7.26 1. _X_ skunk
2. _X_ snacked
3. ___ target [tʰɑrgət˺]
4. ___ brave [breɪv]
5. ___ toga [tʰoʊgə]
6. _X_ guarded
7. ___ person [pʰɝsən]
8. _X_ carefully
9. ___ slope [sloʊp˺]
10. ___ great [greɪtʰ]

7.27 1. ___ mean 4. _X_ string
2. _X_ boon 5. ___ slam
3. ___ buddy 6. _X_ thong

7.28 1. [kɛt̚l̩] 3. [wɑɾɚ] 6. [bæt̚l̩d]

7.29 1. [pju̥rɚ] 5. [hi dʌʐ]
2. [kl̥ɪrlɪ] 6. [rɪd̥ʒ strit]
3. [hiʐ stʌbɚn] 7. [aɪ luʐ]
4. [beɪð̥ pæm] 8. [ðeɪɣ pleɪd̥]

7.30 1. x 6. k'
2. pf 7. ʊ
3. ʕ 8. ɖ
4. β 9. ɤ
5. ɫ 10. ɱ

Review Exercises

A. 1. d   6. d
    2. c   7. b
    3. a   8. c
    4. b   9. d
    5. a   10. a

B. 1. R   6. P
    2. R   7. P
    3. R   8. P
    4. P   9. R
    5. R   10. P

C. 1. c   6. d
    2. d   7. b
    3. a   8. c
    4. e   9. b
    5. a   10. e

D. 1. c   5. a, c
    2. a   6. a, c
    3. b   7. b
    4. b   8. a

E. 1. a, b, c   5. b, d
    2. a, b   6. b, d
    3. a, c   7. a, d
    4. b, d   8. a, b, c

F. 1. /sip/ or /lip/
    2. /græg/
    3. /dɑr/
    4. /wɛmən/ or /jɛmən/
    5. /beɪp/
    6. /ʒɛlɪ/
    7. /bʌv/
    8. /taɪn/
    9. /teɪm/
   10. /groʊ/

G. 1. No   7. No
   2. No   8. Yes
   3. Yes   9. Yes
   4. Yes   10. No
   5. Yes   11. Yes
   6. No   12. No

H. 1. reiterated articulation
   2. bidental median fricative
   3. velar nareal fricative
   4. labioalveolar plosive
   5. linguolabial median fricative
   6. whistled [s]
   7. interdental trill
   8. lateral + median voiced alveolar fricative

I. 1. wɑb̥ster   14. hæmɚ
   2. nɝ·s   15. wɑrm kwɑk
   3. souldʒɚ   16. vækjum kwinɚ
   4. æstrənɑt   17. ɛlfənt
   5. titʃɚ   18. taɪgɚ
   6. trʌk draɪvɚ   19. skwɝl
   7. dɛntɪst   20. paɪrɚ
   8. frɪdʒɚɛɾɚ   21. jaɪən
   9. tɛlfon   22. dɑlfɪn
  10. wæmp   23. kæŋgru
  11. tusbwəʃ   24. ɑktəpʊs̥
  12. bæftəb   25. jɔɪjɚ
  13. tɔɪwət

J. 1. tʃɛrɪz̥   8. pænkeks̥   15. dʒinz̥
   2. s̥ɛlɚi   9. ɛgz̥   16. s̥wɛrɚ
   3. tʃiz̥   10. s̥paɪrɚ   17. pədʒæməz̥
   4. s̥ɪrɪəl   11. ɑktəpʊs̥   18. s̥ændl̥z̥
   5. greɪps̥   12. s̥kwɝl̩   19. mɪʔn̥z̥
   6. aɪs̥krim   13. s̥neɪk   20. s̥lɪpɚz̥
   7. piz̥   14. s̥kʌŋk

21. We went to Ben Franklin's and looked at the toys.
    /wiwɛnt˺tubɛnfræŋklɪnz̥ | ænd lʊktætðətɔɪz̥ ‖ /

22. I saw some dolls that I liked.
    /aɪs̥ɑs̥əmdɑlz̥ðætaɪlaɪkt ‖ /

23. They traveled to Maine from Nebraska.
    /ðeɪtrævl̩dtumeɪn | frʌmnəbras̥kə ‖ /

24. We do spelling and math.
/widuṣpɛlɪŋænmæθ‖/

25. Sometimes we play mystery games.
/ṣʌmtaɪmẓwipleɪmɪṣtrigeɪmẓ‖/

K. 1. frɑg
    2. ẓibrə
    3. kʊkɪẓ
    4. hæmbʊgʊ
    5. ṣkʌŋk
    6. strɔbɛrɪẓ
    7. pɛəkit
    8. kɛətṣ
    9. ṣɪrɪəl
    10. hɑtdɑg
    11. pænkekṣ
    12. ṣɛlɚ
    13. dʒɚæf
    14. lɑmpṣtə
    15. ɚæbɪt
    16. ṣpaɪdə
    17. ɛləfənt
    18. aɪṣkrim
    19. bʌtʌ
    20. tʃɛrɪẓ
    21. ṣkwʊl
    22. ɑrəndʒ
    23. hɔṣ
    24. pəteɪtoʊ
    25. tʌtʊl

L. 1. [pʰ]
    2. [u̯]
    3. [r̥]
    4. [gʷ]
    5. [zˡ or ɮ]
    6. [õ]
    7. [w̥]
    8. [k̚]
    9. [ŋ̃]
    10. [l̟]

M. Possible answers include:
    1. [st⁼ɔr]
    2. [m̃aɪ]
    3. [rʌb̚]
    4. [hɛ̃n]
    5. [bɛt̬ɚ]
    6. [tɛn̪θ]
    7. [d̥rɪŋk]
    8. [kɑɫ]
    9. [ɪɱfɔrm]
    10. [kɪʔn̩]

N. 1. clue   [kʰlu]
    2. lymph   [lɪɱf]
    3. money   [mɅ̃nɪ]
    4. coop   [kʰupʰ]
    5. trial   [tʰr̥aɪɫ]
    6. skunk   [sk⁼Ʌ̃ŋkʰ]
    7. menthol [mɛ̃n̪θɑɫ]
    8. sweet   [sʷw̥itʰ]

Chapter 8

Chapter Exercises

8.2 1. lid   /lɪd/   [lɪd]
     2. when   /wɛn/   [wɛ̃n]
     3. rub   /rʌb/   [rʌb]
     4. caught /kɔt/   [kɔt] or /kɑt/ (if pronounced as /kɑt/)
     5. bag   /bæg/   [bæg]

8.3   1. may   /me/   [me̥]   4. like   /laɪk/   [laɪ̥k]
      2. lick   /lɪk/   [lḭk]   5. weed   /wid/   [wḭd]
      3. cat   /kæt/   [kæ̰t]

8.4   These vowels will vary, based on your dialect.

8.5   1. diphthongization   6. vowel merger
      2. ɪ/ə substitution   7. derhotacization
      3. laxing of vowels   8. monophthongization
      4. deletion of postvocalic /r/   9. tensing of vowels
      5. monophthongization   10. derhotacization

8.6   1. laxing of /u/   6. lack of vowel merger (lowering of /ɛ/)
      2. backing of /æ/   7. rhotacization
      3. derhotacization   8. derhotacization
      4. derhotacization   9. fronting of /ɑ/
      5. backing of /æ/   10. deletion of postvocalic /r/; derhotacization

8.7   1. /ræ̃ː/   6. /jɛlɪn/
      2. /wɪf/   7. /brʌvə/ or /brʌðə/
      3. /kɛʊl/   8. /haɪnd/
      4. /wiz/   9. /dɪnɪ/
      5. /wʌdn̩t/   10. /pɪkʊ/

8.8   1. cluster reduction   6. stopping
      2. ɑ/ʌ substitution   7. affrication
      3. deaffrication   8. stopping
      4. affrication   9. devoicing
      5. epenthesis   10. cluster reduction

8.9   Cantonese
      1. /sɪŋk/   think   Japanese
      2. /suz/   shoes   5. /zɪs/   this
      3. /waɪn/   vine   6. /hri/   free
      4. /bæz/   badge   7. /ʃip/   ship

      Tagalog
      8. /paɪn/   fine
      9. /tsɛk/   check
      10. /bæt/   vat

8.10 1. u/ʊ substitution   5. stopping
      2. gliding   6. dentalization; epenthesis
      3. devoicing; ɑ/æ substitution   7. devoicing; ɑ/ʌ substitution
      4. frication   8. fronting; i/ɪ substitution

8.11 _X_ 1. devoicing   _X_ 5. i/ɪ substitution

    _X_ 2. voicing   _X_ 6. devoicing

    ___ 3.   _X_ 7. epenthesis

    _X_ 4. deaffrication   ___ 8. win

Review Exercises

A. 1. /stɪl/   6. /fɔt/
    2. /stɪə/   7. /kɔːl/
    3. /fɛrɪ/   8. /trɛʒə/
    4. /diu/   9. /lanz/
    5. /meɪʃ/   10. /wɪn/

B. 1. lemon   7. heel
    2. sport   8. worthy
    3. precious   9. chair
    4. pure   10. stew
    5. wish   11. cart
    6. watch   12. carry

C. 1. /biwɛə/   6. /stɔə/
    2. /staːt/   7. /skwɜːt/
    3. /hæŋə/   8. /glɛə/
    4. /səvɪə/   9. /dɑktə/
    5. /klɜːdʒɪ/   10. /kaːbən/

D. 1. can't   6. explore
    2. broom   7. charter
    3. marrow   8. largest
    4. bath   9. demand
    5. parrot   10. conspire

E. 1. /mɑf/   6. /dɛm/
    2. /kʌz/   7. /mand/
    3. /ðɪn/   8. /weɪsəz/
    4. /kæ̃ː/   9. /əlɛbn̩/
    5. /hʊld/   10. /skreɪt/

F. _X_   1. final stop deletion

    ___   2.

    _X_   3. deletion of unstressed initial syllable

    _X_   4. cluster reduction

    _X_   5. glottal stop substitution

    _X_   6. /ɛ/-/ɪ/ merger

<u>X</u>   7. monophthongization

<u>X</u>   8. /l/ (liquid) deletion

___   9.

<u>X</u> 10. fronting

___ 11.

<u>X</u> 12. final nasal deletion

G. 1. stopping
    2. i/ɪ substitution
    3. deaffrication
    4. a/ʌ substitution
    5. affrication and ɑ/ʌ substitution
    6. cluster reduction
    7. u/ʊ substitution
    8. dentalization
    9. affrication of a fricative
   10. stopping
   11. stopping
   12. epenthesis

H. 1. Mandarin, Korean, Japanese
    2. Cantonese, Mandarin, Japanese
    3. Vietnamese, Korean, Japanese, Tagalog
    4. Cantonese, Vietnamese, Korean, Japanese, Tagalog
    5. Korean
    6. Vietnamese, Tagalog
    7. Cantonese
    8. Japanese, Tagalog
    9. Korean, Japanese
   10. Japanese

I. 1. Arabic   voicing
    2. Russian   gliding
    3. Russian   stopping
    4. both   u/ʊ substitution
    5. both   a/ʌ substitution
    6. Russian   fronting
    7. Russian   devoicing
    8. Arabic   epenthesis
    9. Russian   voicing
   10. Arabic   epenthesis
   11. both   r/ɹ substitution
   12. Arabic   pronouncing silent letters

J. 1. /ma | aɪ garə gorə ðəstɔː wɪθ pɔl tədeɪ ‖/
    2. /wərəju tɔkɪŋ əbaʊʔ ‖ fəgɛt əbaʊt ɪt ɔlrɛdɪ ‖/
    3. /kaːlɪ | waɪ dəju hæftə run ɛvrɪθɪŋ ‖/
    4. /aɪ hævə dɛntɪst əpɔɪʔmənt æt sɪks θɜˑɾɪ ‖/
    5. /rɔbət nidz təgoʊrə ðə bɔbə | hɪz hɛrz tu lɔŋ ‖/
    6. /aɪ wɔkt ovətə ðə mɔl jɛstədeɪ æftənun tə gɛtənu pɛrə ʃuʐ ‖/
    7. /maɪ dɔg laɪks tərən ɔl əraʊnd ðə jɑːd n̩ bɑːk ‖/
    8. /wɛn aɪ wəz pleɪŋ bæskətbɔl| aɪ ræn ɔlovə ðəkɔːt ‖/
    9. /aɪ garəgofudʃapən‖aɪ nid wɔrəmɛlən | kɔn | n̩ soʊdə ‖/
   10. /maɪ frɛn mɛrɪzə wiədoʊ | ʃidontwɑnəlimiəloʊn ‖/

K. 1. /pɑk ðə kɑ ɪnðə gəraʒ ‖ /
    2. /əmgoʊənə ðəmɑkət ɪn bɔstən ‖ /
    3. /aɪ lʌvrə ʃɔp hɑvəd skwɪə ‖ /
    4. /hæv juz gaɪz bɪnə ðəkeɪp ɔ mɑθədz vɪnjəd fə ðəsʌmə ‖ /
    5. /doʊnt fəgɛrəbrɪŋ jə pɔkətbʊk ‖ /
    6. /danɚ lʌvztə drɪŋk tɔnɪk ‖ /
    7. /kɪn ju wɪə jə dʌŋgəriz n̩ snikəz ‖ /
    8. /gɛrəfɑk fə ðæt judʒ hɛlpənə pɑstəŋgreɪvɪ ‖ /
    9. /gəhɛdŋ̩gɪvmʌmɪ səm dʒɪmɪz fɚɚ bənænɚ splɪt ‖ /
    10. /dʒɔn mɪlə ɪzə disənt jumən biən ‖ /

L. 1. /ʃiz drɑvɪn tu luziænə təmarə mɔrnɪn ‖ /
    2. /əmgʊnə bɔːl ədəzən ɛgz fɚ ɪstɚ ‖ /
    3. /læs naɪt | aɪwəz tɑkən təma frɛn mɛrɪlɪn ‖ /
    4. /əmfɪksən təhævrə bɑ səm tarz fəməkar ‖ /
    5. /əmlʊkənfɚma blu bɑl pɔɪʔ pɛn ‖ /
    6. /ju bɛrə kʌvɚ ðæt brɔːlən pæn wɪθ əlumɪnəm fɔːl ‖ /
    7. /weɪrəmɪnətleɪɪ | a nid ənə ðɚ mɪnət təmeɪkəpma mand ‖ /
    8. /a lɛft ðə tʃɪkən aʊt an ðə kaʊnɚ ænd ɪt spɔːld ‖ /
    9. /ðə junɪvɚsəɪɪ əv tɛnəsi ɪz ɪn nɑksvəl ‖ /
    10. /hɜːɪkənz n̩ tɔrnaɪɾəz arbʊθ lardʒ dæmədʒɪn wɪnstɔrmz ‖ /

M. 1. /də bɔɪ nid moʊ mʌnɪ ‖ /
    2. /wi fɪksəntə gotudə stoʊ ‖ /
    3. /hi bi pleɪən bɑl ætdəpark ‖ /
    4. /ðɛr ar foʊ nu kɪːz ɪn maɪ klæs/
    5. /maɪ sɪstə æn brʌvə wəzætdæt kɑnsɚt ‖ /
    6. /maɪ fæmlɪ goʊ tə tʃɜtʃ ɛrː ɪ sʌndeɪ ‖ /
    7. /joʊ mɑməkarɪnəmɪl̩əðəʃtriːʔ ‖ /
    8. /ʃi faʊn faɪː kwoʊrəz ɪnɚ pɜs ‖ /
    9. /kwɑnzə gɑt hɚ hɛr dən ‖ /
    10. /ðə studənts hɛlpt dɛmsɛlvz tu brɛkfəs ‖ /

N. 1. /pliʐ | pʊt dəflaʊɚʐ ɪndə beɪs ‖ /
    2. /it wəs ə βɛrɪ əspɛʃəl okeɪzjən ‖ /
    3. /ju sʊd kwɪt dʒɛlɪŋ æt jɔr marɚ ‖ /
    4. /aɪ wəs nat sʊɚ | aɪ wʊt bi eɪb̩ltu hɛlp ‖ /
    5. /maɪ feɪβɚɪtːɪtʃɚʐ neɪmis mɪstɚ dʒonʐ ‖ /
    6. /doʊnt lɛt jɔr dɑk pleɪ ɪn maɪ djart ‖ /
    7. /waɪ dont ju pʊt dis kloʊðz ɪn də gʌraʒ ‖ /
    8. /jɛstɚdeɪ | aɪ wɛntːu ðə su wɪθ dɑk ‖ /
    9. /sɛlɪ pʊt ðə poteɪtoʊ tʃips an ðə loʊɚ sɛlf ‖ /
    10. /aɪwəʐ bɛrɪ ɛksaɪtət əbaʊt winɪŋ də futbɑl geɪm ‖ /

O. 1. /aɪ hæv wʌn jʌŋgɚ brʌzɚ ɪn maɪ fæməɹɪ ‖/
   2. /aɪwʊd raɪkə grɪld tʃiz sandwɪtʃ fɔr:ʌntʃ priz ‖/
   3. /ɪt ɪz səpoʊs tu reɪn hɛvɹɪ fɔr mʌtʃ əvðəwik ‖/
   4. /zə rɪvɚ ɪz hɛvɹɪ pʊrutəd ‖/
   5. /maɪ θɪstɚ kjoʊkoʊ wɪl bi twɛnɪsri jɪrzold nɛksθɚsdeɪ ‖/
   6. /wʊdʒu raɪk tu goʊ ʃɒpɪŋ wɪsmi æftɚaɪ gɛt af wɚk ‖/
   7. /wʊd jɔr ʌðɚ brʌzɚ hɛlp mi lɪft ðɪθ ‖ ɪts hɛvɪ ‖/
   8. /sæŋk ju bɛrɪ mʌtʃ fɔr zə bjutɪfʊl fraʊɚz ‖/
   9. /aɪ hæv ə hard taɪm dɪstɪŋgwɪʃ bɪtʰwin zə sɪŋgjurɚ ænd prɚəl fɔrmz ‖/
  10. /ðɪ oʊnɹɪ konɛktɪŋ fraɪt ɪs: ru pɔrtrənd ɔrəgɒn ‖/

P. 1. /taɪpɪŋ imeɪlz hɛlps mi fɪŋk ɪn ɪŋgrɪʃ ‖/
   2. /aɪ wɛnt tudə ʒu tu si də nu pændə bɪrs ‖/
   3. /wʌt duju θɪŋkəvdə nu tɛrəvɪʒn̩ ʃoʊ ‖/
   4. /aɪ hæb tu ɔr θri frɛnz hu ar goʊɪŋ tu də sakɚ geɪm ‖/
   5. /juzəlɪ | si ɪs nat | so fɔrgɛtʰfʊl ‖/
   6. /aɪ bɛt ju dæt aɪ wɪl wɪn də reɪs ‖/
   7. /maɪ gɚlfrɛnd sɛnt mi fraʊɚz last wik fɔr maɪ bɚfdeɪ ‖/
   8. /dɛr ar sɛvrəl pipəl aɪ nid tu gɛt tu noʊ ‖/
   9. /də leɪaʊt əʒ dis:ɪrɪ ɪs nat vɛrɪ kanvinɪənt ‖/
  10. /aɪ præn tu goʊ tu pɚdu fɔr maɪ mæstɚʒ digri ‖/

Q. 1. /aɪwʊd laɪk e wɔdkə ænd tɔnɪk pliʒ/
   2. /pʊt de bʊks ovɚ dɛr an də teɪbl̩/
   3. /ɪt wʌʒ difikʊlt fɔr mi tu lʊrn də kərɛkt pronaʊnseɪʃən/
   4. /aɪ hæv bɪn livɪŋ ɪn də junaɪɾəd steɪts sɪns last ɔgəst/
   5. /xi xæʒ mɛni prabləmz wɪθ hɪz vokæbələrɪ/
   6. /də rʌʃən ikɔnəmi dipɛnz ɔn də karənt praɪs əv ɔɪl/
   7. /maɪ jʌŋgɚ brʌdɚ aləgzandɚ ɪz stʌdɪŋ mɛtəlʊrdʒi æt mɔskoʊ steɪt junivɚsiti/
   8. /di aʊtɚ əv də bʊk wʊz e feɪməs raɪtʊr/
   9. /aɪ hɛd sɛvɔrəl wizɪtɚz frəm vʊrdʒɪnɪə last manθ/
  10. /haʊ mɛni ʌðɚ pipʊl nidəd tu teɪk di klɛs/

R. 1. /bliz juz dæt wʊrd ɪn e sɛntəns/
   2. /aɪ nid ʃugɚ səbɪstɪtut fɔr maɪ kɔfi/
   3. /dʊktɚ kubɚ tɔld mi tu meɪk e kɔbi əv ðə hoʊmwɚk əsaɪnmənt/
   4. /ðɛr frɛnd robɪn gat mɛrɪd tu fɪktɔr maɪ nekst dɔr neɪbɔr/
   5. /aɪ wʌz dib̩rɛst bikʊz wi hæv had soʊ mʌtʃ bæd wɛd̩ɚ/
   6. /bit gɔt ə prɛzn̩ sɪntɪns bikʊz hi hɛd ðə polismɛn/
   7. /maɪ feɪfərɪt kɔtən ʃɚt ʃrʌŋk ɪn ðə lɔndərɪ/
   8. /bɪnɪ fɪzɪtəd hɚ fiɑnseɪ an fraɪdeɪ/
   9. /aɪ nid tu stʌdɪ ɪŋgəlɪʃ fonəloʊdʒɪ tu ɪmbruv maɪ pronaʊnzieɪʃən/
  10. /aɪ gru e bɪrd so ðæt aɪ wʊd əbɪr oʊldɚ/

Audio CDs to Accompany Fundamentals of Phonetics: A Practical Guide for Students, 3rd Ed.

CD One

Track #	Chapter	Track Title	Text Page #
1	2	Intro. to Word Stress	25
2	2	Stress Word List 1	26
3	2	Stress Word List 2	26
4	2	Stress Word List 3	26
5	2	Stress Word List 4	26
6	2	Stress Word List 5	26
7	2	Stress Word List 6	26
8	2	Stress Word List 7	26
9	2	Stress Word List 8	27
10	2	Stress Word List 9	27
11	2	Stress Word List 10	27
12	2	Stress Word List 11	27
13	2	Stress Word List 12	27
14	2	Exercise 2.17	27
15	2	Exercise 2.18	28
16	2	Exercise 2.19	28
17	2	Review Exercise J	31
18	2	Review Exercise K	31
19	2	Review Exercise L	32
20	4	Review Exercise E	101
21	4	Review Exercise F	101
22	4	Review Exercise G	102
23	4	Review Exercise L	104
24	4	Review Exercise M	105
25	4	Assignment 4-1	107
26	4	Assignment 4-2	109
27	4	Assignment 4-3	111
28	4	Assignment 4-4	113

CD Two

Track #	Chapter	Track Title	Text Page #
1	5	Review Exercise H	165
2	5	Review Exercise I	166
3	5	Assignment 5-1	169
4	5	Assignment 5-2	171
5	5	Assignment 5-3	173
6	5	Assignment 5-4	175
7	5	Assignment 5-5	177
8	5	Assignment 5-6	179
9	5	Assignment 5-7	181
10	6	Exercise 6.4	190
11	6	Exercise 6.5	192
12	6	Exercise 6.6	193
13	6	Exercise 6.7	194
14	6	Exercise 6.8	194
15	6	Exercise 6.9	195
16	6	Exercise 6.11	197
17	6	Exercise 6.12	198
18	6	Exercise 6.13	199–200
19	6	Exercise 6.14	202

CD Three

Glossary

abduction a movement of the vocal folds away from the midline (closed) position

accent modification therapy for a non-native speaker of English, designed to increase speech intelligibility, without jeopardizing the integrity of the individual's first dialect

acoustic phonetics the study of the auditory aspects of speech including frequency, intensity, and duration (length)

addition the insertion of an extra phoneme in the production of a word, usually used in reference to disordered speech; *epenthesis*

adduction a movement of the vocal folds toward the midline (closed) position

affricate a consonant characterized as having both a fricative and a stop manner of production, e.g., /tʃ and dʒ/

African American English (AAE) a dialect of English, spoken throughout the United States, traced back to the dialects of English spoken in Britain and brought to America by British settlers; also referred to as Black English, Black English Vernacular, African American Vernacular English, and Ebonics

allograph differing letter sequences that represent the same phoneme, e.g., h<u>ea</u>t, k<u>ey</u>, and r<u>ee</u>d

allophone variant production of a phoneme, e.g., [pʰ] and [p˺]

alveolar referring to the alveolar ridge; a consonant produced with a constriction formed by the tongue apex or blade and the alveolar ridge, e.g., /t, d, n, s, z, and l/

alveolar assimilation an assimilatory phonological process that occurs when a non-alveolar consonant is produced with an alveolar place of production due to the presence of an alveolar phoneme elsewhere in the word

alveolar ridge the gum ridge of the maxilla located directly behind the upper front teeth

antiresonance a negative resonance (brought about when the velum lowers during production of nasal sounds) that cause a decrease in the intensity of nasal and vowel formants

apex the tip of the tongue

approximant a consonant, such as a glide or liquid, produced with an obstruction in the vocal tract, less than that associated with the obstruents or nasals but greater than that associated with the vowels

articulation modification of the airstream by the speech organs in production of spoken language

articulation disorder difficulty in coordinating the articulators in production of a limited set of phonemes; difficulty with the motoric aspects of speech production

arytenoid cartilages paired cartilages of the larynx that attach to the superior portion of the cricoid cartilage; each vocal fold attaches to one arytenoid cartilage

aspiration the production of a frictional noise (similar to /h/) following the release of a voiceless stop consonant

assimilation the process by which phonemes take on the phonetic character of neighboring sounds due to coarticulation; refers to articulatory changes that result in the production of an allophone, or of a completely different phoneme

assimilatory processes phonological processes that involve an alteration in phoneme production due to phonetic environment

back (of the tongue) the portion of the tongue body posterior to the front of the tongue; it lies inferior to the velum

Back Upglide Shift a chain shift associated with the South; affects production of /ɔ/ and /aʊ/

Bernoulli effect a drop in air pressure, created by an increase in airflow through a constriction; helps to explain, in part, vocal fold adduction

bilabial *see* labial

blade the part of the tongue located just posterior to the tip

body (of the tongue) the portion of the tongue posterior to the blade, comprising the front and the back of the tongue

bound morpheme a morpheme that must be linked to another morpheme in order to convey meaning; e.g., <u>pre</u>date and think<u>ing</u>

bunched   one method of /r/ production in which the tongue apex is lowered as the tongue blade is raised to form one constriction with the palate, while the tongue root forms a second pharyngeal constriction; *see also* retroflexed

central incisor   any of the four front teeth, located in both the upper and lower jaws

chain shift   a dialectal modification in the pronunciation of English vowels, reflecting an alteration in their place of production; the change in the articulatory target for one vowel has a relative effect on the targets for other vowels, e.g., *Northern Cities Shift* and *Southern Shift*

citation form   the pronunciation of a word as a single, isolated item

clinical phonetics   the study and transcription of speech sound disorders

closed syllable   a syllable with a consonant phoneme in the final position

close internal juncture   two syllables in the same intonational phrase with no transitional pause between them, e.g., /aɪskrim/

cluster reduction   a syllable structure phonological process that results in the deletion of a consonant from a cluster

coarticulation   an articulatory process whereby individual phonemes overlap one another due to timing constraints and ease of production

coda   the consonants that follow a vowel in any syllable; not all syllables have a coda

cognates   phonemes that differ only in voicing, e.g., /t/ and /d/

complementary distribution   allophone production that is tied to a particular phonetic environment

connected speech   an utterance consisting of two or more continuous words

consonant   a phoneme produced with a constriction in the vocal tract; usually found at the beginning and end of a syllable; *generally* shorter in duration and having higher frequency spectra than vowels

consonant cluster   two or three contiguous consonants in a syllable, e.g., strike, please, and leapt

content word   a word that contains the most salient information in an utterance; e.g., a noun, verb, adjective, or adverb

creole   a pidgin language that is passed on to a new generation of users

cricoid cartilage   the most inferior cartilage of the larynx, shaped like a class ring

damping   the reduction in amplitude of energy (intensity) of a vibrating system

deaffrication   a substitution phonological process that involves the replacement of a fricative for an affricate

denasality (hyponasality)   production of nasal phonemes with raised velum

dental (interdental)   referring to the teeth; a consonant produced with a constriction formed by the tongue apex and the teeth, e.g., /θ and ð/

dentalization   production of an alveolar phoneme as linguadental, that is, with the tongue tip more forward than normal

derhotacization   the loss of r-coloring of the central vowels /ɜ/ and /ɚ/, and postvocalic /r/

devoicing   an assimilatory phonological process (voicing assimilation) that involves the replacement of a voiceless phoneme for a normally voiced, syllable-final consonant preceding a pause or silence

diacritic   a specialized phonetic symbol used in both systematic and impressionistic transcription to represent both allophone production as well as suprasegmental features of speech

dialect   a variation in speech or language related to geographic area, social class, or ethnic group

diaphragm   the major muscle that separates the abdomen from the thorax

digraph   pair of letters that represent one sound; the letters may be the same or different, e.g., look, think, and ear

diphthong   a single phoneme consisting of two vowel elements, the first termed the onglide and the second termed the offglide

diphthong simplification   *see* monophthongization

distortion   a characteristic of disordered speech involving the production of an allophone of an intended phoneme

dorsum   the body of the tongue, comprised primarily of the front and back; also, the back of the tongue

Eastern American English   a regional dialect of English spoken in the New England states and in New York, New Jersey, and Pennsylvania

ejective   a non-pulmonic consonant produced with a large glottalic air pressure release; brought about by raising the larynx, causing a decreased area between the closed vocal folds and the constriction in the oral cavity

elision   the omission of a phoneme from a word as a result of a historical change, or from coarticulation associated with connected speech

English language learner (ELL)   an individual who is attempting to master English as a second language

epenthesis   the addition of a phoneme to a word during speech production as a result of coarticulation, dialect, or a speech disorder

epiglottis   a cartilaginous structure that protects the larynx from food and drink during swallowing

ethnolect   a dialect associated with a particular ethnic group

eustachian tube   a tube, composed of cartilage and bone, that connects the nasopharynx with the middle ear; important for equalization of changes in air pressure and in drainage of middle ear fluids

experimental phonetics   the laboratory study of physiologic, perceptual, and acoustic phonetics

external intercostal muscles   muscles located between the ribs that aid in inhalation; the internal intercostals are deep to the external intercostals

external juncture   a pause serving to connect two intonational phrases in connected speech

extIPA an extension to the IPA that has become the official diacritic set for the transcription of disordered speech; adopted by the International Clinical Phonetics and Linguistics Association in 1994

falling intonational phrase a fall, or declination, in the pitch of the voice across the length of an intonational phrase; usually associated with complete statements and commands, as well as wh-questions

final consonant deletion a syllable structure phonological process that involves the deletion of the final consonant in a syllable, resulting in an open syllable (CV)

formal standard English the English of dictionaries, grammar books, and most printed manner; the idealized form of English used in teaching English

formant a resonant frequency of the vocal tract

formant transition dynamic change in the resonant frequencies of the vocal tract over time, signaling modifications in the place of articulation of speech sounds (as seen on a spectrogram)

free morpheme a morpheme that can stand alone yet still carry meaning

free variation refers to allophone production that is not tied to a particular phonetic environment

frequency the number of cycles a vibrating body completes in one second

fricative a consonant produced by forcing the breath stream through a narrow channel formed by two separate articulators in the vocal tract

front (of the tongue) the part of the tongue body anterior to the back of the tongue; it lies inferior to the (hard) palate

fronting a substitution phonological process that involves the replacement of an alveolar consonant for a velar or palatal consonant

function word a word that contributes little to the meaning of an utterance, e.g., a pronoun, article, preposition, or conjunction

fundamental frequency the basic rate of vibration of the vocal folds

General American English sometimes used synonymously with Standard American English to denote a form of English devoid of any regional pronunciation; may be used when comparing regional or ethnic dialects to a national "standard"

given information previous exchange of words, or shared world knowledge between two conversational participants

glide a consonant characterized by a continued, gliding motion of the articulators into the following vowel; also referred to as a semi-vowel, e.g., /j/ and /w/

gliding a substitution phonological process that involves the replacement of a glide for a liquid

glottal referring to the glottis; a phoneme produced with a constriction formed at the level of the vocal folds, e.g., /h/

glottal stop an allophonic variation of /t/ or /d/, produced when the release of the stop is at the level of the vocal folds instead of at the alveolar ridge, i.e., /ʔ/

glottis the space between the vocal folds

grapheme a printed alphabet letter used in the representation of an allograph

habitual pitch the inherent fundamental frequency of a given individual

hard palate the structure, also known as the "roof of the mouth," that separates the oral and nasal cavities

historical phonetics the study of sound changes in words over time

homorganic two consonants sharing the same place of articulation, e.g., time and neck

hyoid bone a "floating bone" that provides structural support for the larynx; attaches inferiorly to the larynx by a broad curtain-like ligament and superiorly to the tongue by muscle tissue

hypernasality the presence of excessive nasality accompanying the production of a non-nasal phoneme due to improper velopharyngeal closure

hyponasality (denasality) production of nasal phonemes with a raised velum

idiolect a speech pattern unique to an individual, based on dialect and personal speaking habit

idiosyncratic process a phonological process that is not typical of the speech behavior of a normally developing child

implosive a non-pulmonic consonant produced with an ingressive glottalic airstream; brought about by lowering the larynx, causing an increased area between the vocal folds and the constriction in the oral cavity

impressionistic transcription allophonic transcription of an unknown speaker or an unknown language

informal standard English based on listener judgments of patterns of spoken English deemed to be acceptable or not

intensity the amplitude (magnitude) of energy associated with a particular sound

interdental *see* dental

internal intercostal muscles muscles located between the ribs that aid in exhalation; the internal intercostals are deep to the external intercostals

International Phonetic Alphabet (IPA) an alphabet used to represent the sounds of the world's languages; created to promote a universal method of phonetic transcription

intervocalic a consonant located between two vowels, e.g., above

intonation the modification of voice pitch associated with varying utterance types (such as a question or a statement), or associated with a speaker's particular mood

intonational phrase the changes in the fundamental frequency of the voice spanning the length of a meaningful utterance (a word, phrase, or sentence)

intraoral pressure the air pressure within the oral cavity, created by a constriction of the articulators during production of stop consonants

juncture the transitional pauses and breaks between syllables and words in speech production

labial (bilabial) referring to the lips; a consonant produced with a constriction formed at the lips, e.g., /p, b, m, and w/

labial assimilation   an assimilatory phonological process that occurs when a nonlabial phoneme is produced with a labial place of articulation due to the presence of a labial phoneme elsewhere in the word

labialization   addition of lip rounding to the articulation of a typically unrounded phoneme

labiodental   a consonant produced with a constriction formed by the lower lip and upper central incisors, e.g., /f and v/

language transfer   the incorporation of native language (L₁) features into the target language (L₂) as the second language is being learned

larynx   cartilaginous and muscular structure that houses the vocal folds; responsible for phonation

lateral   a manner of production in which the airstream is directed over the sides of the tongue, e.g., /l/

lateralization   production of a non-lateral phoneme (any phoneme except /l/) with a lateral place of production; e.g., producing /s/ or /z/ as /ɬ/ or /ɮ/, respectively

lax   the description of a vowel produced with a reduction in muscular effort; a lax vowel does not appear in the final position of an open monosyllable, e.g., /ɪ, ɛ, æ, ʊ, ɚ, ʌ, and ə/

lexical stress   *see* word stress

lingual   referring to the tongue; a consonant produced with the tongue as the major articulator

liquid   a generic label used to classify two English approximant consonants, /r/ and /l/

loudness   the perceptual correlate of intensity

Low Back Merger   a dialectal variation reflecting a change in the articulatory targets for /ɔ/ and /ɑ/, so that no differentiation occurs in their production; characteristic of certain Western, Midwestern, and New England speakers

mandible   the lower jaw

manner of production   the way in which the airstream is modified as it passes through the vocal tract in production of consonants; English manners of production include stop, fricative, affricate, nasal, glide, and liquid

maxilla   the upper jaw

metathesis   the transposition of phonemes in a word due to a speech error, dialectal variation, or speech disorder

minimal contrast   *see* minimal pair

minimal pair   a pair of words that vary by only one phoneme, e.g., cook/book and passed/last; *minimal contrast*

misarticulation   an articulatory error, classically categorized as an omission, substitution, distortion, or addition

monophthong   a vowel phoneme consisting of one distinct articulatory element (as opposed to a diphthong, which has two elements)

monophthongization   the process of producing a diphthong as a monophthong, e.g., "fire" /far/; *diphthong simplification*

morpheme   the smallest unit of language capable of carrying meaning

nares   the nostrils

nasal emission   the audible escape of air through the nares due to improper velopharyngeal closure or to a cleft in the palate or the velum

nasal murmur   radiation of acoustic energy outward through the nasal cavity (due to a lowered velum) during production of nasal consonants

nasal phoneme   a consonant produced with complete closure in the oral cavity along with a lowered velum to allow airflow through the nasal cavity; the only nasal phonemes in English are /m, n, and ŋ/

nasalization   production of an oral phoneme with accompanying nasal resonance, due to a lowered velum, e.g., [mɛ̃n]

nasal plosion   the release of a stop consonant through the nasal cavity, as opposed to the oral cavity, as in the word /sʌdn̩/

natural phonology   Stampe's theory that supports the idea that children are born with innate processes necessary for the development of speech

new information   an exchange of words between two conversational participants that adds to the knowledge already shared

nonlinear phonology   a method of phonological analysis that involves performing an inventory of a child's speech sound system on multiple levels including words, syllables, segments, and features; phonemes are identified without consideration of what is phonemic or contrastive in the target language (adult system), but rather which consonants and vowels are used contrastively in particular contexts in the child's system

non-resonant consonants (non-resonants)   *see* obstruent consonants

non-sibilant consonants   the fricatives /f, v, θ, ð, and h/; perceived as being less intense when compared to the sibilant consonants /s, z, ʃ, and ʒ/

Northern Cities Shift   an ongoing change in the production of vowels, causing a shift from their standard place of articulation in the vowel quadrilateral; seen in the northern tier of the United States in cities such as Cleveland, Detroit, and Buffalo

nuclear accent   see tonic accent

nuclear syllable   see tonic syllable

nucleus   the part of a syllable with the greatest acoustic energy; usually, but not always, a vowel

obstruent consonants   a class of sounds (with a noise source) including the stops, fricatives, and affricates; also referred to as non-resonant consonants; produced with a constriction in the oral cavity that results in turbulence in the airstream coming from the larynx

offglide   the second element of a diphthong

omission   the deletion of a phoneme in a word, usually related to disordered speech

onglide   the first element of a diphthong

onset   all consonants preceding a vowel in any syllable; not all syllables contain an onset

open internal juncture   a transitional pause between two syllables within the same tone group, e.g., /aɪ + skrim/

open syllable a syllable with a vowel phoneme in the final position

oral phoneme a phoneme produced with a raised velum (velopharyngeal closure) so that the airstream is directed through the oral cavity; all English phonemes are oral except for /m, n, and ŋ/

palatal referring to the hard palate; a consonant produced with a constriction formed by the tongue blade and the hard palate, e.g., /ʃ, ʒ, tʃ, dʒ, r, and j/

palatoalveolar a consonant produced with a constriction formed by the tongue blade and the hard palate, slightly posterior to the constriction formed during production of alveolar consonants; often used to describe the place of production of /ʃ and ʒ/; also referred to as *postalveolar*

perceptual phonetics the study of listeners' perception of speech sounds in terms of pitch, loudness, perceived length, and quality

pharynx a muscular tube-like structure that connects the larynx and the oral cavity; the throat

phonation the vibration of the vocal folds in creation of a voiced sound

phoneme a speech sound capable of differentiating morphemes

phonetic alphabet an alphabet that contains a separate letter for each individual sound in a language, e.g., the IPA

phonetics the study of the speech sounds, their acoustic and perceptual characteristics, and how they are produced by the speech organs

phonological disorder a difficulty in speech sound production resulting in multiple speech sound errors ultimately involving the sound system of a language; also used to describe articulation disorder

phonological processes simplifications used by children not capable of producing adult speech patterns

phonology the systematic organization of speech sounds in the production of language; the study of the linguistic rules that specify the manner in which phonemes are organized and combined into syllables, words, and sentences

physiological phonetics the study of the function of the speech organs and their role in speech production

pidgin a language that results when individuals speaking two different languages begin to communicate; typically characterized as having a reduced vocabulary and grammar

pitch the perceptual correlate of frequency

place of articulation refers to the specific articulators employed in the production of a particular phoneme; the location of the constriction in the vocal tract in production of a consonant

point vowel one of four extreme corner vowels of the vowel quadrilateral, i.e., /i, æ, u, and ɑ/

postalveolar *see* palatoalveolar

postvocalic consonant a consonant following a vowel, e.g., a<u>t</u>

prevocalic consonant a consonant preceding a vowel, e.g., <u>m</u>e

prevocalic voicing an assimilatory phonological process (voicing assimilation) that involves the voicing of a normally unvoiced consonant preceding the nucleus of a syllable

progressive assimilation a modification in the identity of a phoneme due to a previously occurring phoneme; left-to-right or perseverative assimilation

quality the perceptual character of a sound based on its acoustic resonance patterns; timbre

r-colored vowel a speech sound consisting of the two elements: vowel + /r/, e.g., /ɪr, ɛr, ʊr, ɔr, and ɑr/; *rhotic diphthong*

reduplication a syllable structure phonological process that involves the repetition of a syllable of a word

regressive assimilation a modification in the identity of a phoneme due to a later occurring phoneme; right-to-left or anticipatory assimilation

resonance the vibratory properties of any sound-producing body

resonant consonants (resonants) *see* sonorant consonants

retroflexed one method of /r/ production in which the tongue tip is raised and curled back toward the alveolar ridge, as the back of the tongue creates a second velar constriction; *see also* bunched

rhotacization production of a phoneme with an /r/ auditory quality, e.g., /r/, /ɝ/, or /ɚ/

rhotic diphthong *see* r-colored vowel

rhyme a syllable segment consisting of an obligatory nucleus (usually a vowel) and an optional coda

rising intonational phrase a general rise in the pitch of the voice across the length of an intonational phrase; usually associated with yes/no questions, tag questions, lists, and incomplete utterances

root the portion of the tongue that attaches to the anterior wall of the pharynx and to the mandible

rounded a rounded lip position during vowel production; the rounded English vowels include /u, ʊ, o, ɔ, ɝ, and ɚ/

sentence stress added emphasis given to a specific word in a sentence due to the importance of that word in conveying meaning, or due to speaker intent; often found in association with the last word in a declarative utterance

sibilant the alveolar and palatal fricatives /s, z, ʃ, and ʒ/, which are perceived as being louder than the other fricatives

sociolect a dialect associated with a particular social class

sonorant consonants (sonorants) a class of sounds produced with resonance throughout the entire vocal tract, e.g., the nasals, glides, and liquids; they are produced with little constriction in the vocal tract and are therefore produced without much turbulence in the airstream coming from the larynx

Southern American English a regional dialect spoken in the Southern and South Midland states

Southern Shift an ongoing change in the production of vowels, causing a shift from their standard place of articulation in the vowel quadrilateral; this shift is seen in the southern, middle Atlantic, and southern mountain states

spectrogram   a graphic representation of the three major parameters that describe the acoustic characteristic of any sound: *time, frequency,* and *intensity*

spectrum   the frequency array, or energy pattern, characteristic of any sound

speech sound disorder   term used to refer to an individual with a phonological or articulation disorder

Standard American English (SAE)   a form of English that is relatively devoid of regional characteristics; the English used in textbooks and by national broadcasters

sternum   the breastbone

stop   a consonant characterized by: (1) a complete obstruction of the outgoing airstream by the articulators, (2) a build-up of intraoral air pressure, and (3) a release; also referred to as a *plosive*

stop gap   the time (in msec.) on a spectrogram that reflects increasing intraoral pressure prior to the release of a stop

stopping   a substitution phonological process that involves the replacement of a stop for a fricative or an affricate

subglottal pressure   the air pressure applied to the inferior surface of the vocal folds (glottis); the air pressure (from the lungs) necessary to blow the vocal folds apart

substitution   the replacement of one phoneme by another in a syllable or word

substitution processes   phonological processes involving the substitution of one phoneme class by another, e.g., *gliding, deaffrication,* or *fronting*

suprasegmental   a feature of speech production, such as stress, intonation, and timing, which transcends the phonemic level

syllabic consonant   a consonant that serves as the nucleus of a syllable, e.g., /l, m, and n/

syllable   a basic unit of speech production and perception generally consisting of a segment of greatest acoustic energy (a peak, usually a vowel) and segments of lesser energy (troughs, usually consonants); a unit of speech consisting of an *onset* and/or a *rhyme*

syllable structure processes   phonological processes that generally simplify the production of syllables, creating a consonant-vowel (CV) pattern

systematic narrow transcription   allophonic transcription of an individual, used when the rules of the language are known; also referred to as *narrow transcription* or *allophonic transcription*

systematic phonemic transcription   phonemic transcription of an individual, used when the rules of a language are known; variant phoneme (i.e., allophone) production is not recorded; also referred to as *broad transcription* or *phonemic transcription*

tap   a manner of consonant production involving a rapid movement of the tongue tip against the alveolar ridge resulting in the creation of a very brief phoneme, i.e., /ɾ/

Telsur Project   a telephone survey conducted by the University of Pennsylania to study variation in vowel production across the United States

tempo   the timing, or durational aspect, of connected speech

tense   the description of a vowel produced with an increased muscular effort; a tense vowel can be located in the final position of an open monosyllable, e.g., /i, e, u, o, ɔ, ɑ, and ɝ/

thoracic cavity (thorax)   the part of the human body between the head/neck and the abdomen; the chest cavity

thyroid cartilage   the most anterior cartilage of the larynx to which the vocal folds attach; the notch of the thyroid cartilage forms the "Adam's apple"

timbre   sound quality

time   (in acoustics) the duration of any particular sound

tongue advancement   a term used to classify vowel production in relation to tongue position along the front/back dimension in the oral cavity

tongue height   a term used to classify vowel production in relation to tongue position along the high/low dimension in the oral cavity

tonic (nuclear) accent   the emphasis given to the tonic (nuclear) syllable in any particular intonational phrase

tonic (nuclear) syllable   the syllable that contains the greatest pitch change in any particular intonational phrase

trachea   a tube, comprised of cartilaginous rings embedded in muscle tissue, that connects the lungs with the larynx; windpipe

unreleased   a stop consonant produced with no audible release burst

unrounded   a spread or retracted lip position during vowel production, e.g., /i, ɪ, e, ɛ, æ, ɑ, ʌ, and ə/

uvula   the rounded, tablike structure located at the posterior tip of the velum

velar   referring to the soft palate (velum); a consonant produced with a constriction formed by the back of the tongue and the velum, e.g., /k, g, and ŋ/

velar assimilation   an assimilatory phonological process that occurs when a non-velar phoneme is produced with a velar place of production due to the presence of a velar phoneme elsewhere in the word

velarization   the backed production of an alveolar phoneme (such as /l/) so that the tongue is more posterior than normal (in the velar region); e.g., [rigl̩]

velopharyngeal closure   a constriction formed by the velum and the rear wall of the pharynx, resulting in a diversion of the airstream into the oral cavity

velum   a muscular structure located directly posterior to the hard palate; the *soft palate*

vernacular dialect   the variety of language spoken by a non-standard speaker of a language

vocal folds   elastic folds of tissue, primarily composed of muscle; the vocal cords

vocalization   the substitution of a vowel for postvocalic or syllabic /l/, postvocalic /r/, or the substitution of a non-rhotic vowel for the central vowels /ɚ/ and /ɝ/

vocal tract the network consisting of the larynx, pharynx, and the oral and nasal cavities

voice bar a low-frequency energy band as seen on a spectrogram (due to the vibrating vocal folds) that occurs during the stop gap phase of voiced stop consonants in non-initial position of words

voiced a sound produced with vocal fold vibration

voiceless a sound produced without vocal fold vibration

voicing the participation of the vocal folds during phoneme production; all vowels are voiced, whereas only certain consonants are voiced

VoQS the voice quality symbols diacritic set; designed to be used in the transcription of individuals with voice disorders

vowel a phoneme produced without any appreciable blockage of airflow in the vocal tract

vowelization *see* vocalization

vowel merger a dialectal modification in which vowels with separate articulations fuse into one similar place of articulation, e.g., /ɑ/ and /ɔ/ both being produced as /ɑ/

vowel quadrilateral a two-dimensional figure (representing tongue height and tongue advancement) that displays the relative position of the tongue during vowel production

vowel reduction an articulatory process associated with connected speech whereby the full form of a vowel is produced with less weight due to a more central production in the oral cavity, often similar to a mid-central vowel

weak syllable deletion a syllable structure phonological process that involves the omission of an unstressed (weak) syllable either preceding or following a stressed syllable

word class also known as "part of speech," e.g., noun, verb, adjective

word stress (lexical stress) the production of a syllable with increased force or muscular energy, resulting in a syllable that is perceived as being louder, longer in duration, and higher in pitch; also known as word accent

Index